Advances in Experimental Medicine and Biology

The Breast Cancer Research Foundation

Larry Norton, MD
Medical Director, Evelyn H. Lauder Breast Center
Memorial Sloan Kettering Cancer Center
Professor of Medicine, Weill Cornell Medical College
Scientific Director, Breast Cancer Research Foundation

Clifford Hudis, MD
Chief, Breast Medicine Service
Memorial Sloan Kettering Cancer Center
Professor of Medicine, Weill Cornell Medical College
Chairman, Scientific Advisory Board, Breast Cancer Research Foundation

Volume 862

More information about this series at http://www.springer.com/series/5584

Patricia A. Ganz
Editor

Improving Outcomes for Breast Cancer Survivors

Perspectives on Research Challenges and Opportunities

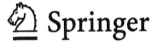 Springer

Editor
Patricia A. Ganz
Distinguished Professor of Health Policy & Management and Medicine
UCLA Fielding School of Public Health
David Geffen School of Medicine at UCLA
Director, Cancer Prevention & Control Research
Jonsson Comprehensive Cancer Center
Los Angeles, CA, USA

ISSN 0065-2598   ISSN 2214-8019   (electronic)
Advances in Experimental Medicine and Biology
ISBN 978-3-319-16365-9   ISBN 978-3-319-16366-6   (eBook)
DOI 10.1007/978-3-319-16366-6

Library of Congress Control Number: 2015938588

Springer Cham Heidelberg New York Dordrecht London

Printed on acid-free paper

Springer International Publishing AG Switzerland is part of Springer Science+Business Media (www.springer.com)

About the Breast Cancer Research Foundation

The Breast Cancer Research Foundation (BCRF) advances the world's most promising research to eradicate breast cancer. Founded by Evelyn H. Lauder in 1993, BCRF has raised more than $550 million to fuel discoveries in tumor biology, genetics, prevention, treatment, survivorship, and metastasis, making it one of the largest nongovernmental funders of breast cancer research in the world. In 2014, BCRF invested $58.6 million in research, including $11.6 million to the international Evelyn H. Lauder Founder's Fund focused on metastasis, to support more than 220 researchers at leading medical institutions across six continents. By spending 91 cents of every dollar on research and public awareness programs, BCRF remains one of the nation's most fiscally responsible nonprofits. BCRF is the only breast cancer organization with an "A+" from CharityWatch and has been awarded Charity Navigator's highest rating of four stars 13 times since 2002. For more information, please visit: www.bcrfcure.org.

Series Editors

Larry Norton, M.D.
Deputy Physician-in-Chief for Breast Cancer Programs; Medical Director,
Evelyn H. Lauder Breast Center; Norna S. Sarofim Chair in Clinical Oncology,
Memorial Sloan Kettering Cancer Center

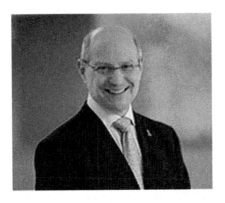

Dr. Norton is a board-certified medical oncologist with broad interests in cancer prevention, diagnosis, and treatment. In his clinical practice, he cares for women with breast cancer and is now Deputy Physician-in-Chief for Breast Cancer Programs at Memorial Sloan Kettering and Medical Director of the Evelyn H. Lauder Breast Center.

His research concerns the basic biology of cancer; the mathematics of tumor causation and growth; and the development of approaches to better diagnosis, prevention, and drug treatment of the disease. He is involved in many areas of research, including identifying the genes that predispose people to cancer or that cause cancer and developing new drugs, monoclonal antibodies that target growth factor receptors, and vaccines. A major milestone in his research career was the development of an approach to therapy called "dose density" or "sequential dose density," which maximizes the killing of cancer cells while minimizing toxicity.

Dr. Norton is currently the principal investigator of a program project grant from the National Cancer Institute (NCI) that is aimed at better understanding breast cancer in the laboratory and in bringing these advances into clinical practice. On a national level, he was formerly the Chair of the Breast Committee of the NCI's Cancer and Leukemia Group B. He was President of the American Society of Clinical Oncology (ASCO) from 2001 to 2002 and was appointed by President Clinton to serve on the National Cancer Advisory Board (the board of directors of The NCI). He has served as Scientific Director of the Breast Cancer Research Foundation since its inception in 1993.

Among many awards over the course of my career, he was honored to receive ASCO's David A. Karnofsky Award and The McGuire Lectureship at the San Antonio Breast Cancer Symposium. He is an author of more than 350 articles and many book chapters; has served as a visiting professor throughout USA, Canada, South America, Europe, Israel, and Asia; and has also trained many cancer doctors and researchers.

Clifford A. Hudis, M.D.
Chief, Breast Medicine Service
Memorial Sloan Kettering Cancer Center

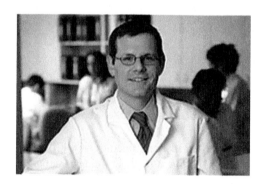

Dr. Hudis is Chief of the Breast Medicine Service and Attending Physician at Memorial Sloan Kettering Cancer Center (MSKCC) in New York City, where he is co-Leader of the Breast Disease Management Team and a Professor of Medicine at the Weill Cornell Medical College. He is the immediate Past President of the American Society of Clinical Oncology (ASCO), Chairman of BCRF Scientific Advisory Board, co-Chair of the Breast Committee of the Alliance (formerly the CALGB), and a member of the Steering Committee of the Translational Breast Cancer Research Consortium (TBCRC).

A 1983 graduate of the Medical College of Pennsylvania (a combined 6-year BA/MD program with Lehigh University), Dr. Hudis trained in Internal Medicine in Philadelphia before completing his fellowship in Medical Oncology at MSKCC. He joined the faculty in 1991.

Dr. Hudis's research includes the development of a wide range of novel drugs and the study of relevant correlative science endpoints in breast cancer. With his collaborators both at MSKCC and elsewhere, his personal research is focused on understanding the mechanisms that link diet, obesity, inflammation, and breast cancer risk and outcomes. Building on their discoveries of low-grade inflammation in association with overweight and obesity, Dr. Hudis and his colleagues are studying interventions that may reduce the risk, and return, of breast cancer. Across his service at MSKCC, his team conducts studies of novel-targeted therapies in advanced disease, of new strategies in the adjuvant and neo-adjuvant settings, and of risk reduction.

Preface

Breast cancer is a heterogeneous disease. There are multiple biological subtypes of breast cancer that dictate diverse therapies whose application results in prolonged survival for the vast majority of patients. The women (and men) who are diagnosed with breast cancer are also heterogeneous. They experience the disease in individual ways that are often dependent on their age, socioeconomic and partnership status, residence in an urban or rural environment, access to care and receipt of appropriate treatment, and receipt of adequate psychosocial support during and after treatment. Breast cancer treatments extend over many months of primary treatment, followed by prolonged endocrine treatments for the majority of women. A segment of the breast cancer population lives with metastatic disease while receiving continuous serial treatments during which time physical, psychosocial, and financial concerns are substantial. Nearly three million US breast cancer survivors must adjust to "the new normal."

In this volume, we focus on the patient-centered outcomes of breast cancer, highlighting specific patient populations, their unique needs and experiences, as well as more general outcomes (symptoms, quality of life, psychosocial concerns) and chronic health risks that are consequences of breast cancer and its treatments. We also focus on opportunities for health and wellness promotion that are essential to facilitating recovery after breast cancer treatment. It was a privilege for me to serve as the editor for this first volume in a series that is a collaboration between the Breast Cancer Research Foundation (BCRF) and Springer. The content of this volume reflects the commitment of both organizations to this area of breast cancer research, as well as the depth of the BCRF research portfolio in this domain. The 16 contributing authors are all funded BCRF investigators and their research reveals the breadth of scientific research on breast cancer outcomes.

We are extremely grateful to Dr. Larry Norton, whose visionary scientific leadership of the BCRF has created a community of investigators dedicated to conducting research along the entire continuum of scientific inquiry—from cells to society. In conceiving of this book series and our work on this volume, Dr. Norton encouraged us to "share our viewpoints, interpretations, and 'gut feelings' about where we are, where we are going, and how we think we should get there. We don't always agree, but creative thought feeds off our opinions, as long as they are evidence based and insightful. This project is an attempt to recapture that spirited conversation. This is your chance to get your ideas, criticisms, questions, predictions, and concepts for how we can make progress faster out there for discussion, maybe debate, and—I would hope—action." Larry, I hope we have delivered on your request!

Finally, as we worked hard during a 12-month period to produce this volume, we were inspired by the memory of the late Evelyn Lauder, as well as the dedicated BCRF staff—Myra Biblowit, Margaret (Peg) Mastrianni, and many others. They have made it possible for this group of investigators to pursue the most innovative and exciting research they can imagine, focused on improving outcomes for patients with breast cancer. We extend our sincere appreciation to the BCRF and its supporters.

Los Angeles, CA   Patricia A. Ganz
March 2015

Contents

About the Editor

Patricia A. Ganz M.D. currently holds an American Cancer Society Clinical Research Professorship and is a Professor in the UCLA Schools of Medicine and Public Health. For over 30 years, Dr. Ganz has been doing systematic research on the health-related quality of life impact of cancer and its treatment. Through her research, she has contributed to the understanding of how women adjust to the diagnosis of breast cancer, including its effects on their physical, emotional, social, and sexual well-being. Her current research focuses on understanding the biological mechanisms associated with the development of posttreatment fatigue and cognitive dysfunction, along with the development and testing of interventions to mitigate these symptoms in breast cancer patients and survivors. Dr. Ganz is a founding member of the National Coalition for Cancer Survivorship (NCCS) and was previously awarded the Breast Cancer Research Foundation's Jill Rose Award and the Susan G. Komen Professor of Survivorship. Dr. Ganz is the first recipient of the ASCO Professorship in Breast Cancer Comparative Effectiveness Research. Dr. Ganz serves as a Deputy Editor for the Journal of the National Cancer Institute and Associate Editor of CA-A Journal for Clinicians. She has also been actively involved in measurement of quality of life endpoints in clinical trials, with leadership roles in the Southwest Oncology Group (SWOG), the National Surgical Adjuvant Breast and Bowel Project (NSABP), and now NRG Oncology. She has published over 390 scientific papers and countless book chapters, and she has also edited three books with Springer. She has received over 23,000 citations in her career.

Chapter 1
Breast Cancer Survivorship: Where Are We Today?

Patricia A. Ganz and Pamela J. Goodwin

Abstract Breast cancer is the most common cancer in women, and survivors with this diagnosis account for almost one fourth of the over 14 million cancer survivors in the US. After several decades of basic and clinical trials research, we have learned much about the heterogeneity of breast cancer and have evolved a complex and multidisciplinary treatment approach to the disease. Increasingly, we are paying attention to the long term and late effects of breast cancer treatment, and this is largely the subject of this volume. In this chapter, the authors introduce the topic of breast cancer survivorship and highlight the organization and content of this volume, briefly describing the contents of the subsequent chapters.

Keywords Breast cancer • Survivorship • Outcomes • Quality of life • Quality of care

Breast cancer is one of the most feared diseases, especially among women in North America, yet it has become an exemplar of success in the war against cancer.[1] Not too long ago, most breast cancers were detected by the woman herself (substantially larger than 2 cm) and had already spread to the axillary lymph nodes. Just 40 years ago we were still using radical surgical approaches for the treatment of breast cancer, declaring that we had "got it all" surgically, even though metastatic disease would appear within a few years after surgery. The concept of adjuvant chemotherapy and endocrine therapy slowly evolved over several decades of systematic investigation through clinical trials, and we even experimented with high dose chemotherapy as adjuvant therapy.

---

[1] Please note, while we acknowledge that men are diagnosed with breast cancer as well, we will focus on the experience of women as so much more information is available on their outcomes.

P.A. Ganz (✉)
UCLA Schools of Medicine and Public Health, Jonsson Comprehensive Cancer Center, Los Angeles, CA, USA
e-mail: pganz@mednet.ucla.edu

P.J. Goodwin
Lunenfeld-Tanenbaum Research Institute, Mount Sinai Hospital, Toronto, ON, Canada
e-mail: pgoodwin@mtsinai.on.ca

© Breast Cancer Research Foundation 2015
P.A. Ganz (ed.), *Improving Outcomes for Breast Cancer Survivors*,
Advances in Experimental Medicine and Biology 862,
DOI 10.1007/978-3-319-16366-6_1

Today, there has been a significant shift in the stage of newly-diagnosed breast cancer to negative node disease, and we have refined our knowledge of the disease biology, such that risk stratification by molecular subtypes allows us to define more tailored and often less toxic therapies. The multidisciplinary clinical approach to the management of breast cancer (surgery, radiology, pathology, medical oncology, radiation therapy, and reconstructive surgery), as well as the translational approach to breast cancer research, are now the models for other cancer sites. While we can argue about whether or not intensive mammographic screening has led to overdiagnosis, identifying low risk conditions that may cause no harm, there is no question that the overall outcomes for women with breast cancer diagnosed today are substantially better than when many of us started our oncology training several decades ago.

As a consequence of the advances, there has been a striking decline in breast cancer mortality over the past two decades (Siegel et al. 2014). A secondary outcome is the growing number of breast cancer survivors who now number nearly 3 million in the US and represent 41 % of female cancer survivors (Desantis et al. 2014). These women live in our communities, share our workplaces, teach our children, and may be a spouse or loved one. Almost everyone has acquaintances who have had breast cancer, and most of those affected are no longer hiding their experience from others, unlike the situation 50 years ago when the first women with breast cancer could not talk about it in public and had trouble finding support for each other. On the other hand, there are still many women living with metastatic breast cancer who are being maintained on treatment for long periods of time and who are hoping for the next therapeutic breakthrough. In the United States, nearly 40,000 women are lost to breast cancer each year, and we clearly need to do a better job eliminating premature death and suffering from this disease.

As survival outcomes improve, many survivors are at risk for non-breast cancer related diseases. One recent study that examined deaths in postmenopausal women with hormone receptor positive breast cancer participating in a trial of extended adjuvant endocrine therapy found that non-breast cancer deaths accounted for 60 % of all deaths; this proportion was higher in women over 70 years of age (72 %) and lower in younger women (48 %) (Chapman et al. 2008). Second cancers and cardiovascular disease were the commonest non-breast cancer causes of death. Because obesity is associated with increased postmenopausal breast cancer risk, survivors may be at increased risk of obesity associated conditions such as diabetes. These observations underscore the importance of maintaining overall health in breast cancer survivors, and suggest that secondary prevention strategies, including adoption of a healthy lifestyle and appropriate management of non-breast cancer related health issues, such as hypertension and lipid disorders, should be considered high priorities. The diagnosis of cancer has been considered a "teachable moment" (Demark-Wahnefried et al. 2005), a time when many women re-evaluate their priorities and may be more amenable to making lifestyle and other changes (including smoking cessation, weight loss, enhanced physical activity, and adoption of a healthy diet) that will lead to improved health. Exploitation of this teachable moment may yield important benefits.

In this volume, we have been given an opportunity to focus on a wide range of outcomes associated with the diagnosis and treatment of breast cancer. This work is the product of an innovative collaboration between the Breast Cancer Research Foundation (BCRF) and Springer, as part of its Advances in Experimental Medicine and Biology series. The charge to the authors was to produce a work that provides perspective and commentary, and not the traditional review article that so often is found in multi-authored edited volumes. All of the authors are BCRF funded researchers who are working in the topic areas that they are writing about. Many of the author teams are active research collaborators, but several of the chapters have brought together scientists who have not previously worked together and were asked to do so for the purpose of this effort. For those of you who may know some of the authors, you will likely hear their personal voice come through—something we encouraged to make this book different and to emphasize the goal of providing a perspective on the field and where the research is today and where it needs to be going. As such, those of you who read this volume will be disappointed if you are expecting a thorough review of a chapter topic—this was not our goal.

The title of this volume—*Improving Outcomes for Breast Cancer Survivors*—actually has two meanings: the word "improving" is both an adjective and a verb as used to describe the book's content. We are faced with a large and growing population of breast cancer survivors whose outcomes are much improved over a generation ago. In the long term, many of these survivors experience quality of life that is comparable to that of women without breast cancer (Hsu et al. 2013), but this experience is not universal. We need to work on improving outcomes for those survivors who suffer from persistent symptoms and side effects after treatment ends, and for those with recurrent or persistent disease who remain on long term therapy. In the section that follows, we briefly highlight how the BCRF authors address specific content areas, so as to direct your attention to the expert opinion this volume contains.

In three early chapters in the book, we have chosen to highlight the needs of several special populations among breast cancer patients and survivors. While the average age of breast cancer diagnosis is 61 years in the United States, and it is still largely a disease of women of European origin in the US and Canada, it affects women of all ages and all ethnic and racial subgroups. In fact, it is the leading cause of cancer in women worldwide. Age at diagnosis can have a tremendous effect on how women cope and adjust to a breast cancer diagnosis, as well as to the toxicities they experience from treatments. In a chapter devoted to younger women (Chap. 2, Ganz et al.) the unique needs and concerns of this population are addressed, including life stage, premature menopause, reproductive and fertility concerns, risk of hereditary cancers, as well as the unique emotional needs of younger women. Importantly, because of the long life span these women face after breast cancer treatment, preventing and reducing the risk for late effects of cancer treatment is critical. In parallel, the older woman with breast cancer may be extremely vigorous or, at the other extreme, burdened with comorbid conditions when cancer is diagnosed. In Chap. 3, Hurria and Muss, highlight the unique needs of older women with breast cancer and how we need more research to better understand how to manage treatment and potential toxicities in this population. The importance of maintaining functional independence in this population is a central goal. For both older and younger patients with breast cancer, there is a paucity of research targeting their specific needs and concerns, and the authors highlight areas that need our attention. Lastly, in Chap. 4 on Disparities in Care Across the Cancer Control Continuum, Paskett alerts us to the many gaps in knowledge related to the experience of vulnerable populations (racial/ethnic groups, older women, women from rural and urban areas) who are most likely to experience disparities in care related to breast cancer. In some settings it is a lack of institutional (health system) resources for early detection and prompt treatment, in others there are patient level factors that lead to poorer outcomes including attitudes, behaviors, culture and limited financial resources/access to care. There is much to be done, and there are important US national efforts that are now focusing on many of these problems.

In the next section of the book, we focus on key symptoms/syndromes that are frequent consequences of breast cancer treatment. In Chap. 5, scientific collaborators Bower and Ganz provide important insights into the biological mechanisms associated with cancer-related fatigue and cognitive dysfunction, both of which are nearly universal during the primary treatment of breast cancer (surgery, radiation, chemotherapy) and are persistent in a about 25 % of survivors long after treatment ends. Their pioneering work has demonstrated a close biological linkage between these two common symptoms, with a focus on the development and evaluation of interventions to mitigate post-treatment fatigue and cognitive complaints. However, much more research needs to be done. Much less is known about the biological mechanisms associated with the development of chemotherapy-induced peripheral neuropathy (Chap. 6 by Schneider et al.). This is especially concerning given the frequent use of taxanes in contemporary adjuvant therapy regimens. Addressing this important gap in knowledge, as well as understanding who is at greatest risk for neuropathy, will be important steps to reducing the frequency with which long-term breast cancer survivors suffer with ongoing symptoms. A lack of animal models for studying this toxicity is an important gap. These authors allude to the fact that we have now traded the rare complications of leukemia and cardiac dysfunction from anthracyclines for the persistent numbness and pain associated with taxane chemotherapy in as many as one quarter of patients, who receive this common adjuvant therapy.

Aromatase inhibitor induced arthralgias are another common symptom experienced by large numbers of breast cancer patients and survivors, and this topic is ably addressed in Chap. 7 by Hershman et al. Musculoskeletal pain and stiffness in association with this widely prescribed endocrine therapy occurs at a much higher rate (40–50 %) than initially described in the phase three randomized trials that led to the approval of these agents. These authors explored potential mechanisms for these symptoms, as well as possible strategies to identify those at high risk. Unfortunately, this symptom co-occurs with many chronic comorbid conditions of aging, compromising the functional independence that is so important among older women. In Chap. 8, Paskett addresses the challenges associated with the prevention, detection and treatment of lymphedema. Fortunately, this is one symptom that has become much less frequent in the past decade with the more widespread use of sentinel node biopsy and less frequent radiation of the axilla when it is not necessary. Nevertheless, for those women who develop swelling of their arm either early or late in the course of survivorship, it is often difficult to manage and the swelling becomes a constant reminder of their cancer and its treatment. There remain many gaps in knowledge of how best to prevent and manage this unfortunate complication of breast cancer treatment. In Chap. 9, Barton and Ganz, highlight the challenges of delivering therapies for breast cancer where these highly effective therapies often precipitate menopause and its associated symptoms, along with infertility and disruptions in sexual health and functioning. There is considerable understanding of the biology of many of these symptoms based on research on the menopause in healthy women, but strategies to mitigate common symptoms may not be appropriate in breast cancer patients. The authors note that "reducing the untoward effects of cancer treatment on the reproductive health of breast cancer survivors is the ultimate goal," and strategies need to be developed to provide more personalized therapies to meet the needs of individual patients.

Several chapters explore comorbidities and other aspects of the woman herself (often called host factors) that may relate to breast cancer outcomes. Some of these host characteristics are amenable to change, potentially leading to improved outcomes, while others are not. Understanding the contributions of these factors to breast cancer outcomes, including treatment toxicities, may impact choice of treatment. When modifiable, change may lead to improved outcomes.

In Chap. 10, Ambrosone et al. review the revolution that has occurred in classifying breast cancers, based on their genetic profiles. This has led, for example, to the recognition of intrinsic subtypes (e.g. luminal A and B, basal, HER2, normal) that have different biology, treatment responsiveness and outcomes. Additional work has explored DNA copy number variations, mutation profiles and expression patterns overall and within these intrinsic subtypes that are of potential utility in the development of targeted treatments. These authors discuss the potential importance of germline factors, such as polymorphisms in the CYP2D6 gene, a gene that is responsible for activation of tamoxifen to endoxifen. Although genotyping for CYP2D6 variants is not widely used (because the link between genotype and tamoxifen benefit has not been convincingly established), the concurrent use of tamoxifen and strong CYP2D6 inhibitors (such as serotonin reuptake inhibitors) can lead to reduced tamoxifen benefit and is not recommended. It is hoped that additional research, including genome wide association studies will identify genetic factors associated with metabolism and toxicity of a broader range of breast cancer drugs. Research into the potential contributions of environmental factors related to DNA methylation and function, and of Vitamin D exposure to cancer outcomes is also discussed. The goal of this broad area of research is the development of more personalized breast cancer treatment, maximizing efficacy while minimizing toxicity.

Hong and colleagues (Chap. 11) address the important issue of comorbidity in breast cancer patients, discussing the impact of comorbidity on treatment selection and outcomes (both breast cancer related and overall). Comorbidity is most common in older survivors, and is associated with less intense treatment, greater treatment toxicity, poorer quality of life and increased risk of death from breast cancer or other causes. Given the growing number of breast cancer survivors who live long periods of time after their diagnosis, proper management of comorbidities is an important clinical issue. Involvement of primary care physicians, and co-ordination of care between oncologists and these physicians is critical to the management of survivors with comorbidities. Many studies of comorbidity have used cancer registries or administrative databases that have restricted availability of information about younger women, disease severity and treatment that may limit the scope of research that can be performed; future research will need to overcome these limitations. Key research priorities include improved management of comorbidities and evaluation of the effect of this improved management on outcomes, evaluation of potential effects of medications used to treat comorbidities (e.g. metformin, NSAIDs) on outcomes, and investigation of comorbidities in susceptible populations.

In Chap. 12, Goodwin et al discuss the potential contribution of modifiable lifestyle factors (weight, diet, physical activity, alcohol) to breast cancer outcomes while in Chap. 13 Irwin and colleagues focus on diet, physical activity and weight management interventions in breast cancer survivors. Together, these chapters highlight the growing recognition that lifestyle may contribute to breast cancer outcomes. Overweight and obesity have been associated with poor outcomes in over 50 studies over the past 35–40 years; more recent work has suggested physical activity may be associated with better outcomes. Lifestyle change, notably increased physical activity, dietary change and weight loss are feasible and may have beneficial effects on fitness, quality of life and treatment-related symptoms. Ongoing intervention research is discussed and potential biologic mediators of lifestyle effects on outcome identified. These chapters discuss ongoing areas of controversy and stress the need for well-designed intervention trials that will formally test the effects of lifestyle interventions, notably weight loss, on breast cancer outcomes. Both groups of authors identify research priorities, including translational biomarker studies, and they advocate for adequately powered intervention trials that will provide definitive evidence regarding effects of lifestyle change on breast cancer outcomes.

The next series of chapters highlights survivorship issues that warrant special attention, including cardiac dysfunction, psychosocial adjustment, quality of care and survivorship in the face of metastatic disease. These broad issues have emerged as important research and clinical priorities, and they will likely continue to be major areas of focus over the next decade.

Fabian discusses the important issue of cardiac dysfunction in breast cancer survivors in Chap. 14. Breast cancer patients may be at increased risk for cardiovascular disease at diagnosis due the presence of risk factors such as obesity and physical inactivity. Two major classes of drugs (anthracyclines and HER-2 targeted agents) that are most commonly associated with cardiac dysfunction are reviewed. Anthracyclines are directly cardiotoxic with age, higher cumulative dose, comorbidity and African American ethnicity being associated with increased cardiac toxicity. In contrast, HER-2 targeted agents can promote reversible cardiotoxicity by interfering with neuregulin binding to HER-2 receptors on cardiac myocytes. Fabian advocates for research to develop a standard nomenclature for cardiac dysfunction (suggesting a decline in LVEF of at least 10 % or to a level below 50 %, as a commonly used definition), to identify cardioprotective treatment regimens and to generate more accurate models to predict risk of cardiac dysfunction, potentially including measures of global left ventricular strain and troponin. She also discussed treatment of cardiotoxicity and preventive approaches that incorporate drugs such as ACE inhibitors and beta-blockers, as well as manpower issues in the burgeoning area of cardio-oncology.

In Chap. 15, Stanton and Bower discuss psychosocial adjustment in breast cancer survivors. In addition to the commonly recognized negative psychosocial sequelae (e.g. depression, anxiety, Post-Traumatic Stress Disorder), they discuss the growing recognition of the potential for positive growth after breast cancer diagnosis. They introduce trajectories of adjustment and recovery during the initial months and years after diagnosis, but comment that anxiety regarding recurrence often persists after other symptoms have resolved. They suggest that greater disease impact and engagement may be important correlates of positive psychological outcomes, including "strengthened inter-personal relationships, life appreciation, commitment to priorities, spirituality, personal regard, and attention to health behaviors". Stanton and Bower discuss key directions for psychosocial and biobehavioral intervention research, prioritizing issues such as understanding biopsychosocial mechanisms of intervention benefits, the use of stepped-care interventions to allow delivery to those who would benefit most, and extending research to less well studied minorities, socially and financially disadvantaged groups.

Ganz and Stanton focus on the complexities of survivorship in women with metastatic breast cancer in Chap. 16, including those who present with metastatic disease at diagnosis and those who develop metastases after initial potentially curative treatment. They estimate that there may be up to 160,000 individuals living with metastatic breast cancer in the US and suggest that younger patients may be disproportionately represented. Although women dealing with metastatic disease face a broad range of issues that are relevant in this population (including life threat and uncertainty, interpersonal challenges, physical symptoms such as pain and fatigue as well as psychological symptoms such as depression, anxiety and adjustment disorders), most attain positive psychological health. Recognizing the profound heterogeneity of the course of disease, with survival ranging from months to decades, these authors advocate for early palliative and psychosocial support in addition to ongoing expert oncologic management. They highlight the need for more systematic research in this population, with a focus on psychosocial, quality of life and symptom endpoints, as well as how to best integrate palliative care into standard disease management and how to best address practical issues such as the costs of medical care, the potential to continue working, and how to deal with family issues. The focus on women living with metastatic breast cancer is an important emerging area in survivorship research—it highlights a somewhat understudied and underserved population of survivors.

Hershman and Ganz close out this volume with a discussion of quality of survivorship care in Chap. 17. They adopt a broad definition of survivorship—from diagnosis through the balance of life, including those close to the woman with cancer—and they discuss challenges in the delivery of quality care, highlighting the contributions of clinical guidelines in the establishment and dissemination of quality care. Examples of common gaps in quality care include discussions of fertility/ premature menopause with younger patients, the potential for long term toxicity, non-adherence to oral endocrine therapy and the need for formal survivorship care planning. Challenges for survivors include the cost of care. The need for evidence-based, cost-effective follow-up, avoiding unnecessary testing and minimizing disparities in treatment and outcomes are discussed. Finally, key areas of ongoing and future research are reviewed, including the need to reduce over-diagnosis and over-treatment as well as appropriate survivorship care planning that focusses on communication, involvement of primary care physicians, attention to psychosocial issues and individualization of the process rather than on a "one size fits all" care plan document.

In summary, this is a very unique volume in that it presents in one place the spectrum of non-mortality outcomes from breast cancer treatment in a comprehensive way, with attention to unique populations (older, younger, living with metastatic disease) and common toxicities. Improving outcomes for breast cancer survivors is the goal, and the contributing authors provide a perspective on what we know and where the research should be heading. The BCRF has invested extensively in funding a broad portfolio of research during the past two decades, and we are pleased to be able to share this portion of the portfolio with the scientific, advocacy and lay community.

References

Chapman JA, Meng D, Shepherd L, Parulekar W, Ingle JN, Muss HB, Goss PE (2008) Competing causes of death from a randomized trial of extended adjuvant endocrine therapy for breast cancer. J Natl Cancer Inst 100(4):252–60. doi:10.1093/jnci/djn014

Demark-Wahnefried W, Aziz NM, Rowland JH, Pinto BM (2005) Riding the crest of the teachable moment: promoting long-term health after the diagnosis of cancer. J Clin Oncol 23(24): 5814–30

Desantis C, Ma J, Bryan L, Jemal A (2014) Breast cancer statistics, 2013. CA Cancer J Clin 64(1):52–62. doi:10.3322/caac.21203

Hsu T, Ennis M, Hood N, Graham M, Goodwin PJ (2013) Quality of life in long-term breast cancer survivors. J Clin Oncol 31(28):3540–8. doi:10.1200/JCO.2012.48.1903

Siegel R, Ma J, Zou Z, Jemal A (2014) Cancer statistics, 2014. CA Cancer J Clin 64(1):9–29

Chapter 2
Special Issues in Younger Women with Breast Cancer

Patricia A. Ganz, Julienne E. Bower, and Annette L. Stanton

Abstract Although women less than 50 years old make up less than 25 % of the patient population with breast cancer in industrialized countries, they have unique clinical and psychosocial issues that must be addressed as part of their oncology care to ensure the best health and psychosocial outcomes after treatment. Preserving fertility is a major issue for many younger women who have either not had children or would like to have additional children after treatment. Dealing with the disruption of a cancer diagnosis at a young age is challenging physically, socially and emotionally, and the health care system does not always address these patients' concerns. Because younger women have the potential for a long life expectancy after cancer treatment, preventing and reducing the risk for late effects of cancer treatment is very important. We discuss these and a range of other issues throughout this chapter.

Keywords Younger women • Fertility • Psychosocial distress • Premature menopause • Hereditary breast cancer

Introduction

In Western industrialized countries, breast cancer is primarily a disease of post-menopausal women, with incidence patterns showing a modest premenopausal peak in the fifth decade of life, but a much more substantial incidence peak in the seventh and eighth decades. For a woman who is age 30, the probability of developing breast cancer in the next 10 years is 0.44 % or 1 in 228, while at age 70 the 10

P.A. Ganz (✉)
UCLA Schools of Medicine and Public Health, Jonsson Comprehensive Cancer Center, Los Angeles, CA, USA
e-mail: pganz@mednet.ucla.edu

J.E. Bower • A.L. Stanton
Departments of Psychology and Psychiatry/Biobehavioral Sciences, Jonsson Comprehensive Cancer Center, University of California, Los Angeles, CA, USA
e-mail: jbower@ucla.edu; astanton@ucla.edu

© Breast Cancer Research Foundation 2015
P.A. Ganz (ed.), *Improving Outcomes for Breast Cancer Survivors*,
Advances in Experimental Medicine and Biology 862,
DOI 10.1007/978-3-319-16366-6_2

9

Table 2.1 Age-specific probabilities of developing invasive female breast cancer[a]

If current age is	The probability of developing breast cancer in the next 10 years is (in %)	Or 1 in:
20	0.06	1,732
30	0.44	228
40	1.45	69
50	2.31	43
60	3.49	29
70	3.84	26
Lifetime risk	12.29	8

Adapted from Desantis et al. (2014) with permission

[a]Among those free of cancer at the beginning of the age interval. Based on cases diagnosed between 2008 and 2010. Percentages and "1 in" numbers may not be numerically equivalent due to rounding. Probabilities derived using the National Cancer Institute DevCan software (version 6.7.0)

years probability is 3.84 % or 1 in 28 (Desantis et al. 2014) (Table 2.1). Thus, when cancer occurs in a very young woman it is a rare and unexpected event. She has no peers who have the disease, and she may be at a time in life where she has not completed her education or professional development, and may or may not be in a long-term partnered relationship. If she is without children, cancer treatment may substantially disrupt her childbearing plans; if she already is a parent, she may fear for her ability to successfully raise her children, and not leave them prematurely. For women who are in their 40s, cancer treatments may precipitate early menopause, and the disruptions of cancer treatments often add stresses to normal mid-life issues and career challenges.

Younger women are a heterogeneous group, at various developmental stages, and as such, their concerns and needs differ substantially from more mature women who have likely had friends who have experienced breast cancer, and for whom years of screening mammography and educational campaigns have alerted them to the possibility of breast cancer occurring. In this chapter, we will provide a description of the diverse characteristics of younger women with breast cancer, including the tumor and treatment variations, the reproductive consequences of treatments, the social and psychological sequelae, and their higher risk of mortality from breast cancer. We subsequently will examine the many research challenges and opportunities that management of this target population requires, including the tailoring of treatments to reduce the burden of long term toxicities, better management of psychological health, as well as better access to fertility preservation, health promotion and cancer prevention.

Who Are the Younger Women with Breast Cancer?

Breast cancer in women younger than 50 makes up about 25 % of the incident breast cancer cases each year (Desantis et al. 2014) (see Table 2.2). Fewer numbers of incident cases occur if one uses earlier age cut-points, as noted previously. In a recent systematic review of the unique psychosocial needs of younger women with breast cancer, we used age 50 years as the cut-point for the review due to the paucity of

Table 2.2 Estimated new female breast cancer cases and deaths by age, United States, 2013[a]

Age	In situ cases	Invasive cases	Deaths
<40	1,900	10,980	1,020
<50	15,650	48,910	4,780
50–64	26,770	84,210	11,970
65+	22,220	99,220	22,870
All ages	64,640	232,340	39,620

Adapted from Desantis et al. (2014) with permission
Source Total estimated cases are based on 1995–2009 incidence rates from 49 states as reported by the North American Association for Central Cancer Registries. Total estimated deaths are based on data from the US mortality data, 1995–2009, National Center for Health Statistics, Centers for Disease Control and Prevention
[a]Rounded to nearest 10

literature focused solely on very young women (Howard-Anderson et al. 2012). 45 years is probably a more appropriate age to use as a cut point for linking to other studies of young adults with cancer, which use 39 years as the upper age limit (Brinton et al. 2008; Tricoli et al. 2011). However, in detailed interviews with younger women with breast cancer, classification of "young" was more often associated with life stage and challenges, rather than chronological age (Dunn and Steginga 2000). While there is no official definition of "young breast cancer patient" we will focus on the diversity of clinical and psychosocial features of women with breast cancer who are less than 50 years at diagnosis. However, a CDC program and federal legislation that has called attention to this group of patients using an age of less than 45 years at diagnosis (http://www.cdc.gov/cancer/breast/young_women/index.htm) Although we acknowledge that younger men may be affected by breast cancer, this is such a small group, for which even less is known, that we confine our discussion to women.

The complexity of discussing this special population relates foremost to the diversity of life stage of development interacting with chronological age. The experience of the rare young woman diagnosed with breast cancer while in college is extremely different from the mother of teenage children who is in her early 40s. However, within these several decades of risk that these two women mark, the emotional, educational, professional and reproductive issues may be similar and be independent of chronological age. The ability to accept the cancer diagnosis, complete treatment, remain adherent to endocrine therapy if required, and continue with education or work, may be more tied to emotional maturity and financial resources, which may or may not be related to chronological age. Also, younger women with breast cancer have a higher likelihood of hereditary breast cancer, where knowledge of the potential risk for the disease is known (i.e., by family history if not by established mutation); however, many women diagnosed at a young age may first learn of having a germ line mutation for breast cancer at the time of cancer diagnosis, without prior knowledge of the disease in any relatives, especially if this is passed through the paternal line. The rate of germ line mutations of *BRCA1* are considerably higher in younger women than in older women, and *TP53* mutations may also be responsible for breast cancer in these

Table 2.3 Predicted probabilities of a *BRCA1* mutation based on age and tumor characteristics

Age (years)	All histologies (%)	ER-negative and high-grade tumors (%)
<30	8	35
31–34	5	26.5
35–39	2	6.6
40–44	1.5	3.7
45–49	1	2.5
50–59	0.3	0.9

ER Estrogen receptor
Adapted from Gabriel and Domchek (2010) with permission

women (Gabriel and Domchek 2010) (Table 2.3). Increasingly, breast cancer gene panels are being used to assess these younger women, and in the future, we may have a better explanation for the occurrence of cancer at such a young age. Also, among these women may be survivors of a prior childhood cancer in which radiation treatment to the thorax or total body was included (Moskowitz et al. 2014). Such women are also among the younger breast cancer patients and survivors.

One of the other challenges among younger women is the co-occurrence of breast cancer and pregnancy—largely due to the later age of marriage and childbearing among well-educated women (Litton et al. 2013; Partridge et al. 2004; Theriault and Litton 2013). Deferring pregnancy until an older age is a recent phenomenon in Western industrialized countries. These breast cancers may be diagnosed during pregnancy or in the first years after childbirth. Large tumors and delays in diagnosis are common due to the natural changes that occur in the breast as part of pregnancy and lactation. Clearly, these cancers are already present in the breast prior to the pregnancy, but come to clinical recognition with the stimulation of hormones during pregnancy. The increased challenge of delivering antineoplastic treatments during pregnancy, as well as the high risk management of the mother and fetus, can add to the stress of the cancer diagnosis and treatment for young women. And of course, for most young women of reproductive age who are diagnosed with breast cancer, the concerns about preserving fertility may influence decision-making about treatments, (Ruddy et al. 2014) including finding clinicians to provide these services in a timely manner, as well as having the financial resources to pay for these services.

Is Breast Cancer Biologically Different in Younger Women?

Genetic and genomic discoveries during the past 15 years have allowed us to subtype breast cancer molecularly and develop classifications that are useful with regard to biology and therapy. Survival outcomes for women younger than 35 have been historically poor (Keegan et al. 2013), although most of the improvements related to introduction of adjuvant chemotherapy were most apparent in younger women. For some time, it has been known that the frequency distribution of hormone receptor positive breast cancer is lower in younger women than post-menopausal women, but

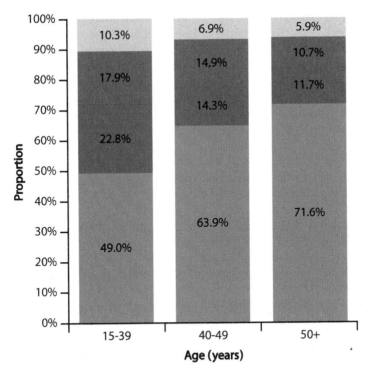

Fig. 2.1 Proportion of breast cancer subtypes among California women by age group, 2005–2009. Hormone receptor (HR) positive and human epidermal growth factor receptor 2 (HER2) negative (*blue*), HR+/HER2+ (*red*), HR-/HER2+ (*green*), and triple negative (*purple*). Adapted from Keegan et al. 2012 with permission

recent gene expression studies have more extensively characterized the distribution of hormone receptor positive, triple negative, double negative and HER2 positive tumors (Keegan et al. 2012) (Fig. 2.1). Also, some of these subtypes vary by race/ethnicity, most notably the high proportion of triple negative and basal cell phenotypes in African American and Latino women, as well as the higher rates of incident breast cancer in African American women before age 40 compared to other ethnic groups (Brinton et al. 2008). In addition, the higher rate of incident stage IV metastatic breast cancer among younger age women compared to older women complicates the initial treatment and management (Johnson et al. 2013).

Treatment of Breast Cancer in Younger Women

All of the age and life stage variables described earlier will influence the treatment of young women, beyond the tumor stage and biological features, which would be the dominant consideration in older women. If the younger woman carries a deleterious *BRCA1/2* mutation, she may opt for bilateral mastectomy at the time of initial surgery, even though breast conservation could be considered. The young woman's treatment decision-making may also be influenced by her marital status and whether she has completed childbearing. In addition, we see some women opting for very aggressive chemotherapy regimens, even in the setting of small tumors with favorable characteristics, due to their desire to stay alive to raise children or pursue other meaningful goals. Other younger women may avoid treatments because they fear their toxicity, such as infertility. Because younger women often have more advanced stage disease at diagnosis, they will more likely be subjected to post-mastectomy or axillary radiation, which may contribute to the burden of survivor-ship symptoms. In our experience, younger women opt for disability during treatment more frequently than older women. The experience can be physically and emotionally overwhelming.

The psychosocial challenges of getting young women through treatment may be considerable. As alluded to earlier, the emotional and financial resources needed to cope with treatments which often last more than a year, are substantial. Finally, adherence to endocrine therapy is a particularly challenging problem, as often chemotherapy has induced transient or permanent amenorrhea, and the addition of tamoxifen increases the likelihood of greater vasomotor symptoms (Ganz et al. 2011), as well as sexual dysfunction in some. Several studies document a relationship between younger age and nonadherence to endocrine therapy. Factors such as low social support, a perceived lack of understanding of endocrine therapy and lack of the opportunity to ask questions at diagnosis, and a greater number of meno-pausal symptoms are associated with nonadherence [e.g., (Cluze et al. 2012)].

Premature menopause and infertility are a frequent consequence of treatments in young women, and prolonged treatments may also interfere with the timing of sub-sequent childbearing. Specifically, the 5 years of endocrine therapy with tamoxifen may make it difficult to fit in a pregnancy, especially if a woman is in her late 30s. Although recent data do not suggest increased risk for breast cancer recurrence with childbearing, (Azim et al. 2012, 2013) this is still a major concern for some women. This is especially an issue for women with DCIS for whom treatment decisions may be quite difficult. We discuss fertility and reproductive concerns in greater detail in the Chap. 10. Premature menopause may lead to other health consequences such as weight gain and menopause-related symptoms.

Risk of Mortality and Late Effects from Breast Cancer and Its Treatments

Breast cancer is the leading cause of death among women 40–59 years (Siegel et al. 2014) so that fear of recurrence and death from cancer is a reality for younger women with breast cancer. This is in spite of the significant advances in treatment with chemotherapy and targeted therapies. Many of the women living for long periods of time with metastatic breast cancer are younger women (see Chap. 15 on metastatic breast cancer survivors). Younger women are also at greatest risk for experiencing the long-term and late effects of cancer treatment, similar to childhood cancer survivors, as they have a long time horizon of survival in which these long-term and late effects may occur. For example, fractures from early osteoporosis, cardiac failure, and second cancers (breast and non-breast) can occur. The extent to which the breast cancer treatments received as a young woman may accelerate various aspects of organ aging is uncertain at this time. Clearly, some of the manifestations of cognitive difficulties may portend accelerated brain aging, and both structural and functional brain changes have been observed in breast cancer survivors several decades later (Koppelmans et al. 2012a, b). Thus, younger women need to be viewed as a high-risk population at risk for future health events, and should be considered for systematic cancer prevention and control interventions. This is particularly true for *BRCA1/2* carriers in whom second cancers of the breast and Fallopian tubes/ovaries can be prevented or their risk reduced.

Quality of Life, Psychological, and Behavioral Concerns

Breast cancer has a more negative impact on quality of life among younger women, particularly in the psychosocial and emotional domains (Cimprich et al. 2002; Ganz et al. 2003; Howard-Anderson et al. 2012; Mor et al. 1994). Younger women with breast cancer report worse mental health-related quality of life than both age-matched women without breast cancer and older women with breast cancer (Howard-Anderson et al. 2012). Younger women also report elevated levels of distress and depressive symptoms following cancer diagnosis, which may persist into survivorship (Avis et al. 2012, 2013). Higher levels of depressive symptoms in younger women are due to a variety of factors, including more aggressive treatment (though differences remain after controlling for type of treatment), a lower sense of peace and meaning in life, and particularly greater illness intrusiveness (Avis et al. 2012, 2013). Indeed, younger women report higher levels of illness intrusiveness in all domains of life, including health, diet, work, recreation, financial situation, relationships, and sex life, which are closely tied to depression. Further, younger women perceive cancer as more threatening (Vinokur et al. 1990) and report greater fear of cancer recurrence (Lebel et al. 2013) than older women.

In terms of physical symptoms, younger women report higher levels of bodily pain, vasomotor symptoms, fatigue, and sleep disturbance (Avis et al. 2012, 2013; Bower et al. 2000; Ganz et al. 2003; Palesh et al. 2010). These symptoms likely contribute to the increased depression and distress observed in younger women, and also have independent (negative) effects on quality of life. Indeed, fatigue is now recognized as one of the most common and distressing side effects of cancer treatment, as discussed in Chap. 6. Fatigue, depression, pain, and sleep problems not only erode quality of life but may also influence adherence to treatment, and possibly survival (Groenvold et al. 2007).

Many women are able to find some benefit from their experience with cancer, including positive changes in relationships with others, an enhanced feeling of self-worth and mastery, and a deepened appreciation for life. Younger women are particularly likely to report these positive changes (Koutrouli et al. 2012), perhaps because breast cancer may be one of the first highly stressful events they have experienced. Among younger women, finding benefit is facilitated by approach-oriented coping strategies and a sense of optimism about the future (Boyle et al. 2015). Thus, although the experience of breast cancer can be particularly devastating for younger women, they may experience more positive life changes in the aftermath of the experience, which prompts an increased appreciation of the preciousness (and fleetingness) of life.

Social Consequences

The experience of breast cancer challenges young women's interpersonal spheres, deepening some relationships and diminishing others. As an "off-time" non-normative event, being diagnosed with breast cancer under age 50 can carry several social consequences (Adams et al. 2011). Specifically, the young woman who has no one among her similarly aged peers who has had breast cancer can feel isolated and have few models for adaptive coping. Moreover, friends and co-workers may not know how to provide effective support, having never encountered another young woman with breast cancer. The threat of mortality might become real for the first time in some social network members, leading even well-intentioned friends to avoid the young woman. Greater social support is associated with better psychological adjustment in young women with breast cancer (see Howard-Anderson et al. 2012 review). Even when among other breast cancer survivors, however, young women can feel alone; younger breast cancer survivors report feeling more isolated and less satisfied with cancer support groups due to their age (Thewes et al. 2004).

When diagnosed in young adult women, breast cancer also prompts developmental interpersonal challenges, as documented in clinical and qualitative reports (Corney et al. 2014; Schnipper 2003). Just as they are attaining adult independence, very young women with breast cancer can find themselves relying on their parents, other family members, and friends for care. At the same time, young breast cancer survivors who are mothers can feel that they are slighting their children's care. Women who have not forged relationships with intimate partners can experience anxiety about doing so and feel that treatments delay precious time for establishing adult relationships. Questions are common about when to raise the issue in a dating relationship, whether potential partners will be rejecting, and how to consider having children.

Existing intimate partner relationships also are affected by the breast cancer experience for young survivors (Baucom et al. 2005; Lewis et al. 2012). The threat of mortality often is paramount, with each partner afraid of the potential losses that can accompany cancer, as the assumption of a long life together is called into question.

Plans for having children can change, as can caretaking for children or elderly parents. Sexual intimacy also is affected. Young, partnered breast cancer survivors are less sexually active and have more body image and sexual problems than are similarly aged healthy women, although it is important to note that approximately a third of young survivors do not report problems in those realms (Fobair et al. 2006). Relationship, sexual, and body image problems all are related to lower quality of life in young survivors, likely with reciprocal causality (Avis et al. 2005). The potential for strengthening the relationship also can occur as the couple faces the cancer experience together.

Research Challenges and Opportunities

In much of the world, breast cancer is primarily a disease of younger women, whereas in North America and Europe, younger women are in the minority because of the high incidence of postmenopausal breast cancer. Understanding the biological and psychosocial context of breast cancer in younger women is one of our central challenges. To the extent that risk factors for poor outcomes after a breast cancer diagnosis can be modulated by interventions directed at biological or behavioral factors, then research needs to focus on identifying those risk factors and developing specific post-treatment cancer control interventions. They may be as simple as providing information regarding normative psychosocial experiences of younger women with breast cancer or more complex, such as reducing tobacco and alcohol use, promoting adherence to endocrine therapy, or providing evidence-based therapy to women or couples to reduce anxiety and depression and enhance well-being. The double-edged sword of the benefits of amenorrhea for reduction in risk of breast cancer recurrence, and its negative consequences for women who want to have children, may interfere with effective treatment strategies.

Among the things we must do for all breast cancer patients, but particularly for younger women, is to tailor cancer treatments so that we do not over treat with very toxic therapies that have no benefit. For example, patients with small tumors and favorable, low risk tumors are unlikely to receive benefit from multi-agent chemotherapy. Yet, that is often the normative treatment for a younger premenopausal woman. Both she and the physician want to do "everything." This may also include prophylactic mastectomy and oophorectomy in women who are not at hereditary risk for breast and ovarian cancer. Finding better ways to clarify actual risk and to communicate it will be critical (Institute of Medicine 2013). In contrast, there are some younger women who will avoid receiving recommended therapies either due to their belief systems or because they are unable to cope with the diagnosis in an effective way (see below for psychological challenges). Patients' active engagement in medical decision-making and care is critical for support of clinical decisions that best fit the needs, values and preferences of the patient. For this patient population, having concomitant expert mental health support as part of the treatment team is crucial in light of the evidence of their heightened psychosocial morbidities (Adler and Page 2007).

Identification of Psychological Risk Groups in Need of Intervention

In light of the evidence that younger breast cancer survivors as a group are more likely than older women to experience cancer as psychologically disruptive, all younger women stand to benefit from education regarding what to expect after diagnosis of and treatment for breast cancer, including strategies for managing the attendant life changes. Patient age does not appear to influence the efficacy of psychosocial interventions for distress and quality of life in adult cancer survivors generally (Faller et al. 2013). However, it is possible that interventions for younger women with breast cancer, specifically directed toward and tailored to address their predominant concerns, might produce more robust effects than current evidence-based approaches for the general population of adults with cancer. Development of effective strategies for promoting healthy behaviors, including physical exercise, healthy eating patterns, and adherence to endocrine therapies, also are warranted for young survivors.

Intervention development for young breast cancer survivors who are at particular risk for untoward psychological outcomes also is needed. Within the group of young breast cancer survivors, a number of psychosocial factors are associated with poorer psychological outcomes, including low social support, more cancer-related intrusive thoughts and feelings regarding cancer, and abruptly experienced menopausal symptoms, among others. Unfortunately, most research regarding risk and protective factors for positive quality of life in young survivors is cross-sectional in design, which precludes causal inference. Targeting survivors who might be in most need of intervention, such as socially isolated or depressed young women, is an important future direction for intervention.

Development of More Specialized Approaches to the Younger Patient in Practice Settings

Just as the geriatric or pediatric cancer patient may need specialized services, so are there a number of critical services that need to be offered to younger women. First, honest and careful discussion of the reproductive health implications of the planned cancer treatment is essential. Just as we consider breast reconstruction as a covered benefit of rehabilitation from cancer treatment, fertility preservation should be organized, available, and potentially financed at an affordable rate. While there are likely only small numbers of patients who will need this service, its availability reinforces to the woman that she is expected to survive and that she may be able to have a family or more children in the future. Fortunately, increasing numbers of younger survivors now are able to have children either naturally or through preservation mechanisms.

We need to provide survivorship care for young women that focuses on their long time horizon after breast cancer, addressing lifestyle, health behaviors, and emotional well-being. Such care can maximize their chance of a healthy life including prevention of cancer recurrence if possible, and early detection of second cancers should they occur. Many younger women avoid mammograms because the first one did not detect their initial cancer. Effective and trusting long-term relationships with oncology professionals and knowledgeable primary care providers are necessary to address the health promotion and disease prevention that is a necessary part of follow-up for younger women. Finally, we should re-assess family history and re-evaluate the need and opportunity for genetic counseling and testing in younger women, as these options may have been overlooked initially in the rush to treat. As survivors, women will benefit from new knowledge about hereditary predisposition syndromes that may affect their future health and that of their family members.

In closing, younger women have been the beneficiaries of the major advances in the treatment of breast cancer, including adjuvant chemo- and hormonal therapies, hereditary predisposition testing, breast reconstruction, and breast conservation treatments. However, they are most at risk for psychological difficulties as a result of a breast cancer diagnosis and can benefit from information and psychosocial resources to help them adapt and cope with the untimely diagnosis. Because of their extended potential life span, they are especially vulnerable to the long term and late consequences of cancer treatment. As a result, cancer survivorship care planning should be an important component of young women's post-treatment care (see Chap. 17), to help mitigate preventable conditions that may result from or be exacerbated by cancer treatments.

References

Adams E, McCann L, Armes J, Richardson A, Stark D, Watson E, Hubbard G (2011) The experiences, needs and concerns of younger women with breast cancer: a meta-ethnography. Psychooncology 20:851–861

Adler NE, Page AEK (2007) Cancer care for the whole patient: meeting psychosocial health needs. Institute of Medicine, National Academies Press, Washington, DC

Avis NE, Crawford S, Manuel J (2005) Quality of life among younger women with breast cancer. J Clin Oncol 23:3322–3330

Avis NE, Levine B, Naughton MJ, Case DL, Naftalis E, Van Zee KJ (2012) Explaining age-related differences in depression following breast cancer diagnosis and treatment. Breast Cancer Res Treat 136:581–591

Avis NE, Levine B, Naughton MJ, Case LD, Naftalis E, Van Zee KJ (2013) Age-related longitudinal changes in depressive symptoms following breast cancer diagnosis and treatment. Breast Cancer Res Treat 139:199–206

Azim HA Jr, Santoro L, Russell-Edu W, Pentheroudakis G, Pavlidis N, Peccatori FA (2012) Prognosis of pregnancy-associated breast cancer: a meta-analysis of 30 studies. Cancer Treat Rev 38:834–842

Azim HA Jr, Kroman N, Paesmans M, Gelber S, Rotmensz N, Ameye L, De Mattos-Arruda L, Pistilli B, Pinto A, Jensen MB, Cordoba O, de Azambuja E, Goldhirsch A, Piccart MJ, Peccatori

FA (2013) Prognostic impact of pregnancy after breast cancer according to estrogen receptor status: a multicenter retrospective study. J Clin Oncol 31:73–79

Baucom DH, Porter LS, Kirby JS, Gremore TM, Keefe FJ (2005) Psychosocial issues confronting young women with breast cancer. Breast Dis 23:103–113

Bower JE, Ganz PA, Desmond KA, Rowland JH, Meyerowitz BE, Belin TR (2000) Fatigue in breast cancer survivors: occurrence, correlates, and impact on quality of life. J Clin Oncol 18:743–753

Boyle C C (2014). A lifespan approach to posttraumatic growth in breast cancer survivors (Unpublished master's thesis). University of California, Los Angeles

Brinton LA, Sherman ME, Carreon JD, Anderson WF (2008) Recent trends in breast cancer among younger women in the United States. J Natl Cancer Inst 100:1643

Cimprich B, Ronis DL, Martinez-Ramos G (2002) Age at diagnosis and quality of life in breast cancer survivors. Cancer Pract 10:85–93

Cluze C, Rey D, Huiart L, Bendiane MK, Bouhnik AD, Berenger C, Carrieri MP, Giorgi R (2012) Adjuvant endocrine therapy with tamoxifen in young women with breast cancer: determinants of interruptions vary over time. Ann Oncol 23:882–890

Corney R, Puthussery S, Swinglehurst J (2014) The stressors and vulnerabilities of young single childless women with breast cancer: a qualitative study. Eur J Oncol Nurs 18:17–22

Desantis C, Ma J, Bryan L, Jemal A (2014) Breast cancer statistics, 2013. CA Cancer J Clin 64:52–62

Dunn J, Steginga SK (2000) Young women's experience of breast cancer: defining young and identifying concerns. Psychooncology 9:137–146

Faller H, Schuler M, Richard M, Heckl U, Weis J, Kuffner R (2013) Effects of psycho-oncologic interventions on emotional distress and quality of life in adult patients with cancer: systematic review and meta-analysis. J Clin Oncol 31:782–793

Fobair P, Stewart SL, Chang S, D'Onofrio C, Banks PJ, Bloom JR (2006) Body image and sexual problems in young women with breast cancer. Psychooncology 15:579–594

Gabriel C, Domchek S (2010) Breast cancer in young women. Breast Cancer Res 12:212

Ganz PA, Greendale GA, Petersen L, Kahn B, Bower JE (2003) Breast cancer in younger women: reproductive and late health effects of treatment. J Clin Oncol 21:4184–4193

Ganz PA, Land SR, Geyer CE, Cecchini RS, Costantino JP, Pajon ER, Fehrenbacher L, Atkins JN, Polikoff JA, Vogel VG, Erban JK, Livingston RB, Perez EA, Mamounas EP, Wolmark N, Swain SM (2011) Menstrual history and quality-of-life outcomes in women with node-positive breast cancer treated with adjuvant therapy on the NSABP B-30 trial. J Clin Oncol 29:1110–1116

Groenvold M, Petersen MA, Idler E, Bjorner JB, Fayers PM, Mouridsen HT (2007) Psychological distress and fatigue predicted recurrence and survival in primary breast cancer patients. Breast Cancer Res Treat 105:209–219

Howard-Anderson J, Ganz PA, Bower JE, Stanton AL (2012) Quality of life, fertility concerns, and behavioral health outcomes in younger breast cancer survivors: a systematic review. J Natl Cancer Inst 104:386–405

Institute of Medicine (2013) Delivering high-quality cancer care: charting a new course for a system in crisis. The National Academies Press, Washington, DC

Johnson RH, Chien FL, Bleyer A (2013) Incidence of breast cancer with distant involvement among women in the United States, 1976 to 2009. JAMA 309:800–805

Keegan T, DeRouen M, Press D, Kurian A, Clarke C (2012) Occurrence of breast cancer subtypes in adolescent and young adult women. Breast Cancer Res 14:R55

Keegan TH, Press DJ, Tao L, DeRouen MC, Kurian AW, Clarke CA, Gomez SL (2013) Impact of breast cancer subtypes on 3-year survival among adolescent and young adult women. Breast Cancer Res 15:R95

Koppelmans V, Breteler MMB, Boogerd W, Seynaeve C, Gundy C, Schagen SB (2012a) Neuropsychological performance in survivors of breast cancer more than 20 years after adjuvant chemotherapy. J Clin Oncol 30:1080–1086

Koppelmans V, de Ruiter M, van der Lijn F, Boogerd W, Seynaeve C, van der Lugt A, Vrooman H, Niessen W, Breteler M, Schagen S (2012b) Global and focal brain volume in long-term breast cancer survivors exposed to adjuvant chemotherapy. Breast Cancer Res Treat 132(3):1099–1106

Koutrouli N, Anagnostopoulos F, Potamianos G (2012) Posttraumatic stress disorder and post-traumatic growth in breast cancer patients: a systematic review. Women Health 52:503–516

Lebel S, Beattie S, Ares I, Bielajew C (2013) Young and worried: age and fear of recurrence in breast cancer survivors. Health Psychol 32:695–705

Lewis PE, Sheng M, Rhodes MM, Jackson KE, Schover LR (2012) Psychosocial concerns of young African American breast cancer survivors. J Psychosoc Oncol 30:168–184

Litton JK, Warneke CL, Hahn KM, Palla SL, Kuerer HM, Perkins GH, Mittendorf EA, Barnett C, Gonzalez-Angulo AM, Hortobagyi GN, Theriault RL (2013) Case control study of women treated with chemotherapy for breast cancer during pregnancy as compared with nonpregnant patients with breast cancer. Oncologist 18:369–376

Mor V, Malin M, Allen S (1994) Age differences in the psychosocial problems encountered by breast cancer patients. J Natl Cancer Inst Monogr 16:191–197

Moskowitz CS, Chou JF, Wolden SL, Bernstein JL, Malhotra J, Friedman DN, Mubdi NZ, Leisenring WM, Stovall M, Hammond S, Smith SA, Henderson TO, Boice JD, Hudson MM, Diller LR, Bhatia S, Kenney LB, Neglia JP, Begg CB, Robison LL, Oeffinger KC (2014) Breast cancer after chest radiation therapy for childhood cancer. J Clin Oncol 32(21):2217–2223

Palesh OG, Roscoe JA, Mustian KM, Roth T, Savard J, Ancoli-Israel S, Heckler C, Purnell JQ, Janelsins MC, Morrow GR (2010) Prevalence, demographics, and psychological associations of sleep disruption in patients with cancer: university of Rochester cancer center-community clinical oncology program. J Clin Oncol 28:292–298

Partridge AH, Gelber S, Peppercorn J, Sampson E, Knudsen K, Laufer M, Rosenberg R, Przypyszny M, Rein A, Winer EP (2004) Web-based survey of fertility issues in young women with breast cancer. J Clin Oncol 22:4174–4183

Ruddy KJ, Gelber SI, Tamimi RM, Ginsburg ES, Schapira L, Come SE, Borges VF, Meyer ME, Partridge AH (2014) Prospective study of fertility concerns and preservation strategies in young women with breast cancer. J Clin Oncol 32:1151–1156

Schnipper HH (2003) Life after breast cancer. J Clin Oncol 21:104s–107s

Siegel R, Ma J, Zou Z, Jemal A (2014) Cancer statistics, 2014. CA Cancer J Clin 64:9–29

Theriault RL, Litton JK (2013) Pregnancy during or after breast cancer diagnosis: what do we know and what do we need to know? J Clin Oncol 31:2521–2522

Thewes B, Butow P, Girgis A, Pendlebury S (2004) The psychosocial needs of breast cancer survivors; a qualitative study of the shared and unique needs of younger versus older survivors. Psychooncology 13:177–189

Tricoli JV, Seibel NL, Blair DG, Albritton K, Hayes-Lattin B (2011) Unique characteristics of adolescent and young adult acute lymphoblastic leukemia, breast cancer, and colon cancer. J Natl Cancer Inst 103:628–635

Vinokur AD, Threatt BA, Vinokur-Kaplan D, Satariano WA (1990) The process of recovery from breast cancer for younger and older patients. Changes during the first year. Cancer 65:1242–1254

Chapter 3
Special Issues in Older Women with Breast Cancer

Arti Hurria and Hy Muss

Abstract The true face of breast cancer is more commonly that of an older woman. The rapid aging of the US population is contributing to an increasing number of breast cancer cases in older adults today, as well as an increase in the number of breast cancer survivors who carry the long-term side effects of breast cancer treatment. The number one problem facing older women with breast cancer today is that they are not receiving the same benefits from treatment advances as younger women. This disparity in outcomes highlights the great need for studies that specially include older women with breast cancer in order to guide informed decisions regarding the most efficacious treatment options. Novel study designs are needed to fill these gaps in knowledge which include metrics that provide a detailed understanding of the individual beyond chronologic age, and which identify areas of vulnerability for which targeted interventions can be employed. In studying cancer therapeutics in older adults, metrics of success, beyond disease-free and overall survival should be included, such as the feasibility of delivering the therapy, as well as the impact of treatment on functional independence and cognition. Ultimately, this framework will lead to evidence-based "personalized" medicine for the older adult.

Keywords Older patient • Breast cancer • Cancer survivors • Cancer and aging • Geriatric assessment

Introduction

Breast cancer is a disease associated with aging. The median age of diagnosis is 61 and the median age of death is 68 [NCI (National Cancer Institute) 2010]. The lifetime risk of developing breast cancer increases dramatically with age, with a cumulative

A. Hurria, M.D. (✉)
City of Hope, 1500 E Duarte Road, Duarte, CA 91010, USA
e-mail: ahurria@coh.org

H. Muss, M.D.
University of North Carolina, Chapel Hill, NC, USA
e-mail: muss@email.unc.edu

© Breast Cancer Research Foundation 2015
P.A. Ganz (ed.), *Improving Outcomes for Breast Cancer Survivors*,
Advances in Experimental Medicine and Biology 1,
DOI 10.1007/978-3-319-16366-6_3

23

lifetime risk of 12 % (Siegel et al. 2014). Although social media often highlights breast cancer in younger women, the true face of breast cancer is more commonly that of an older woman. This will become even more apparent over the next 20 years as the cancer incidence rises with the aging of the US population (Smith et al. 2009).

The baby boomers began to turn age 65 in the year 2011, leading to rapid growth in the number of individuals age 65 and older. From 2010 to 2050, this population is projected to increase from 40 million (13 % of the US population) to 89 million individuals (20 % of the US population) (Smith et al. 2009). Together, the association of breast cancer with aging and the aging of the US population will contribute to an increased number of breast cancer cases in older adults, as well as an increase in the number of breast cancer survivors who carry the long-term side effects of breast cancer treatment (Fig. 3.1) (Smith et al. 2009; Parry et al. 2011; Siegel et al. 2012, 2014; DeSantis et al. 2014).

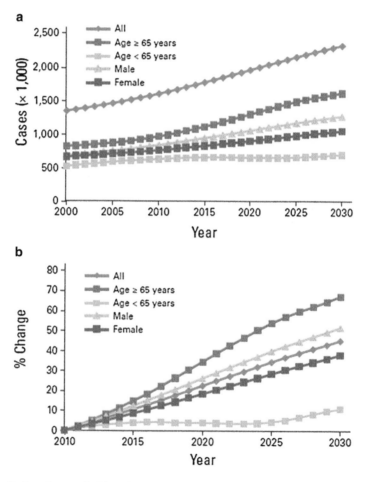

Fig. 3.1 Projected cases of all invasive cancers in the United States by age and sex [Reproduced with permission from Smith et al. (2009)]

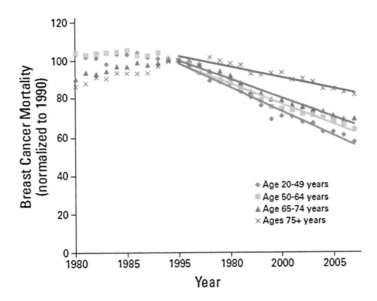

Fig. 3.2 US breast cancer death rates from 1980 to 2007. Larger decrease in breast cancer mortality seen in younger vs. older patients [Reproduced with permission from Smith et al. (2011)]

Although breast cancer is associated with aging, older women are not receiving the same benefits from treatment advances as younger women (Smith et al. 2009, 2011). Breast cancer death rates decreased by 1.14 % per year in women age ≥75 from 1990 to 2007, compared with 2.49 % a year in women age 20–49 (Fig. 3.2) (Smith et al. 2011). Although overall breast cancer death rates are decreasing, the improvements in mortality are driven by greater decreases in younger not older women, and highlight the age-related disparities in breast-cancer outcomes. In this manuscript, we review the key knowledge gaps in treatment of older women with breast cancer and their survivorship issues; and propose ways for future research to fill these gaps to improve the overall health and well-being of older adults who are breast cancer survivors.

Describing Older Women with Breast Cancer

Older women with breast cancer are a heterogeneous group. With aging there is a decline in physiologic function and an accumulation of comorbid conditions, breast cancer often being one of many other competing health problems (Kimmick et al. 2014). For early stage disease in particular, older women are more likely to die of a comorbid condition other than breast cancer (Fig. 3.3). Therefore, a key part of decision-making is weighing the risk of morbidity and mortality from breast cancer vs. other diseases (Patnaik et al. 2011). Tools such as e-prognosis can help

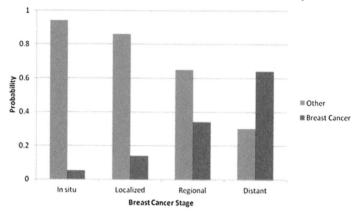

Fig. 3.3 Causes of death for patients age 70 and older with breast cancer based on stage [Adapted from Schairer (2004)]

estimate overall life expectancy; however, these tools have not been validated among patients with breast cancer (Yourman et al. 2012). Tools such as Adjuvant Online can calculate the risk of breast cancer recurrence and mortality, but do not include a detailed assessment of the specific competing comorbid illnesses facing the older adult. A single tool that synthesizes the risk of breast cancer mortality versus mortality from other causes, as well as the potential benefits and risks of treatment in the face of competing comorbidities is not currently available and is a key area for research.

Aging is a heterogenous process associated with decline in organ function and physical function; however, the rate of decline is unique to each individual, and chronological age is a poor measure of overall fitness. Older women with breast cancer vary widely in their functional states, ranging from an 80-year-old marathon runner to a 70-year-old patient with dementia and degenerative joint disease. A more detailed assessment of an older adult, as captured by a geriatric assessment, is needed in order to derive an understanding of physiologic or functional age (Freyer et al. 2005; Hurria et al. 2011; Dale et al. 2012; Extermann et al. 2012; Aparicio et al. 2013; Mandelblatt et al. 2013). This assessment evaluates individual functional status, comorbidity, cognitive function, psychological state, social support, nutritional status, medications, and socioeconomic status. Taken together, this assessment provides a detailed understanding of the individual beyond chronologic age, and identifies areas of vulnerability for which targeted interventions can be employed. Performing this assessment is a key part of "knowing" an older patient with breast cancer.

Is Breast Cancer Biologically Different in an Older Adult?

Overall there are several favorable changes that occur in breast cancer biology with increasing age: an increase in proportion of tumors that are lower grade, estrogen and progesterone receptor positive, and HER2 negative (Diab et al. 2000). However, these age-related differences are modest, and as in younger patients, tumor biology should be utilized to drive decision-making regardless of age. For older women with hormone-receptor positive, HER2 negative tumors, the tumor phenotype found in about 70 % of older women, gene-based assays (Oncotype and others), which are independent of patient age, can be utilized to estimate the risk of breast cancer relapse and the benefits of adjuvant chemotherapy in addition to endocrine therapy (Paik et al. 2004). Among triple-negative cancers, older adults derive survival benefits from chemotherapy, because the risk of relapse is highest in the first 3 years, a timeframe in which other comorbid illness are unlikely to impact life expectancy, except in the very sick (Elkin et al. 2006; Muss et al. 2009). In addition and as with younger patients, a review of the older patient's personal and family history of cancer is essential in order to appropriately refer the patient for a genetics consultation to evaluate for a hereditary predisposition.

Therapeutic Considerations for Management of Breast Cancer in Older Adults

The main therapeutic options for the treatment of breast cancer are the same across the aging spectrum. However, specific studies have guided the approach to care of the older adult and whether therapeutic decisions could be altered based on patient age and tumor type. The key motivators driving the development of these studies include: (1) determining whether alternative strategies can be utilized that would produce similar efficacy with a lower risk of toxicity, and (2) evaluating whether treatment would be associated with a meaningful decrease of breast cancer morbidity or mortality during the patient's remaining life span.

Local Therapy

The approaches to local therapy are similar between younger and older adults. The surgical treatment of early stage breast cancer is an integral part of therapy, given a low risk of surgical morbidity in all age groups. A key consideration in many older adults is whether to recommend breast radiation after breast-conserving surgery. Radiation is known to decrease the risk of local recurrence; however, its overall benefit must be considered in the context of competing comorbidities and life expectancy. This question was studied among patients age ≥70 who were treated with breast-conserving therapy and endocrine therapy for stage I disease and tumors that were hormone receptor positive and node negative. In patients randomized to radiation therapy or none, after 12 years of follow-up the omission of radiation was associated with a modest increase in the risk of a local recurrence (10 % versus 2 %) but no difference in overall survival. The majority of deaths were caused by comorbidities other than breast cancer (Hughes et al. 2010). However, gaps in knowledge remain regarding this approach in older patients with larger tumors. Of note, despite the results of this randomized trial, translation into clinical care has been limited, and most women continue to receive postoperative radiation (Soulos et al. 2012). Additional studies are needed to determine how to expedite the translation of research findings into practice, and to pinpoint the barriers to translation.

Among those where radiation therapy is warranted, barriers and challenges to receipt of radiation need to be considered including whether the patient has transportation, and whether a caregiver is needed to accompany the patient. These challenges can be amplified in an older adult who is dependent on others for transportation or who has difficulty attending a daily appointment because they are the primary caregiver for another family member such as a spouse. Randomized studies have evaluated the role of hypofractionated breast radiation therapy, and demonstrate the efficacy of such an approach (Haviland et al. 2013; Eblan et al. 2014). Additional studies are needed to identify which older patients truly need radiation therapy and whether shorter courses could yield similar benefits with less resource requirement.

Systemic Treatment Considerations

Chemotherapy CALGB 49907 is a landmark study evaluating adjuvant treatment in the care of older adults. This randomized trial in women age 65 and older evaluated the efficacy and toxicity of standard chemotherapy (AC or CMF) versus single-agent capecitabine (Muss et al. 2009). Compared with most adjuvant treatment studies, which evaluate whether more treatment improves efficacy (i.e., if AB is the standard, is AB+C superior to AB?), CALGB 49907 evaluated whether less therapy (i.e., single-agent, orally administered capecitabine) was as effective as standard-of-care intravenous polychemotherapy. The study results demonstrated a superiority of standard adjuvant intravenous polychemotherapy (AC or CMF) for both disease-free and overall survival, thus reinforcing the importance of utilizing standard regimens among patients age 65 and older.

There were several unique components in this study, including the consideration of drug dosing based on organ function, additional safety parameters to decrease the risk of toxicity, and a rich correlative component evaluating the impact of therapy on quality of life, adherence, and geriatric assessment parameters (such as function, comorbidity, and cognition) (Partridge et al. 2010; Kornblith et al. 2011; Freedman et al. 2013).

A novel component in the design of CALGB 49907 was the development of a parallel registry study, CALGB 366901, led by Dr. Jeanne Mandelblatt. The rationale for this observational cohort study was to understand the factors, including patient preferences, that influenced adjuvant treatment decisions in older adults with breast cancer. This study demonstrated that patient preference for chemotherapy and a higher rating of physician communication were associated with chemotherapy receipt (Mandelblatt et al. 2010). Furthermore, physician decision styles also influenced the treatment chosen. In particular, the oncologists' preference for chemotherapy was associated with patients' subsequent receipt of chemotherapy treatment. Those patients who preferred to have more of the oncologist's input in treatment decisions were more likely to receive chemotherapy. Both patient and physician decision styles were independently associated with chemotherapy use (Mandelblatt et al. 2012). The measures included in CALGB 49907 were similar to those utilized in 369901, allowing for a comparison of characteristics and outcomes of patients who enrolled in these two studies with inclusion of detailed geriatric assessment measures.

Additional studies of adjuvant chemotherapy for breast cancer in older adults are needed. This is particularly true because the risks of adjuvant breast cancer treatment are greater in older adults. An evaluation of four adjuvant breast cancer trials performed in the Cancer and Leukemia Group B over a quarter of a century demonstrated that although patients age 65 and older received the same benefits as younger patients from more versus less aggressive chemotherapy regimens, older women had a higher risk of treatment toxicity, a greater likelihood of not being able to complete the treatment course, and an increased risk of treatment-related mortality (Crivellari et al. 2000; Muss et al. 2007). These risks must be weighed in the decision-making process, and studies of novel regimens are needed. CALGB 49907 can serve as a model for future studies in terms of design, implementation, and successful execution of an adjuvant treatment trial in older adults. Trials designed specifically for older patients should be expanded.

Trastuzumab The gaps in knowledge regarding the selection of adjuvant regimens in patients with pre-existing comorbidities are particularly relevant for novel targeted therapies that are introduced in the adjuvant setting, as they seldom have been evaluated in older adults. For example, adjuvant trastuzumab, in conjunction with chemotherapy, is now the standard of care for most patients with Her2 positive breast cancer. However, the studies that set this standard included few older adults, and patients with cardiac comorbidities were excluded (Piccart-Gebhart et al. 2005; Romond et al. 2005; Slamon et al. 2011). Furthermore, among those patients enrolled, older age and comorbidities common to the older patient population (pre-existing hypertension, high body mass index, and low/normal baseline left ventricular ejection fraction) have been noted to be risk factors for toxicity (Tan-Chiu et al. 2005; Suter et al. 2007; Perez et al. 2008). Studies of the late cardiac effects of chemotherapy have been performed in the cooperative group setting (Ganz et al. 2008). Similar studies are needed with targeted therapies which carry a risk of long-term cardiac complications. (This topic is covered in detail by Fabian in Chap. 13).

Endocrine Therapy Endocrine therapy remains a mainstay of therapy for hormone-receptor positive disease, and the efficacy is similar across the aging spectrum [Early Breast Cancer Trialists' Collaborative Group (EBCTCG) 2005]. Adherence to therapy is necessary in order to derive optimal benefit, suggesting that this should be an area of focus for older individuals where polypharmacy is common. For an older adult, the main treatment considerations and survivorship issues for aromatase inhibitors revolves around the impact of therapy on comorbidities including bone health, joint pain and musculosketal symptoms, and potential cardiac risk; while for tamoxifen the major risks are thromboembolism and endometrial cancer (Perez et al. 2006; Cuppone et al. 2008; Eastell et al. 2008; Amir et al. 2011; Mieog et al. 2012). As the benefits of prolonged endocrine therapy beyond 5 years are becoming apparent, studies of the long-term side effects of prolonged therapy and interventions to decrease these side effects are needed, especially in older women whose life expectancy can dramatically decrease with increasing age (Goss et al. 2005).

Approach to Metastatic Disease

Overall, the goals of treatment for metastatic disease are the same across all age groups. Since breast cancer is treatable but not curable, the goals of treatment include preserving function, minimizing symptoms, maintaining quality of life, and prolonging survival. Just as with younger patients, there is an overall desire to integrate new therapies, but the challenge is the low representation of older adults on FDA registration trials, and therefore limited guidelines on how to dose these medications in the geriatric population (Talarico et al. 2004; Scher and Hurria 2012). Furthermore, there have been almost no studies performed in frail older adults, leading to a major gap in knowledge.

Research Needs

Overcoming Barriers to the Enrollment of Older Adults in Clinical Trials

As with most cancers, older adults continue to be underrepresented on clinical research studies; as a result there is scant evidence-based data regarding treatment and survivorship issues facing older adults with breast cancer (Lewis et al. 2003; Murthy et al. 2004; Unger et al. 2006). This is particularly true among older patients with breast cancer enrolling in adjuvant treatment trials. Among four cooperative group adjuvant trials for node-positive breast cancer conducted over a quarter of a century, only 8 % of participants were age ≥ 65, and only 2 % were age ≥ 70 (Muss et al. 2005). Furthermore older adults are underrepresented on FDA registration trials, so there is inadequate evidence-based data available on how to dose these drugs in older patients (Talarico et al. 2004; Scher and Hurria 2012).

A study performed in Cancer and Leukemia Group B evaluated the barriers to clinical trial enrollment in a matched sample of patients (older vs. younger adults) with breast cancer who had the same treating physician. This study demonstrated that older adults were less likely to be offered a clinical trial but were as likely to accept enrollment if offered (Kemeny et al. 2003). A survey of treating physicians highlighted concerns regarding treatment-related toxicity and the need for specific trials in older adults with safety parameters in place (Kornblith et al. 2002). Education regarding the potential benefits of clinical trial enrollment in older adults is needed, but a multicenter study showed that education alone will not increase clinical trial enrollment, and a multifaceted approach is necessary (Kimmick et al. 2005).

Understanding the Impact of Treatment on Functional and Cognitive Aging

Traditional clinical trials focus on metrics of disease-free and overall survival. For an older adult, the impact of treatment on functional status and cognition may be as, if not more, important to their decision-making process (Braithwaite et al. 2010; Dale et al. 2012; Mandelblatt et al. 2013; Sehl et al. 2013). Measures of functional status, as captured in a geriatric assessment pre-treatment, predict cancer treatment toxicity and survival. Furthermore, among older adults with breast cancer, a decline in functional status in the 2 years following diagnosis has been associated with poorer overall survival (Sehl et al. 2013).

There is a biologic rationale for concern that cancer treatment may accelerate the aging process. Aging and chemotherapy, in particular, are associated with a variety of similar biologic changes including DNA damage, inflammation, oxidative stress, and cellular senescence. A cross-sectional study of breast cancer survivors demonstrated that prior chemotherapy was associated with an increase in p16 *INK4a* expression, a potential molecular marker of aging, which equated to approximately 10 years of chronological aging (Muss et al. 2009; Sanoff et al. 2014). The potential medical, functional, and social impact of these biologic findings is unknown, and further research is needed to address this knowledge gap (Pallis et al. 2014).

There is emerging data suggesting that receipt of cancer therapy may be associated with decrements in cardiopulmonary function, which persist throughout the survivorship years. A study of breast cancer survivors, who were on average 7 years post diagnosis demonstrated reductions in cardiovascular fitness in comparison to a non-cancer control group (mean 55 years; SD 10 years) (Lakoski et al. 2013). Furthermore, another study demonstrated that patients with breast cancer have a marked impairment in peak oxygen consumption (a measure of aerobic consumption) in the survivorship years (Jones et al. 2012). These data demonstrate that adjuvant chemotherapy is likely associated with aging of the cardiopulmonary system.

These findings are seen across the aging spectrum and are especially germane to older patients.

There is a dearth of knowledge regarding cancer treatment impact on cognitive aging, as the majority of studies to date have been performed in younger adults (Hurria et al. 2006; Yamada et al. 2010; Koppelmans et al. 2012; Mandelblatt et al. 2013). Studying the cognitive effects of cancer therapy in older adults is complex because breast cancer is only one of many other factors (such as comorbid medical conditions, lifestyle, and genetics) that can affect cognitive function. However, emerging literature is demonstrating an interaction of cancer treatment, aging, and cognitive function/reserve which highlights the importance of studying the cognitive effects of cancer therapy in older adults (Ahles et al. 2010). The age at which an individual is treated (i.e., the more vulnerable brain with decreased cognitive reserve) may also have an impact on the risk of cognitive decline. Research is needed to understand how cancer therapy affects cognitive aging both during the acute post-treatment phase and in the survivorship years. Interventions to maintain or minimize therapy's potential harm to cognition are needed.

Clinical and biological markers of functional age and cognition (as captured in a geriatric assessment) are vital components to be included in breast cancer trial design, at baseline as well as longitudinally. Interventions to maintain function and independence, such as home-based exercise interventions, have proven efficacious, and additional research is needed to understand both the physical and cognitive impact of such interventions and to evaluate the "dose" of the intervention that is needed to obtain and sustain a positive effect (Demark-Wahnefried, et al. 2006).

Social, Emotional, and Financial Considerations of Breast Cancer in Older Adults

There are unique social considerations for the older adult with breast cancer. Questions that arise during the treatment planning process usually include: If the older adult lives alone, who would bring them to the hospital in the event of an emergency? Can the patient and family afford caregiver support? Is the patient a caregiver for someone else (spouse, children, grandchildren)? Who would provide that care if the patient is unable to do so? Does the patient still drive? If not, who will provide transportation for treatment-related visits? These questions are not necessarily unique to patients with breast cancer, and need to be considered when caring for any older adult with cancer. However, studies are needed among patients with breast cancer to more accurately quantify the potential impact of a treatment course on both the patient's and caregiver's well-being, and on patients and families planning for treatment.

The emotional impact of breast cancer in older adults is related to the patient's physical function, mental function, and psychosocial adjustment. For example, after surgery, older women with impaired mental health, physical functioning, and emotional social support have poorer psychosocial adjustment and self-perceived health 1 year later (Ganz et al. 2003). Other studies demonstrate that emotional wellbeing is associated with enhanced physical function, emotional social support, and the quality of the medical interactions (Clough-Gorr et al. 2007). Therefore studying the emotional impact of cancer therapy in an older adult requires a thorough understanding of the other potential factors that play a role in the patient's emotional wellbeing.

Preparing to Care for an Aging Population with Breast Cancer

The challenge facing the field of medical oncology is the projected shortage of individuals to care for this growing population of older adults with cancer. By 2020, the demand for oncologists (driven primarily by the aging population and increase in cancer survivors) will grow by 48 %; however, the supply of healthcare workers will only grow by 14 % (Hortobagyi 2007). At the same time, the number of geriatricians is predicted to decline, despite the aging of the US population (IOM 2008). This workforce shortage will lead to a limited number of physicians with expertise in geriatrics able to provide collaborative care. In order to bridge that gap, the recommendations from the Institute of Medicine (IOM) titled *"Retooling for an Aging America: Building the Health-Care Workforce"* state "…to meet the health-care needs of the next generation of older adults, the geriatric competence of the entire workforce needs to be enhanced…innovative models need to be developed and implemented…"(IOM 2008) The report concludes that all members of the healthcare team must have knowledge of geriatrics in order to meet the needs of the aging patient. Key members of the team are "informal caregivers," often family members, who play an integral and often unrecognized role in the healthcare team.

Research is needed to develop an educational curriculum containing the key principles of geriatric care that are needed across all disciplines, as well as the specific principles that are unique to the discipline being educated. Furthermore, competencies need to be developed to serve as a metric as to whether that content has been successfully learned. Novel means of delivering content to an expanding workforce will need to be evaluated. In particular, special attention must be paid to caregivers, who are a critical part of the healthcare team but require both education and ongoing guidance in order to participate in the care of an older adult. These issues are not unique to patients with breast cancer; however, they are a major component for providing quality cancer care across the trajectory of the disease (Institute of Medicine 2013).

Conclusions

In summary, although progress has been made in the treatment of older adults with breast cancer, several gaps in knowledge exist. A biopsychosocial model can be utilized to summarize some of the key gaps in knowledge. Specifically, markers of risk for adverse treatment outcomes are needed which include biological, functional, and psychosocial factors. These markers, in addition to an understanding of the patient's physiology and organ function, could lead to more refined therapies that are targeted to the "stage of aging" in addition to the stage and biology of the tumor (Dale 2009). This framework could be utilized to evaluate the risks and benefits of treatment regimens in frail, pre-frail, and healthy older patients. An evaluation of the risks includes quantifying the impact of therapy on function and cognition, metrics which may be more important to older adults than disease-specific parameters. With any treatment plan, the feasibility of delivering the treatment is a key outcome. Feasibility should be assessed in terms of both whether treatment toxicity and/or psychosocial factors limit treatment delivery. Ultimately, this framework will lead to evidence-based "personalized" medicine for the older adult.

References

Ahles TA, Saykin AJ et al (2010) Longitudinal assessment of cognitive changes associated with adjuvant treatment for breast cancer: impact of age and cognitive reserve. J Clin Oncol 28(29):4434–4440

Amir E, Seruga B et al (2011) Toxicity of adjuvant endocrine therapy in postmenopausal breast cancer patients: a systematic review and meta-analysis. J Natl Cancer Inst 103(17): 1299–1309

Aparicio T, Jouve JL et al (2013) Geriatric factors predict chemotherapy feasibility: ancillary results of FFCD 2001-02 phase III study in first-line chemotherapy for metastatic colorectal cancer in elderly patients. J Clin Oncol 31(11):1464–1470

Braithwaite D, Satariano WA et al (2010) Long-term prognostic role of functional limitations among women with breast cancer. J Natl Cancer Inst 102(19):1468–1477

NCI (National Cancer Institute) (2010) SEER cancer statistics factsheet: breast cancer. http://seer.cancer.gov/statfacts/html/breast.html. Retrieved 12 Mar 2014

Clough-Gorr KM, Ganz PA et al (2007) Older breast cancer survivors: factors associated with change in emotional well-being. J Clin Oncol 25(11):1334–1340

Crivellari D, Bonetti M et al (2000) Burdens and benefits of adjuvant cyclophosphamide, methotrexate, and fluorouracil and tamoxifen for elderly patients with breast cancer: the international breast cancer study group trial VII. J Clin Oncol 18(7):1412–1422

Cuppone F, Bria E et al (2008) Do adjuvant aromatase inhibitors increase the cardiovascular risk in postmenopausal women with early breast cancer? Meta-analysis of randomized trials. Cancer 112(2):260–267

Dale W (2009) "Staging the aging" when considering androgen deprivation therapy for older men with prostate cancer. J Clin Oncol 27(21):3420–3422

Dale W, Mohile SG et al (2012) Biological, clinical, and psychosocial correlates at the interface of cancer and aging research. J Natl Cancer Inst 104(8):581–589

Demark-Wahnefried W, Clipp EC et al (2006) Lifestyle intervention development study to improve physical function in older adults with cancer: outcomes from project LEAD. J Clin Oncol 24(21):3465–3473

DeSantis C, Ma J et al (2014) Breast cancer statistics, 2013. CA Cancer J Clin 64(1):52–62

Diab SG, Elledge RM et al (2000) Tumor characteristics and clinical outcome of elderly women with breast cancer. J Natl Cancer Inst 92(7):550–556

Early Breast Cancer Trialists' Collaborative Group (EBCTCG) (2005) Effects of chemotherapy and hormonal therapy for early breast cancer on recurrence and 15-year survival: an overview of the randomised trials. Lancet 365(9472):1687–1717

Eastell R, Adams JE et al (2008) Effect of anastrozole on bone mineral density: 5-year results from the anastrozole, tamoxifen, alone or in combination trial 18233230. J Clin Oncol 26(7):1051–1057

Eblan MJ, Vanderwalde NA et al (2014) Hypofractionation for breast cancer: lessons learned from our neighbors to the north and across the pond. Oncology 28(6):536

Elkin EB, Hurria A et al (2006) Adjuvant chemotherapy and survival in older women with hormone receptor-negative breast cancer: assessing outcome in a population-based, observational cohort. J Clin Oncol 24(18):2757–2764

Extermann M, Boler I et al (2012) Predicting the risk of chemotherapy toxicity in older patients: the chemotherapy risk assessment scale for high-age patients (CRASH) score. Cancer 118(13):3377–3386

Freedman RA, Pitcher B et al (2013) Cognitive function in older women with breast cancer treated with standard chemotherapy and capecitabine on cancer and leukemia group B 49907. Breast Cancer Res Treat 139(2):607–616

Freyer G, Geay JF et al (2005) Comprehensive geriatric assessment predicts tolerance to chemotherapy and survival in elderly patients with advanced ovarian carcinoma: a GINECO study. Ann Oncol 16(11):1795–1800

Ganz PA, Guadagnoli E et al (2003) Breast cancer in older women: quality of life and psychosocial adjustment in the 15 months after diagnosis. J Clin Oncol 21(21):4027–4033

Ganz PA, Hussey MA et al (2008) Late cardiac effects of adjuvant chemotherapy in breast cancer survivors treated on Southwest oncology group protocol s8897. J Clin Oncol 26(8):1223–1230

Goss PE, Ingle JN et al (2005) Randomized trial of letrozole following tamoxifen as extended adjuvant therapy in receptor-positive breast cancer: updated findings from NCIC CTG MA.17. J Natl Cancer Inst 97(17):1262–1271

Haviland JS, Owen JR et al (2013) The UK standardisation of breast radiotherapy (START) trials of radiotherapy hypofractionation for treatment of early breast cancer: 10-year follow-up results of two randomised controlled trials. Lancet Oncol 14(11):1086–1094

Hortobagyi GN (2007) A shortage of oncologists? The American society of clinical oncology workforce study. J Clin Oncol 25(12):1468–1469

Hughes K, Schnaper L et al (2010) Lumpectomy plus tamoxifen with or without irradiation in women age 70 or older with early breast cancer [abstract]. J Clin Oncol 28(Suppl 15)

Hurria A, Rosen C et al (2006) Cognitive function of older patients receiving adjuvant chemotherapy for breast cancer: a pilot prospective longitudinal study. J Am Geriatr Soc 54(6): 925–931

Hurria A, Togawa K et al (2011) Predicting chemotherapy toxicity in older adults with cancer: a prospective multicenter study. J Clin Oncol 29(25):3457–3465

Institute of Medicine (2013) Delivering high-quality cancer care: charting a new course for a system in crisis. The National Academies Press, Washington, DC

IOM (2008) Retooling for an aging America: building the healthcare workforce. The National Academies Press, Washington, DC

Jones LW, Courneya KS et al (2012) Cardiopulmonary function and age-related decline across the breast cancer survivorship continuum. J Clin Oncol. 30(20):2530–2537

Kemeny MM, Peterson BL et al (2003) Barriers to clinical trial participation by older women with breast cancer. J Clin Oncol 21(12):2268–2275

Kimmick GG, Peterson BL et al (2005) Improving accrual of older persons to cancer treatment trials: a randomized trial comparing an educational intervention with standard information: CALGB 360001. J Clin Oncol 23(10):2201–2207

Kimmick G, Fleming ST et al (2014) Comorbidity burden and guideline-concordant care for breast cancer. J Am Geriatr Soc 62(3):482–488

Koppelmans V, Breteler MM et al (2012) Neuropsychological performance in survivors of breast cancer more than 20 years after adjuvant chemotherapy. J Clin Oncol 30(10):1080–1086

Kornblith AB, Kemeny M et al (2002) Survey of oncologists' perceptions of barriers to accrual of older patients with breast carcinoma to clinical trials. Cancer 95(5):989–996

Kornblith AB, Lan L et al (2011) Quality of life of older patients with early-stage breast cancer receiving adjuvant chemotherapy: a companion study to cancer and leukemia group B 49907. J Clin Oncol 29(8):1022–1028

Lakoski SG, Barlow CE et al (2013) The influence of adjuvant therapy on cardiorespiratory fitness in early-stage breast cancer seven years after diagnosis: the Cooper Center Longitudinal Study. Breast Cancer Res Treat. 138(3): 909–916

Lewis JH, Kilgore ML et al (2003) Participation of patients 65 years of age or older in cancer clinical trials. J Clin Oncol 21(7):1383–1389

Mandelblatt JS, Sheppard VB et al (2010) Breast cancer adjuvant chemotherapy decisions in older women: the role of patient preference and interactions with physicians. J Clin Oncol 28(19):3146–3153

Mandelblatt JS, Faul LA et al (2012) Patient and physician decision styles and breast cancer chemotherapy use in older women: cancer and leukemia group B protocol 369901. J Clin Oncol 30(21):2609–2614

Mandelblatt JS, Hurria A et al (2013) Cognitive effects of cancer and its treatments at the intersection of aging: what do we know; what do we need to know? Semin Oncol 40(6):709–725

Mieog JS, Morden JP et al (2012) Carpal tunnel syndrome and musculoskeletal symptoms in postmenopausal women with early breast cancer treated with exemestane or tamoxifen after 2-3 years of tamoxifen: a retrospective analysis of the intergroup exemestane study. Lancet Oncol 13(4):420–432

Murthy VH, Krumholz HM et al (2004) Participation in cancer clinical trials: race-, sex-, and age-based disparities. JAMA 291(22):2720–2726

Muss HB, Woolf S et al (2005) Adjuvant chemotherapy in older and younger women with lymph node-positive breast cancer. JAMA 293(9):1073–1081

Muss HB, Berry DA et al (2007) Toxicity of older and younger patients treated with adjuvant chemotherapy for node-positive breast cancer: the cancer and leukemia group B experience. J Clin Oncol 25(24):3699–3704

Muss HB, Berry DA et al (2009) Adjuvant chemotherapy in older women with early-stage breast cancer. N Engl J Med 360(20):2055–2065

Paik S, Shak S et al (2004) A multigene assay to predict recurrence of tamoxifen-treated, node-negative breast cancer. N Engl J Med 351(27):2817–2826

Pallis AG, Hatse S et al (2014) Evaluating the physiological reserves of older patients with cancer: the value of potential biomarkers of aging? J Geriatr Oncol 5(2):204–218

Parry C, Kent EE et al (2011) Cancer survivors: a booming population. Cancer Epidemiol Biomarkers Prev 20(10):1996–2005

Partridge AH, Archer L et al (2010) Adherence and persistence with oral adjuvant chemotherapy in older women with early-stage breast cancer in CALGB 49907: adherence companion study 60104. J Clin Oncol 28(14):2418–2422

Patnaik JL, Byers T et al (2011) The influence of comorbidities on overall survival among older women diagnosed with breast cancer. J Natl Cancer Inst 103(14):1101–1111

Perez EA, Josse RG et al (2006) Effect of letrozole versus placebo on bone mineral density in women with primary breast cancer completing 5 or more years of adjuvant tamoxifen: a companion study to NCIC CTG MA.17. J Clin Oncol 24(22):3629–3635

Perez EA, Suman VJ et al (2008) Cardiac safety analysis of doxorubicin and cyclophosphamide followed by paclitaxel with or without trastuzumab in the north central cancer treatment group N9831 adjuvant breast cancer trial. J Clin Oncol 26(8):1231–1238

Piccart-Gebhart MJ, Procter M et al (2005) Trastuzumab after adjuvant chemotherapy in HER2-positive breast cancer. N Engl J Med 353(16):1659–1672

Romond EH, Perez EA et al (2005) Trastuzumab plus adjuvant chemotherapy for operable HER2-positive breast cancer. N Engl J Med 353(16):1673–1684

Sanoff HK, Deal AM et al (2014) Effect of cytotoxic chemotherapy on markers of molecular age in patients with breast cancer. J Natl Cancer Inst 106(4):dju057

Schairer C, Mink PJ et al (2004) Probabilities of death from breast cancer and other causes among female breast cancer patients. J Natl Cancer Inst 96(17):1311–1321

Scher KS, Hurria A (2012) Under-representation of older adults in cancer registration trials: known problem, little progress. J Clin Oncol 30(17):2036–2038

Sehl M, Lu X et al (2013) Decline in physical functioning in first 2 years after breast cancer diagnosis predicts 10-year survival in older women. J Cancer Surviv 7(1):20–31

Siegel R, DeSantis C et al (2012) Cancer treatment and survivorship statistics, 2012. CA Cancer J Clin 62(4):220–241

Siegel R, Ma J et al (2014) Cancer statistics, 2014. CA Cancer J Clin 64(1):9–29

Slamon D, Eiermann W et al (2011) Adjuvant trastuzumab in HER2-positive breast cancer. N Engl J Med 365(14):1273–1283

Smith BD, Smith GL et al (2009) Future of cancer incidence in the United States: burdens upon an aging, changing nation. J Clin Oncol 27(17):2758–2765

Smith BD, Jiang J et al (2011) Improvement in breast cancer outcomes over time: are older women missing out? J Clin Oncol 29(35):4647–4653

Soulos PR, Yu JB et al (2012) Assessing the impact of a cooperative group trial on breast cancer care in the medicare population. J Clin Oncol 30(14):1601–1607

Suter TM, Procter M et al (2007) Trastuzumab-associated cardiac adverse effects in the herceptin adjuvant trial. J Clin Oncol 25(25):3859–3865

Talarico L, Chen G et al (2004) Enrollment of elderly patients in clinical trials for cancer drug registration: a 7-year experience by the US food and drug administration. J Clin Oncol 22(22):4626–4631

Tan-Chiu E, Yothers G et al (2005) Assessment of cardiac dysfunction in a randomized trial comparing doxorubicin and cyclophosphamide followed by paclitaxel, with or without trastuzumab as adjuvant therapy in node-positive, human epidermal growth factor receptor 2-overexpressing breast cancer: NSABP B-31. J Clin Oncol 23(31):7811–7819

Unger JM, Coltman CA Jr et al (2006) Impact of the year 2000 medicare policy change on older patient enrollment to cancer clinical trials. J Clin Oncol 24(1):141–144

Yamada TH, Denburg NL et al (2010) Neuropsychological outcomes of older breast cancer survivors: cognitive features ten or more years after chemotherapy. J Neuropsychiatry Clin Neurosci 22(1):48–54

Yourman LC, Lee SJ et al (2012) Prognostic indices for older adults: a systematic review. JAMA 307(2):182–192

Chapter 4
Breast Cancer Among Special Populations: Disparities in Care Across the Cancer Control Continuum

Electra D. Paskett

Abstract Disparities in breast cancer risk factors, access, and treatment patterns are responsible for disparities in incidence, mortality and other measures of the impact of breast cancer among different population groups. Moreover, differences in culture and role definition impact various areas of aging and quality of life. Populations most impacted by disparities include women of racial/ethnic groups, older women, and women from rural and urban areas. More research is needed to document and address disparities across the cancer control continuum among a variety of populations that suffer disparities.

Keywords Breast cancer • Special populations • Cancer control continuum • Breast cancer disparities

Introduction

While Breast Cancer (BC) is relatively a "rare" disease, some populations suffer from a disproportionate burden of incidence, mortality, risk factors, or late stage disease. These populations, the elderly, racial/ethnic minorities, rural, low socioeconomic status (SES) populations, women in developing nations, and lesbian/gay/transgender women, face disparities. Disparities, or differences that should not exist, that impact BC survival are evident across the cancer control continuum, from

E.D. Paskett (✉)
Division of Cancer Prevention and Control, Department of Internal Medicine,
College of Medicine, Columbus, OH 43201, USA

Division of Epidemiology, College of Public Health, Columbus, OH 43201, USA

Comprehensive Cancer Center, Ohio State University,
Suite 525, 1590 North High Street, Columbus, OH 43201, USA
e-mail: electra.paskett@osumc.edu

© Breast Cancer Research Foundation 2015
P.A. Ganz (ed.), *Improving Outcomes for Breast Cancer Survivors*,
Advances in Experimental Medicine and Biology 862,
DOI 10.1007/978-3-319-16366-6_4

39

etiology through survivorship. This chapter will focus on first, highlighting disparities across and within many of these populations, second, discuss research that examines/ addresses these disparities, and finally, suggest challenges and directions for future research to reduce/eliminate breast cancer disparities.

Breast Cancer Disparities

Worldwide, the incidence of BC is higher in more developed countries, such as The United States (U.S.) and Canada, Australia/New Zealand, as well as countries in Western Europe compared to less developed nations including those in Middle/ Eastern Africa as well as Eastern Asia (Age-standardized rate (ASR) = 71.7/100,000 women vs. 29.3/100,000 women, respectively); however, the ratio of the mortality rate to incidence rate is higher in less developed regions compared to more developed regions (0.4 vs. 0.24, respectively) (Youlden et al. 2012). Similarly, 5 year relative survival between developed and less developed nations show vast differences (e.g. 89.2 % in the U.S. vs. 38.8 % in Algeria) (Youlden et al. 2012). These disparities are probably the most striking and are due to the lack of population-based mammographic screening in less developed regions, as well as differences in access to state-of-the-art treatments and cultural barriers impacting detection and treatment, respectively. Economic conditions greatly impact access to early detection and treatment services. Unstable economic conditions lead to difficulty in obtaining an adequate oncology workforce in addition to problems in securing resources such as electricity as well as equipment necessary for early detection and treatment. Survivorship and palliative care services are almost non-existent in these developing regions, making estimates nearly impossible (Coughlin and Ekwueme 2009; Harford et al. 2011; American Cancer Society 2013).

Even in the U.S., our model for a developed nation, breast cancer disparities are evident across the cancer control continuum. The most reported disparities are among those of racial/ethnic minority groups (See Table 4.1), older women, women from lower SES groups, and women who reside in urban areas (Table 4.2).

Table 4.1 Examples of breast cancer disparities across the cancer control continuum

Etiology	Prevention	Early detection	Follow-up	Treatment	Survivorship
• Biology and	• Chemo-prevention	• Mammography	• Access	• Adjuvant chemotherapy	• Treatment side effects
• Risk factors		• MRI	• Quality	• Radiation therapy	• Adherence to adjuvant hormone therapy
		• Self-exam	• Timeliness of therapy	• Surgery	• Coping skills
					• Body image
					• Social support
					• Acculturation
					• Quality of life

Table 4.2 Average annual (2006–2010), age-adjusted invasive female breast cancer incidence and mortality rates per 100,000 women, and 5-year relative survival probabilities among race groups and Hispanics/Latinos

Population	Incidence rate (per 100,000)	Mortality rate (per 100,000)	5-year survival probability (%)
White	127.4	22.1	90.4
African-American	118.4	30.8	78.9
Asian/Pacific Islander	84.7	11.5	91.4
Hispanic/Latino	91.1	14.8	87
American Indian/Alaska Native	90.3	15.5	85.4

Source Cancer statistics review, 2013

However, due to limitations in the definition of SES and rural residence, limited data are available across the continuum. Thus, this chapter is limited by available data.

Disparities Across the Cancer Control Continuum

Etiology and Prevention

An examination of risk factors for poor-outcome disease can provide some clues to these disparities. For example, modifiable risk factors, e.g. obesity, pregnancy, and postmenopausal hormone use, are differentially distributed among populations where we see disparities, e.g. African American and Hispanic women are more likely to be overweight/obese vs. white women, however, most of the literature in this area has provided inconclusive results. Furthermore, what we know about the uptake of chemoprevention, diet, exercise and prophylaxis, including genetic testing and surgery, in most of these minority populations is lagging behind that of white women as well as women residing in more urban, as opposed to rural, areas. Studies of non-modifiable risk factors, e.g. genetics, have provided more conclusive results. Germline mutations, for example, *BRCA1* mutations, result in higher risk for triple negative cancers (American Cancer Society 2013). Despite advancements in genetic testing leading to reductions in morbidity and mortality associated with breast cancer, research suggests that African American and minority women are significantly less likely to receive genetic counseling and testing in comparison to white women (Howlander et al. 2014). Health care reform now requires that insurance cover the cost of genetic testing. However, for populations of women who are not covered by health insurance, genetic testing is incredibly expensive, typically costing around $3,400. Exorbitant costs associated with genetic testing clearly place minority and impoverished women at a certain disadvantage for breast cancer outcomes (Hall and Olopade 2006; Johns Hopkins Medicine Breast Center; Susan G. Komen Testing for *BRCA1* & *BRCA2* Mutations).

Triple Negative Breast Cancer (TNBC), accounts for 10–20 % of invasive BC, but has poorer prognosis than luminal tumors and treatment options are more limited (Boyle 2012). Risk of TNBC is roughly three times higher among non-Hispanic black women and pre-menopausal women (Boyle 2012). Moreover, a study from Ghana found that there might be a genetic predisposition to TNBC among women of African ancestry (prevalence of TNBC 82 % in Ghana, 33 % among African American women and 10 % among white American women) (Boyle 2012). Similarly, among Asian/Pacific Islander women, the risk of ER/PR positive tumors is higher among Korean women vs. Hawaiian women (Li et al. 2002). Both Hispanic and American Indian/Alaskan Native women have larger tumors and more advanced disease at diagnosis (Mejia de Grubb et al. 2013; Von Friederichs-Fitzwater et al. 2010).

Screening Behavior

While guidelines have changed over time, clearly average-risk women over age 50 should have a mammogram every 2 years; moderate to high risk women should consult with their physician as to when to start screening, what modality (MRI vs. mammography) and how often. In addition, access to high quality imaging services and prompt/proper follow-up of abnormalities found should be available to all populations. Access to breast cancer screening as well as differences in quality of care among black and white women have contributed greatly to observed disparities in breast cancer mortality. For example, from 1999 to 2003 in Chicago, the mortality rate for breast cancer was 49 % higher among black women compared to white women. In 2003, the mortality rate increased to 68 % higher among black women compared to white women (Hirschman et al. 2007). Explanations for this observed disparity have focused on gaps in education, access to screening, as well as differences in quality of care between black and white women. Research suggests that white women in Chicago are more likely than black women to attend academic and private healthcare facilities, as well as more likely to have their mammograms read by specially trained radiologists (Ansell et al. 2009).

Disparities in mammography use are hard to determine because of the reliance on self-reported use in the most commonly used metric for screening utilization, the Behavioral Risk Factor Surveillance System (BRFSS). Self-reports of recent mammography use are actually highest among African-American women (77 %) than white women (75 %), however, verification of self-reports drop these rates to 59 % vs. 65 %, respectively [Frieden and Centers for Disease Control and Prevention (CDC) 2012]. For example, in Chicago, self reported mammogram screening rates have been similar for blacks and whites since 1996 despite the dramatic difference in breast cancer mortality rates. However, poor and black women tend to over-report screening by as much as 30 % (Hirschman et al. 2007). Asian Pacific/Islander women in general have a 74 % prevalence rate (self-reported); however, disparities exist in mammography prevalence among Asian subgroups e.g. South Asian women

(40 %) vs. Japanese Women (71 %) (Frieden and Centers for Disease Control and Prevention (CDC) 2012; Lee et al. 2002). For American Indians/Alaskan Natives (AI/AN), rates are at 69 %, and geographical differences have also been noted, i.e. AI/AN women from Alaska had higher screening rates than those living in the Southwest [Centers for Disease Control and Prevention (CDC) 2012; Schumacher et al. 2008]. Hispanic women also report moderate screening rates, 70 %; compared to non-Hispanic women (Lim et al. 2009; Lopez-Class et al. 2011; Native American Cancer Research Corporation Native Americans and Cancer). The women from these other racial/ethnic groups are more likely to face cultural barriers to receiving screening, e.g. prefer traditional holistic medicine to Western medicine or have modesty concerns. Ultimately, no single intervention will have the ability to reduce mortality associated with breast cancer in disparity stricken areas such as Chicago. Only through a multifaceted approach that addresses issues such as cultural differences, increased health education, access to care and decreasing barriers to screening, will the mortality gap begin to narrow.

Stage at Diagnosis

Stage at diagnosis is an indicator of both quality of care (e.g. good mammography use and follow-up), as well as outcomes following treatment. Many studies have demonstrated that women living in rural areas are diagnosed at later stages compared to urban breast cancer patients (Monroe et al. 1992; Nguyen-Pham et al. 2014; Amey et al. 1997; Howe et al. 1992). Moreover, rural African-American women are diagnosed at later stages compared to rural white and urban white and African-American women (Amey et al. 1997). Asian women, on the other hand, are more likely to be diagnosed at Stage 1 compared to African-American women, American Indian/Alaskan Native, and Hispanic women; however, again within Asian subgroups there are disparities in not only stage of diagnosis, but age at diagnosis, and tumor grade (see Tables 4.3) (Li et al. 2002; Mejia de Grubb et al. 2013; Von Friederichs-Fitzwater et al. 2010; Yi et al. 2012).

Follow-up for Abnormal Screening Tests

Prompt and proper follow-up for any abnormalities detected on screening is crucial to improving outcomes. Issues such as access (e.g. facilities, proper technology, insurance coverage, transportation), quality state-of-the-art facilities, proper testing, and competent providers are crucial to the receipt of follow-up care. Studies have documented longer intervals for follow-up after an abnormal mammogram for African-American women, even with similar insurance status, compared to white women [Centers for Disease Control and Prevention (CDC) 2012]. Language barriers also contribute to disparities in follow-up in non-English speaking women

Table 4.3 Average annual (2007–2011), age-adjusted invasive female breast cancer incidence rates per 100,000 women, percent late (regional and distant) stage at diagnosis, and 5-year relative survival probabilities according to metropolitan/non-metropolitan residence

Population	Incidence rate (per 100,000)	Percent late stage (%)[a]	5-year survival probability (%)
Metropolitan	122.1	73.6	89.1
Non-metropolitan	111.2	72.5	86.9

Source For incidence and stage: Surveillance, Epidemiology, and End Results (SEER) program (www.seer.cancer.gov) SEER*Stat Database: Incidence—SEER 18 regs research data + Hurricane Katrina impacted Louisiana cases, Nov 2013 sub (2000–2011) "Katrina/Rita population adjustment"—linked to county attributes—total U.S., 1969–2012 counties, National Cancer Institute, DCCPS, surveillance research program, surveillance systems branch, released April 2014, based on the November 2013 submission; for survival: Surveillance, Epidemiology, and End Results (SEER) Program (www.seer.cancer.gov) SEER*Stat Database: Incidence—SEER 18 regs research data + Hurricane Katrina impacted Louisiana cases, Nov 2013 sub (1973–2011 varying)—linked to county attributes—total U.S., 1969–2012 counties, National Cancer Institute, DCCPS, surveillance research program, surveillance systems branch, released April 2014, based on the November 2013 submission (National Cancer Institute Surveillance)
[a]Percent late stage excluded unstaged/unknown stage tumors

(Karliner et al. 2012; Austin et al. 2002; Janz et al. 2009; Sammarco and Konecny 2010; Nápoles et al. 2011; Yanez et al. 2011). Rural women are less likely to receive follow-up testing, probably due to lack of access and facility factors (Schootman et al. 2000; Goldman et al. 2013). Finally, a study among Medicare beneficiaries found that facilities serving more vulnerable populations had lower follow-up rates for women with abnormal screening tests.

Interventions to Address Disparities

Important policy interventions occurred in the 1990s to improve mammography use among vulnerable populations. First, the Centers for Disease Control and Prevention (CDC) started the National Breast and Cervical Cancer Early Detection Program (NBCCEDP) which made free or low-cost mammograms available to low-income, under and uninsured women. Between 1991 and 2006, 1.8 million received breast cancer screening through the NBCCEDP (Hoerger et al. 2011). This program also provides follow-up care after abnormal testing and initial treatment. A recent analysis of data indicated that NBCCEDP is doing a good job in getting women in for timely and quality follow-up [Centers for Disease Control and Prevention (CDC) 2012]. One problem with NBCCEDP is that only a fraction (fewer than 20 %) of eligible women in the U.S. utilize NBCCEDP due to the funding caps on this program (NBCCEDP Breast Cancer Expert Panel 2005).

Secondly, the National Cancer Institute (NCI) developed the Cancer Control Plan, Link, Act, Network with Evidence-based Tools (PLANET) Research-Tested Intervention Programs (RTIPs) which stores research-tested interventions for improving the use of screening (including breast cancer screening) in underserved populations (Sood et al. 2007). For example, the North Carolina—Breast Screening Program (NC-BSP) and Forsyth County Cancer Screening Project (FoCaS) are two programs on RTIPs that provide interventions for improving breast cancer screening among African-American women (Earp et al. 2002; Paskett et al. 1999). Other RTIPs programs are available for Alaskan Native, American Indian, Asian, Hispanic, Pacific Islander and non-Hispanic White women. Programs are free to download; however, few data exist on the effect of diffusion and implementation of RTIPs.

Other successful interventions for reaching vulnerable populations for improving mammography use include utilizing patient navigators (PN) to reduce barriers such as modesty and cultural issues, and including spiritual and religious themes (Freeman 2006; Paskett et al. 2012). For women living in rural areas, mobile mammography (Gardner et al. 2012), free/reduced services (Lane and Martin 2012), as well as agents of change (e.g. lay advisors, PN, public health nurses) (Paskett et al. 2006) have proven successful to improve uptake of mammography. Funding to continue these efforts is a significant challenge.

Treatment

Disparities in treatment have been well-documented. African-American, American Indian and Hispanic women are less likely to have surgery, more likely to refuse surgery, and less likely to receive radiation therapy (RT) compared to non-Hispanic white women (Li et al. 2003). Women from Appalachia (a predominately rural area) have higher rates of mastectomy and lower rates of RT after breast cancer surgery compared to non-Appalachian women (Freeman et al. 2012). Women >70 years and women without insurance were also less likely to receive adjuvant RT (Freeman et al. 2012). Disparities also exist within Asian/Pacific Islander groups for receipt of surgery and RT (Yi et al. 2012). Quality of treatment is also a factor. Fewer African-American women start treatment within 30 days (69 %) compared to white women (82 %); and receive lower quality treatment (Centers for Disease Control and Prevention (CDC) 2012). This is a significant problem, as a modeling study estimated that up to 19 % of the mortality difference between African-American and non-Hispanic white women could be eliminated if the same treatment was provided to both groups (Centers for Disease Control and Prevention (CDC) 2012). Differences in response to treatments, such as Tamoxifen, may also be responsible for some of the disparities in outcomes (American Cancer Society 2013). This area needs to be further explored.

Issues of Survivorship

Issues of survivorship include side effects of treatment, adherence to adjuvant hormone therapy, coping skills, body image, social support, acculturation and quality of life. Hispanic women have been found to suffer more from pain, fatigue, depression, and financial hardship related to treatment compared to non-Hispanic women

(Fu et al. 2009; Graves et al. 2012). American Indian/Alaskan Native women also report problems related to pain, fatigue, depression and hair loss (Burhansstipanov et al. 2010). Latina Spanish speaking women are more likely to discontinue adjuvant hormone therapy compared to white women (Livaudais et al. 2012).

Coping skills allow women to adjust to both physical and emotional distress during and following a cancer diagnosis and treatment. There are significant ethnic, racial and cultural differences in coping strategies used to respond to these stressors. For example, positive and negative forms of coping were more common among women of color than white women; negative coping was more likely to be associated with increased levels of distress and poorer survival (Yoo et al. 2014). Rural breast cancer patients are more likely to use behavioral disengagement, which is related to depressive symptoms compared, to urban patients (Schlegel et al. 2009; Collie et al. 2005).

Factors significantly related to coping strategies, such as religion and spiritual practices, are actually more relevant for minority and rural women. Some practices, e.g. spirituality and family support, actually are helpful in African-American populations, whereas spirituality has little impact on most non-Hispanic white women or negative effects in Asian/Pacific Islander, Hispanic, and American Indian/Alaskan Native women (Austin et al. 2002; Gaston-Johansson et al. 2013; Ashing-Giwa et al. 2013a; Daley et al. 2012; Ndikum-Moffor et al. 2013).

Body image and femininity are domains often impacted by breast cancer diagnosis and treatment. Most studies have been conducted among African-American women, and indicate that body image concerns were very important to their treatment decisions (Yoo et al. 2014; Hawley et al. 2009). Asian/Pacific Islander women report negative feelings towards their bodies after cancer surgery, so much so, that they report loss of self-worth, unhappiness and depression, and avoid looking at their bodies in the mirrors (Ashing-Giwa et al. 2013a). American Indian/Alaskan Native women associate hair loss due to chemotherapy as a sign of loss of spiritual strength which could result in isolation from the tribe (Burhansstipanov et al. 2010).

Social support is seen different in vulnerable populations—more African-Americans report receiving social support from God whereas non-Hispanic whites report receiving support from family and friends (Gaston-Johansson et al. 2013). In Asian culture, women are seen as nurturers not dependents, thus Asian breast cancer survivors may have unmet social support needs (Ashing-Giwa et al. 2013a). Latina women report the family as the main source of social support, however, with a breast cancer diagnosis, women report less acceptance by their husbands, possibly due to a change in gender roles and perceived femininity, resulting in lower perceived social support (Lopez-Class et al. 2011; Ashing-Giwa et al. 2004).

Acculturation also impacts survivorship. Lower acculturated Latinas report poorer health after breast cancer and more functional limitations and poorer mental health (Janz et al. 2009; Sammarco and Konecny 2010; Nápoles et al. 2011; Yanez et al. 2011). Native American languages have no word for cancer, but it translates to "the disease for which there is no cure."(Native American Cancer Research Corporation Native Americans and Cancer) Language barriers compound acculturation issues and produce long-lasting problems with access and adherence (Graves et al. 2012; Ashing-Giwa et al. 2013b).

Studies of quality of life among survivors are rare in populations other than white and African-American women (Ashing-Giwa et al. 2013a). Most African-American survivors report a positive growth from their breast cancer experience which favorably impacted their quality of life compared to white survivors (Russell et al. 2008). Differences were found among Asian/Pacific Islander survivors. For example, Chinese-American survivors had significantly greater medical concerns that negatively impacted their quality of life compared to Japanese-American survivors (Ashing-Giwa et al. 2013a). Hispanic breast cancer survivors report lower mean quality of life compared to women of other races/ethnicities. One study reported 53 % of Hispanic survivors have elevated depressive symptoms (Ashing-Giwa et al. 2013b). Rural women also report high levels of helplessness/hopelessness and at higher risk for lowered quality of life (Reid-Arndt and Cox 2010; Koopman et al. 2001).

Future Research Opportunities and Challenges

There are opportunities and challenges at every point across the cancer control continuum among vulnerable populations. Overall, our progress suffers due to inconsistent and poorly utilized definitions of SES, race/ethnicity and rural residence. For example, in many medical settings, race/ethnicity is not captured correctly or completely, limiting our ability to effectively understand and identify disparities. Secondly, access to preventive, detection and treatment services for all populations is problematic. This concern is reflected in the Institute of Medicine (IOM) report: Delivering high-quality cancer care: charting a new course for a system in crisis, which outlines the difficulties of providing adequate cancer care in an age of growing need, due to complexities of cancer treatment, a shrinking workforce, and increasing costs [*IOM* (Institute of Medicine) 2013]; thus, this is a huge challenge to vulnerable populations. Unfortunately, the ACA may not be able to fully remove barriers to access for all populations.

In terms of research, there are many opportunities to reduce disparities across the cancer continuum. As discussed earlier in this chapter, there are gaps in our knowledge regarding etiology, prevention, and chemoprevention strategies in many vulnerable populations. While diet, exercise, chemoprevention with tamoxifen/raloxifene, and prophylactic mastectomy have been examined for efficacy, few studies have either (1) tested these options in large samples of vulnerable populations to extend efficacy claims; or (2) examined ways to promote uptake of successful strategies, (i.e. tamoxifen in vulnerable populations, dietary strategies, etc.) Questions about what dietary components are protective or causative, what type of exercise is important and how much one needs to exercise, as well as when weight matters—e.g. adolescence, young adulthood or post menopausal—must also be further explored in all populations. Studies into the acceptability and impact of prophylactic mastectomy/oophrectomy for mutation carriers in different racial/ethnic groups need to be conducted.

Early detection strategies mainly center on mammography. The role of magnetic resonance imaging (MRI) and even the role of self-examination in certain cultures need to be explored. All populations are under the Healthy People 2020 goals for regular mammography screening, however, more accurate assessments of the prevalence of regular mammography need to be found rather than relying on self-reports from the BRFSS, as these self-reports may be less reliable in vulnerable populations [Centers for Disease Control and Prevention (CDC) 2012; U.S. Department of Health and Human Services (1953)]. Access to quality mammography, financial barriers, cultural issues, and awareness of the need for regular exams are pressing issues among vulnerable populations. More dissemination and implementation of successful evidence-based interventions needs to occur systematically, such as wider availability of the NBCCEDP to all eligible women.

Treatment is impacted by biology and access. More research, as well as more representation in clinical trials, is needed into biological responses to treatment across all vulnerable populations However, the state-of-the-art treatments are less likely to be available in those vulnerable populations. Thus, access, whether because of availability or financial limitations, must be assured. The use of PN's who can remove barriers to timely and quality care, should be universally accepted by the health care system to address disparities in treatment. As evidenced by the Delaware Experiment for colorectal cancer, PN's and universal access to screening, follow-up and treatment do eliminate disparities (Grubbs et al. 2013).

Furthermore, survivorship is a large area, mainly unexplored in the vulnerable populations discussed in this chapter. Quality of life, adherence to treatment regimens, coping, social support and body image are only some of the areas where more research is needed, especially in subgroups, to identify and intervene on disparities. Survivorship plans may be an intervention to test, as these can be tailored to the needs of each woman and followed with the assistance of a PN.

A large gap in our knowledge is at the end of the cancer control continuum. Little is known about palliative, hospice and end of life care in vulnerable populations. While it is known that the demands for these services exceeds the supply, little is known about what vulnerable populations know about these services, their specific needs, and what special access problems they face (Lewis et al. 2011). These are all areas where future research can be directed.

In summary, while many of the statistics documenting disparities in BC incidence, mortality, and stage of diagnosis are well-known, the reasons for all disparities noted are not as well studied. Moreover, interventions need to be tested and implemented, with policy and diffusion strategies, for BC disparities across the cancer control continuum to be reduced and eventually eliminated.

References

American Cancer Society (2013) Breast cancer facts & figures 2013–2014. American Cancer Society, Atlanta, GA

Amey CH, Miller MK, Albrecht SL (1997) The role of race and residence in determining stage at diagnosis of breast cancer. J Rural Health 13:99–108

Ansell D, Grabler P, Whitman S et al (2009) A community effort to reduce the black/white breast cancer mortality disparity in Chicago. Cancer Causes Control 20:1681–1688. doi:10.1007/s10552-009-9419-7

Ashing-Giwa KT, Padilla G, Tejero J et al (2004) Understanding the breast cancer experience of women: a qualitative study of African American, Asian American, Latina and Caucasian cancer survivors. Psychooncology 13:408–428. doi:10.1002/pon.750

Ashing-Giwa K, Tapp C, Brown S et al (2013a) Are survivorship care plans responsive to African-American breast cancer survivors?: voices of survivors and advocates. J Cancer Surviv 7:283–291. doi:10.1007/s11764-013-0270-1

Ashing-Giwa K, Rosales M, Lai L, Weitzel J (2013b) Depressive symptomatology among Latina breast cancer survivors. Psychooncology 22:845–853. doi:10.1002/pon.3084

Austin LT, Ahmad F, McNally MJ, Stewart DE (2002) Breast and cervical cancer screening in Hispanic women: a literature review using the health belief model. Womens Health Issues 12:122–128

Boyle P (2012) Triple-negative breast cancer: epidemiological considerations and recommendations. Ann Oncol 23(6):vi7–vi12. doi:10.1093/annonc/mds187

Burhansstipanov L, Krebs LU, Seals BF et al (2010) Native American breast cancer survivors' physical conditions and quality of life. Cancer 116:1560–1571. doi:10.1002/cncr.24924

Centers for Disease Control and Prevention (CDC) (2012) Vital signs: racial disparities in breast cancer severity–United States, 2005–2009. MMWR Morb Mortal Wkly Rep 61:922–926

Collie K, Wong P, Tilston J et al (2005) Self-efficacy, coping, and difficulties interacting with health care professionals among women living with breast cancer in rural communities. Psychooncology 14:901–912. doi:10.1002/pon.944, discussion 913–914

Coughlin SS, Ekwueme DU (2009) Breast cancer as a global health concern. Cancer Epidemiol 33:315–318. doi:10.1016/j.canep.2009.10.003

Daley CM, Kraemer-Diaz A, James AS et al (2012) Breast cancer screening beliefs and behaviors among American Indian women in Kansas and Missouri: a qualitative inquiry. J Cancer Educ 27(1):S32–S40. doi:10.1007/s13187-012-0334-3

Earp JA, Eng E, O'Malley MS et al (2002) Increasing use of mammography among older, rural African American women: results from a community trial. Am J Public Health 92:646–654

Freeman HP (2006) Patient navigation: a community centered approach to reducing cancer mortality. J Cancer Educ 21:S11–S14. doi:10.1207/s15430154jce2101s_4

Freeman AB, Huang B, Dragun AE (2012) Patterns of care with regard to surgical choice and application of adjuvant radiation therapy for preinvasive and early stage breast cancer in rural Appalachia. Am J Clin Oncol 35:358–363. doi:10.1097/COC.0b013e3182118d27

Frieden TR, Centers for Disease Control and Prevention (CDC) (2012) Use of selected clinical preventive services among adults–United States, 2007–2010. MMWR Morb Mortal Wkly Rep 61(Suppl):1–2

Fu OS, Crew KD, Jacobson JS et al (2009) Ethnicity and persistent symptom burden in breast cancer survivors. J Cancer Surviv 3:241–250. doi:10.1007/s11764-009-0100-7

Gardner T, Gavaza P, Meade P, Adkins DM (2012) Delivering free healthcare to rural central Appalachia population: the case of the Health Wagon. Rural Remote Health 12:2035

Gaston-Johansson F, Haisfield-Wolfe ME, Reddick B et al (2013) The relationships among coping strategies, religious coping, and spirituality in African American women with breast cancer receiving chemotherapy. Oncol Nurs Forum 40:120–131. doi:10.1188/13.ONF. 120-131

Goldman LE, Walker R, Hubbard R et al (2013) Timeliness of abnormal screening and diagnostic mammography follow-up at facilities serving vulnerable women. Med Care 51:307–314. doi:10.1097/MLR.0b013e318280f04c

Graves KD, Jensen RE, Cañar J et al (2012) Through the lens of culture: quality of life among Latina breast cancer survivors. Breast Cancer Res Treat 136:603–613. doi:10.1007/s10549-012-2291-2

Grubbs SS, Polite BN, Carney J Jr et al (2013) Eliminating racial disparities in colorectal cancer in the real world: it took a village. J Clin Oncol 31:1928–1930. doi:10.1200/JCO.2012.47.8412

Hall MJ, Olopade OI (2006) Disparities in genetic testing: thinking outside the BRCA box. J Clin Oncol 24:2197–2203. doi:10.1200/JCO.2006.05.5889

Harford JB, Otero IV, Anderson BO et al (2011) Problem solving for breast health care delivery in low and middle resource countries (LMCs): consensus statement from the breast health global initiative. Breast 20(2):S20–S29. doi:10.1016/j.breast.2011.02.007, Edinburgh, Scotland

Hawley ST, Griggs JJ, Hamilton AS et al (2009) Decision involvement and receipt of mastectomy among racially and ethnically diverse breast cancer patients. J Natl Cancer Inst 101:1337–1347. doi:10.1093/jnci/djp271

Hirschman J, Whitman S, Ansell D (2007) The black:white disparity in breast cancer mortality: the example of Chicago. Cancer Causes Control 18:323–333. doi:10.1007/s10552-006-0102-y

Hoerger TJ, Ekwueme DU, Miller JW et al (2011) Estimated effects of the national breast and cervical cancer early detection program on breast cancer mortality. Am J Prev Med 40:397–404. doi:10.1016/j.amepre.2010.12.017

Howe HL, Katterhagen JG, Yates J, Lehnherr M (1992) Urban-rural differences in the management of breast cancer. Cancer Causes Control 3:533–539

Howlander N, Noone A, Krapcho M et al (2014) SEER cancer statistics review, 1975–2011. National Cancer Institute, Bethesda

IOM (Institute of Medicine) (2013) Delivering high-quality cancer care: charting a new course for a system in crisis. The National Academies Press, Washington, DC

Janz NK, Mujahid MS, Hawley ST et al (2009) Racial/ethnic differences in quality of life after diagnosis of breast cancer. J Cancer Surviv 3:212–222. doi:10.1007/s11764-009-0097-y

Johns Hopkins Medicine Breast Center. Frequently asked questions about genetic testing. http://m.hopkinsmedicine.org/avon_foundation_breast_center/treatments_services/breast_cancer_diagnosis/breast_ovarian_surveillance_service_genetic_testing/faqs.html. Accessed 10 Jun 2014

Karliner LS, Ma L, Hofmann M, Kerlikowske K (2012) Language barriers, location of care, and delays in follow-up of abnormal mammograms. Med Care 50:171–178. doi:10.1097/MLR.0b013e31822dcf2d

Koopman C, Angell K, Turner-Cobb JM et al (2001) Distress, coping, and social support among rural women recently diagnosed with primary breast cancer. Breast J 7:25–33

Lane AJ, Martin M (2012) Characteristics of rural women who attended a free breast health program. Online J Rural Nurs Health Care 5:12–27

Lee HY, Ju E, Vang PD (2002) Lundquist M (2010) Breast and cervical cancer screening disparity among Asian American women: does race/ethnicity matter [corrected]? J Womens Health 19:1877–1884. doi:10.1089/jwh.2009.1783

Lewis JM, DiGiacomo M, Currow DC, Davidson PM (2011) Dying in the margins: understanding palliative care and socioeconomic deprivation in the developed world. J Pain Symptom Manage 42:105–118. doi:10.1016/j.jpainsymman.2010.10.265

Li CI, Malone KE, Daling JR (2002) Differences in breast cancer hormone receptor status and histology by race and ethnicity among women 50 years of age and older. Cancer Epidemiol Biomark Prev 11:601–607

Li CI, Malone KE, Daling JR (2003) Differences in breast cancer stage, treatment, and survival by race and ethnicity. Arch Intern Med 163:49–56

Lim J, Gonzalez P, Wang-Letzkus MF, Ashing-Giwa KT (2009) Understanding the cultural health belief model influencing health behaviors and health-related quality of life between Latina and Asian-American breast cancer survivors. Support Care Cancer 17:1137–1147. doi:10.1007/s00520-008-0547-5

Livaudais JC, Hwang ES, Karliner L et al (2012) Adjuvant hormonal therapy use among women with ductal carcinoma in situ. J Womens Health 21:35–42. doi:10.1089/jwh.2011.2773

Lopez-Class M, Perret-Gentil M, Kreling B et al (2011) Quality of life among immigrant Latina breast cancer survivors: realities of culture and enhancing cancer care. J Cancer Educ 26:724–733. doi:10.1007/s13187-011-0249-4

Mejia de Grubb MC, Kilbourne B, Kihlberg C, Levine RS (2013) Demographic and geographic variations in breast cancer mortality among U.S. Hispanics. J Health Care Poor Underserved 24:140–152. doi:10.1353/hpu.2013.0043

Monroe AC, Ricketts TC, Savitz LA (1992) Cancer in rural versus urban populations: a review. J Rural Health 8:212–220

Nápoles AM, Ortíz C, O'Brien H et al (2011) Coping resources and self-rated health among Latina breast cancer survivors. Oncol Nurs Forum 38:523–531. doi:10.1188/11.ONF. 523-531

National Cancer Institute Surveillance, Epidemiology, and End Results Program (SEER). http://seer.cancer.gov/

Native American Cancer Research Corporation. Native Americans and Cancer. http://natamcancer.org/page12.html.

NBCCEDP Breast Cancer Expert Panel (2005) White pater on technologies for the early detection of breast cancer. Centers for Disease Control and Prevention, Atlanta, GA

Ndikum-Moffor FM, Braiuca S, Daley CM et al (2013) Assessment of mammography experiences and satisfaction among American Indian/Alaska Native women. Womens Health Issues 23:e395–e402. doi:10.1016/j.whi.2013.08.003

Nguyen-Pham S, Leung J, McLaughlin D (2014) Disparities in breast cancer stage at diagnosis in urban and rural adult women: a systematic review and meta-analysis. Ann Epidemiol 24:228–235. doi:10.1016/j.annepidem.2013.12.002

Paskett ED, Tatum CM, D'Agostino R Jr et al (1999) Community-based interventions to improve breast and cervical cancer screening: results of the Forsyth county cancer screening (FoCaS) project. Cancer Epidemiol Biomark Prev 8:453–459

Paskett E, Tatum C, Rushing J et al (2006) Randomized trial of an intervention to improve mammography utilization among a triracial rural population of women. J Natl Cancer Inst 98:1226–1237. doi:10.1093/jnci/djj333

Paskett ED, Katz ML, Post DM et al (2012) The Ohio patient navigation research program: does the american cancer society patient navigation model improve time to resolution in patients with abnormal screening tests? Cancer Epidemiol Biomarkers Prev 21:1620–1628. doi:10.1158/1055-9965.EPI-12-0523

Reid-Arndt SA, Cox CR (2010) Does rurality affect quality of life following treatment for breast cancer? J Rural Health 26:402–405. doi:10.1111/j.1748-0361.2010.00295.x

Russell KM, Von Ah DM, Giesler RB et al (2008) Quality of life of African American breast cancer survivors: how much do we know? Cancer Nurs 31:E36–E45. doi:10.1097/01.NCC.0000339254.68324.d7

Sammarco A, Konecny LM (2010) Quality of life, social support, and uncertainty among Latina and Caucasian breast cancer survivors: a comparative study. Oncol Nurs Forum 37:93–99. doi:10.1188/10.ONF. 93-99

Schlegel RJ, Talley AE, Molix LA, Bettencourt BA (2009) Rural breast cancer patients, coping and depressive symptoms: a prospective comparison study. Psychol Health 24:933–948. doi:10.1080/08870440802254613

Schootman M, Myers-Geadelmann J, Fuortes L (2000) Factors associated with adequacy of diagnostic workup after abnormal breast cancer screening results. J Am Board Fam Pract 13:94–100

Schumacher MC, Slattery ML, Lanier AP et al (2008) Prevalence and predictors of cancer screening among American Indian and Alaska native people: the EARTH study. Cancer Causes Control 19:725–737. doi:10.1007/s10552-008-9135-8

Sood R, Ho P, Tornow C, Frey W (2007) Cancer control P.L.A.N.E.T. Evaluation Report. Rockville, MD

Susan G. Komen Testing for BRCA1 & BRCA2 Mutations. http://ww5.komen.org/BreastCancer/GeneMutationsampGeneticTesting.html. Accessed 10 Jun 2014

U.S. Department of Health and Human Services. Office of Disease Prevention and Health Promotion. Healthy People 2020. Washington, DC. Available at www.healthypeople.gov/2020/topics-objectives/topic/cancer/objectives. Accessed 10 June 2014.

Von Friederichs-Fitzwater MM, Navarro L, Taylor SL (2010) A value-based approach to increase breast cancer screening and health-directed behaviors among American Indian women. J Cancer Educ 25:582–587. doi:10.1007/s13187-010-0111-0

Yanez B, Thompson EH, Stanton AL (2011) Quality of life among Latina breast cancer patients: a systematic review of the literature. J Cancer Surviv 5:191–207. doi:10.1007/s11764-011-0171-0

Yi M, Liu P, Li X et al (2012) Comparative analysis of clinicopathologic features, treatment, and survival of Asian women with a breast cancer diagnosis residing in the United States. Cancer 118:4117–4125. doi:10.1002/cncr.27399

Yoo GJ, Levine EG, Pasick R (2014) Breast cancer and coping among women of color: a systematic review of the literature. Support Care Cancer 22:811–824. doi:10.1007/s00520-013-2057-3

Youlden DR, Cramb SM, Dunn NAM et al (2012) The descriptive epidemiology of female breast cancer: an international comparison of screening, incidence, survival and mortality. Cancer Epidemiol 36:237–248. doi:10.1016/j.canep.2012.02.007

Chapter 5
Symptoms: Fatigue and Cognitive Dysfunction

Julienne E. Bower and Patricia A. Ganz

Abstract Fatigue and cognitive complaints commonly occur during adjuvant chemotherapy treatment of breast cancer. Fatigue is also associated with radiation therapy, and can occur with surgery alone. Both of these symptoms may persist beyond the initial treatment of breast cancer and they have taken on greater prominence with the growing number of breast cancer survivors. These symptoms are most troublesome when patients try to resume their pre-illness activities (e.g., work, household responsibilities) and find that they are limited. Recovery may take months to years, but in some women these symptoms persist indefinitely and can be very distressing. In this chapter we review what is known about the etiology and biology of these two common symptoms, discuss potential interventions, and describe future research challenges.

Keywords Fatigue • Cognitive complaints • Breast cancer • Chemotherapy • Radiation therapy • Inflammation

Overview of the Problem

Fatigue and cognitive complaints are two of the most common and distressing symptoms reported by women with breast cancer. After two decades of research on cancer-related fatigue, we have a good understanding of the characteristics, prevalence, and course of this symptom and are beginning to elucidate mechanisms, risk factors, and effective treatments among women with breast cancer (Bower et al. 2000, 2006; Bower 2005, 2014). We also have a growing appreciation of the complexity of fatigue, which shows significant inter-individual variability in its severity

J.E. Bower (✉)
Departments of Psychology and Psychiatry/Biobehavioral Sciences, Jonsson Comprehensive Cancer Center, University of California, Los Angeles, CA, USA
e-mail: jbower@ucla.edu

P.A. Ganz
UCLA Schools of Medicine and Public Health, Jonsson Comprehensive Cancer Center, Los Angeles, CA, USA
e-mail: pganz@mednet.ucla.edu

© Breast Cancer Research Foundation 2015
P.A. Ganz (ed.), *Improving Outcomes for Breast Cancer Survivors*,
Advances in Experimental Medicine and Biology 862,
DOI 10.1007/978-3-319-16366-6_5

and expression. In parallel, cognitive complaints emerged as a frequent post-treatment problem in the late 1990s, particularly in women who received high-dose chemotherapy (Ganz 1998; van Dam et al. 1998). Our understanding of the etiology, characteristics, prevalence, and course of cognitive difficulties is not as advanced as the knowledge-base related to fatigue; however, recent advances in neuroimaging have accelerated our understanding of the impact of breast cancer treatments on cerebral functioning. Importantly, research that the authors have jointly conducted over the past decade has begun to identify a common biology for both of these clinical symptoms that is associated with inflammation. In this chapter, we will briefly review descriptive research on cancer-related fatigue and treatment associated cognitive changes in breast cancer patients, provide an overview of research on mechanisms, and highlight key issues to be addressed in future research.

Description of Cancer-Related Fatigue

Research on cancer-related fatigue began with qualitative descriptions of this symptom in the late 1980s and then progressed to more quantitative examination of its prevalence, course, and correlates. Studies conducted with breast cancer patients have documented increases in fatigue during treatment with radiation (Irvine et al. 1998) and with chemotherapy (Jacobsen et al. 1999), although chemotherapy-induced fatigue is somewhat more severe. Fatigue typically improves in the year after treatment completion, although a significant minority of patients continue to experience fatigue for months or years after successful treatment (Bower et al. 2000; Cella et al. 2001). In a survey study we conducted with almost 2000 breast cancer survivors who were between 1 and 5 years post-diagnosis, we found that one-third reported elevated fatigue (Bower et al. 2000). In a follow-up study with this sample, we found that 20 % of study participants continued to report elevated fatigue up to 10 years after breast cancer diagnosis (Bower et al. 2006). Fatigue has a negative impact on work, social relationships, mood, and daily activities and causes significant impairment in overall quality of life during and after treatment among women with breast cancer (Andrykowski et al. 1998; Bower et al. 2000; Broeckel et al. 1998; Curt et al. 2000). Fatigue also predicted shorter recurrence-free and overall survival in a sample of breast cancer patients (Groenvold et al. 2007).

Patient reports suggest that cancer-related fatigue is more severe, more persistent, and more debilitating than "normal" fatigue caused by lack of sleep or overexertion and is not relieved by adequate sleep or rest (Poulson 2001). Indeed, studies have confirmed that the intensity and duration of fatigue experienced by cancer patients and survivors is significantly greater than healthy controls and causes greater impairment in quality of life (Andrykowski et al. 1998; Cella et al. 2002; Forlenza et al. 2005; Jacobsen et al. 1999). Cancer-related fatigue is multidimensional and may have physical, mental, and emotional manifestations including generalized weakness, diminished concentration or attention, decreased motivation or interest to engage in usual activities, and emotional lability (Cella et al. 2001). Fatigue is strongly correlated with depressive symptoms as well as sleep disturbance, pain, and cognitive function, although patients experience fatigue as a distinct and central symptom.

Description of Cognitive Complaints After Breast Cancer Treatments

The first reports of cognitive complaints associated with breast cancer treatments began with the more widespread use of adjuvant chemotherapy, accentuated by the adoption of high dose adjuvant chemotherapy (Phillips and Bernhard 2003). In an early review of this problem (Phillips and Bernhard 2003), Phillips and Bernhard note the strong association of post-treatment cognitive impairment with adjuvant chemotherapy, primarily in cross-sectional studies, with lack of clarity regarding the extent to which premature menopause or adjuvant tamoxifen may have contributed to patient reported complaints. In addition, they raise the question regarding the extent to which these complaints overlap with psychological factors. In a cross-sectional study from a clinical trial comparing neuropsychological tests and quality of life in women who had received either high dose or standard dose adjuvant chemotherapy, those exposed to the high dose chemotherapy were 8.2 times more likely to have cognitive impairment than breast cancer patients who did not receive chemotherapy, and 3.5 times higher than patients receiving standard adjuvant chemotherapy (van Dam et al. 1998). These results were not affected by depression, fatigue, or time since treatment, and suggested a dose response effect for the neuropsychological changes. These women were in their 40s and almost all became menopausal and were receiving tamoxifen. A neurophysiological study done in a subgroup of these patients also reflected changes consistent with a dose effect (Schagen et al. 2001). Additional studies, with small numbers of patients, and with cross-sectional designs (reviewed by Phillips and Bernhard), suffered from similar limitations in being able to determine causal attribution of neurocognitive test abnormalities to chemotherapy exposure, change in menstrual status, or use of tamoxifen. These studies and others (Castellon et al. 2004, 2005) also failed to find significant relationships between self-reported cognitive complaints and neurocognitive testing, and raised the issue of anxiety and depression as confounding factors.

Given these emerging findings, and lack of consensus about how best to study this increasing clinical problem, a group of investigators working in the field came together in April 2003, spurred on by patient advocates who were becoming alarmed about increasing reports of cognitive impairment after treatment. This workshop led to a report (Tannock et al. 2004) that summarized the state of current research, including a number of longitudinal investigations underway or planned, designed to identify prospective changes in cognitive function associated with chemotherapy treatments. In addition, there was a call for more studies to elucidate mechanisms, as well as the addition of assessments in the setting of clinical trials. Breast cancer survivors and advocates emphasized the impact of cognitive impairment on quality of life and recovery after treatments. Subsequently, this group of investigators, supported in part by funding from an advocate organization, formed the International Cognition and Cancer Task Force, which has met every second year, and has provided a forum for scientific discussion that has moved the field forward substantially (Vardy et al. 2008; Wefel et al. 2011).

Several excellent reviews summarize the findings with regard to cognitive impairment after breast cancer (Ahles 2012; Ahles et al. 2012; Jim et al. 2012). Most studies confirm only subtle changes in cognitive function after exposure to adjuvant chemotherapy on neurocognitive testing, most often manifest as a failure to demonstrate improvement with repeated testing (practice effects) that are seen in control subjects. The domains most often affected as shown in a meta-analysis are verbal ability and visuo-spatial ability (Jim et al. 2012). However, classification of neurocognitive tests into specific domains varies across papers. Other studies have identified processing speed as an affected domain, especially in association with aging and tamoxifen (Ahles et al. 2010). Abnormalities associated with cerebral function have also been corroborated in a series of brain imaging studies in breast cancer patients studied longitudinally, prior to and after chemotherapy administration (Deprez et al. 2011, 2012; McDonald et al. 2010, 2012). Most recently, there is convincing evidence that self-reported cognitive complaints are also manifested in cerebral imaging changes in breast cancer patients (Deprez et al. 2012, 2014; Kesler et al. 2011). Our own studies have demonstrated that about 20 % of non-depressed, younger post-treatment early stage breast cancer patients have higher memory and executive function cognitive complaints than healthy controls, and that this is associated with both chemotherapy and radiation treatments as well as significant differences in domain specific verbal memory and executive function neurocognitive performance (Ganz et al. 2013b). In further studies of this same group of patients, we have found that the initiation of endocrine therapy is associated with increased language and communication complaints (Ganz et al. 2014). For this group of patients, there was a strong association of these complaints with past hormone therapy, as well as an interaction between past hormone therapy and breast cancer targeted endocrine treatment. Further work needs to be done to understand the relative contribution of endocrine therapy to post treatment cognitive complaints. However, overall, these data suggest that patient reports of cognitive difficulties are genuine and reflect changes in brain function that can be identified with sensitive neuroimaging procedures. What are the best self-report tools to capture these complaints, and how to separate them from fatigue and depressive symptoms that may overlap, is an important future research question (discussed below).

The pattern and trajectory of cognitive complaints and clinical cognitive decline post-treatment may be influenced by multiple factors and are dependent on initial cognitive reserve, influence of acute and chronic anxiety (as at time of diagnosis and with initial treatments), followed by changes in hormonal mileu as well as influenced by potential direct toxicities of treatments, and persistent elevations of inflammatory markers. Underlying this may be genetic susceptibility to cognitive decline from known markers (i.e. APOE4) as well as other factors (Ahles 2012; Ahles et al. 2012; Mandelblatt et al. 2014).

The major obstacle associated with more regularly assessing cognitive function as a treatment toxicity or for symptom management, has been the perceived burden of assessing cognitive function with extensive batteries of neurocognitive tests. However, the emerging research demonstrating the validity of self-reported complaints may help to advance the regular assessment of this treatment toxicity along with other patient reported outcomes.

Mechanisms for Fatigue and Cognitive Dysfunction: Focus on Inflammation

Fatigue in breast cancer patients is multi-factorial and may be influenced by a variety of demographic, medical, psychosocial, and biological factors. We have found that younger, unmarried women who have a lower household income report higher levels of fatigue (Bower et al. 2000), suggesting that contextual factors (e.g., absence of partner who can provide instrumental and emotional support) may influence the experience of this symptom. Other potential contributing factors include medical comorbidities, medications, nutritional issues, physical symptoms, and physical deconditioning, among others (Mitchell 2010). For example, we found that heart disease was a significant predictor of persistent post-treatment fatigue in a large sample of breast cancer survivors (Bower et al. 2006). However, fatigue often occurs in patients who are otherwise healthy and have few if any of these contributing factors, suggesting that other processes may also be at work. Of note, treatment-related factors (e.g., type of treatment, dose-intensity) are not consistently associated with fatigue, particularly in the post-treatment period.

A variety of biological mechanisms for cancer-related fatigue have been proposed and investigated over the past two decades (Barsevick et al. 2010; Morrow et al. 2002). These include anemia, cytokine dysregulation, hypothalamic-pituitary-adrenal (HPA) axis dysregulation, five hydroxy tryptophan (5-HT) neurotransmitter dysregulation, and alterations in adenosine triphosphate and muscle metabolism, among others (Barsevick et al. 2010). With respect to cognitive function, Ahles and Saykin (2007) reviewed potential mechanisms for the development of cancer-related cognitive changes, which included endocrine factors (reductions in estrogen and testosterone), DNA damage and telomere length, cytokine dysregulation and disruption in the blood brain barrier. The mechanism that is common across both conditions is cytokine dysregulation, and specifically inflammation.

The possibility that inflammatory processes may be involved in the etiology of cancer-related fatigue and cognitive problems draws from basic research on neural-immune signaling. This body of work has demonstrated that peripheral inflammatory cytokines can signal the central nervous system to generate symptoms of fatigue and other behavioral changes (Dantzer et al. 2008; Haroon et al. 2012; Miller et al. 2008) (see Fig. 5.1). Signals from the peripheral immune system are conveyed to the central nervous system through several routes, including direct neural activation via the afferent vagus nerve, transport of peripheral cytokines across

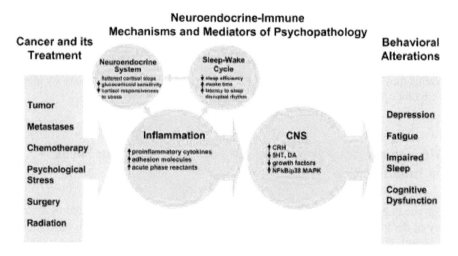

Fig. 5.1 Model for explaining the influence of cancer and its treatments on common behavioral alterations including fatigue and cognitive dysfunction [Reproduced with permission from Miller et al. (2008)]

the blood-brain barrier via carrier molecules, and interaction of circulating cytokines with brain cytokine receptors in areas that lack a functional blood-brain barrier (i.e., circumventricular organs) and with brain vascular endothelial cells that release second messages to stimulate cytokine production in the brain (Irwin and Cole 2011). Cytokine signaling leads to changes in neural activity, physiological processes (e.g., fever), and behavior, including changes in energy/fatigue and cognitive function (Miller et al. 2013). In animal models, induction of pro-inflammatory cytokines leads to decreased motor activity (presumably a behavioral manifestation of fatigue) and altered cognition, as well as reduced food and water intake, social withdrawal, and anhedonia.

These behavioral changes have been collectively described as "sickness behavior" and are thought to represent a motivational shift designed to facilitate recovery and prevent the spread of infection (Dantzer and Kelley 2007; Irwin and Cole 2011). In humans, pharmacologic doses of cytokines given for treatment of cancer or hepatitis C are associated with significant increases in fatigue, cognitive problems, and other markers of sickness (depressed mood, sleep disturbance) (Capuron et al. 2000; Kirkwood 2002; Valentine et al. 1998). Experimental studies of cytokine induction in healthy individuals have documented similar effects, with subjects reporting increased fatigue and cognitive disturbance following endotoxin administration that are correlated with elevations in circulating concentrations of pro-inflammatory cytokines (Reichenberg et al. 2001; Spath-Schwalbe et al. 1998). Further, pharmacologic agents that block the pro-inflammatory cytokine TNFα lead to reduced fatigue among individuals with inflammatory conditions (Tyring et al. 2006), and in pilot studies with cancer patients (Monk et al. 2006) (though fatigue can also be a side effect of these agents in certain patient populations). Together, this evidence provides a strong biological rationale for inflammation as a potential mechanism underlying cancer-related fatigue and cognitive disturbance.

Studies of Inflammation and Fatigue in Cancer Patients

In the cancer context, investigators have proposed that tumors and the treatments used to eradicate them can activate the pro-inflammatory cytokine network, leading to symptoms of fatigue and cognitive disturbance (Cleeland et al. 2003; Miller et al. 2008; Seruga et al. 2008). In the pre-treatment period, the tumor itself may be a source for pro-inflammatory cytokines (Aggarwal et al. 2009; Coussens and Werb 2002) while during treatment, cytokines may be produced in response to tissue damage from surgery, radiation, or chemotherapy (Aggarwal et al. 2009; Stone et al. 2003). The inflammatory response may persist well after treatment completion as the host tries to deal with persisting pathogenesis and alterations in homeostasis.

A growing number of studies have examined the association between circulating markers of inflammation and fatigue during and after breast cancer treatment. In a study of breast cancer patients assessed prior to chemotherapy (but after surgery), fatigue was associated with elevations in CRP, a marker of systemic inflammation (Pertl et al. 2013). In a study of breast and prostate cancer patients undergoing radiation therapy, we found that patients reported increases in fatigue that were correlated with increases in circulating inflammatory markers (CRP, IL-1 receptor antagonist) (Bower et al. 2009). Similarly, increases in fatigue were correlated with increases in the inflammatory cytokine IL-6 among breast cancer patients undergoing chemotherapy (Liu et al. 2012). Documenting an association between inflammatory markers and on-treatment-related fatigue is complicated by dynamic changes in the cellular immune system and inflammation that occur during the acute phase of cancer treatment. Investigators have found more reliable associations between inflammatory activity and fatigue after treatment completion. In a series of cross-sectional studies with breast cancer survivors, we have documented elevations in inflammatory markers among women who report elevated fatigue at 1 month (Bower et al. 2011b), 2 years (Collado-Hidalgo et al. 2006), and 5 years (Bower et al. 2002) post-treatment. Consistent with these results, several other groups have found significant elevations in CRP among breast cancer survivors with persistent fatigue (Alexander et al. 2009; Alfano et al. 2012; Orre et al. 2011). At the molecular level, leukocytes from fatigued breast cancer survivors show increased expression of genes encoding proinflammatory cytokines and other mediators of immunologic activation, as well increased activity of proinflammatory NF-κB/Rel transcription factors, which might structure the observed differences in the expression of inflammation-related genes (Bower et al. 2011a).

Studies of Inflammation and Cognitive Function in Breast Cancer Patients

In parallel to the studies of fatigue, there are increasing reports that have focused on the potential role of inflammation in the etiology of cognitive impairment after breast cancer. Early reviews of potential mechanisms identified inflammation as a possible etiology (Ahles and Saykin 2007) and studies in rodents provide strong support for inflammatory mechanisms (Seigers and Fardell 2011). While some chemotherapeutic agents may cross the blood brain barrier and cause direct toxicity (e.g., especially the CMF regimen, with methotrexate and fluorouracil), the mechanism by which both chemotherapy and radiation cause injury is likely through the production of reactive oxygen species and tissue damage, that result in systemic inflammation as well as stimulation of local microglial inflammation within the brain. Indeed, several studies of breast cancer patients have demonstrated relationships between systemic levels of inflammation and brain imaging structural and metabolic changes (Kesler et al. 2013b; Pomykala et al. 2013). Animal models studies support these findings (Seigers et al. 2013), and an inflammatory basis of cognitive changes associated with cancer treatments would be consistent with age related cognitive changes of which this may be a manifestation (Ahles 2012). Since only a subgroup of patients with breast cancer appear to be vulnerable to cognitive difficulties, as with age-related variation in cognitive decline, similar host factors and susceptibilities may be relevant (see below).

To develop an understanding of the potential role of inflammation and cognitive dysfunction in women with breast cancer, we recruited a cohort of women with newly diagnosed breast cancer who had completed primary adjuvant chemotherapy and/or radiation therapy, but enrolled prior to the start of endocrine therapy if planned. The Mind Body Study (MBS) cohort of 191 patients was less than 66 years of age, and excluded women with significant depressive symptoms, history of central nervous system disorders, conditions with chronic inflammation, or with use of immunosuppressive therapy (see details in Bower et al. 2011b; Ganz et al. 2013a, b). We observed post-treatment elevations of soluble TNFα receptor II (sTNFR2) levels at study enrollment that declined over the subsequent 12 months of follow-up, with elevations only noted in the patients who had received chemotherapy (Ganz et al. 2013a). We should note that there was a parallel association between fatigue and sTNFR2 in this same sample at the baseline assessment (Bower et al. 2011b), and we see the co-occurrence of these two symptoms in the longitudinal follow-up of this sample (unpublished data). The changes in TNF over the 12 months were correlated with self-reported memory complaints, as well as changes in PET scan glucose metabolism in a small subgroup of patients, with normalization of metabolism in the inferior frontal gyrus as TNF levels decreased between baseline and 12 months later. More detailed evaluation of sTNFR2 and other proinflammatory cytokines in the PET scan study are reported separately in an additional publication, where we observed positive correlations between metabolism in the medial prefrontal cortex and anterior temporal cortex with both memory complaints and cytokine markers only in patients who received chemotherapy (Pomykala et al. 2013). Of note, Kesler et al. (2013b) have found an association between decreased hippocampal volume on MRI in breast cancer survivors and elevated TNFα and IL-6, along with decreased verbal memory performance on cognitive testing, in comparison to a healthy control group.

Host Factors that May Increase Risk for Fatigue

Although cancer-related fatigue is common, it does not affect all patients (see Table 5.1). Clinicians have no doubt observed that certain patients are more susceptible to fatigue, and empirical studies have now documented considerable variability in reports of fatigue before, during, and after treatment. This variability was nicely illustrated in a longitudinal prospective study of breast cancer patients who were followed for 6 months after cancer treatment (Donovan et al. 2007). Using growth mixture modeling, two groups of patients were identified on the basis of their fatigue scores. One group, which comprised approximately 30 % of the sample, reported consistently low levels of fatigue across the assessment period, including in the immediate aftermath of treatment. The other group reported elevated fatigue at treatment completion, which declined over the assessment period but remained significantly higher than the low fatigue group. Of note, disease- and treatment-related factors did not determine group membership in this study; instead, body mass index and coping strategies were significant predictors of group membership. Other studies have similarly found no evidence that cancer-related fatigue is associated with

Table 5.1 Host factors associated with fatigue and cognitive dysfunction	*Fatigue*
	Pre-treatment fatigue
	Pre-treatment sleep disturbance
	History of depression
	Loneliness
	Early life stress
	Physical inactivity
	High body mass index
	Catastrophizing coping style
	Genetic factors (e.g., SNPs in inflammation-related genes)
	Neuroendocrine dysregulation
	Cognitive dysfunction
	Pre-treatment diminished cognitive reserve, low educational status
	History of head trauma
	Comorbid conditions (e.g., diabetes, vascular disease)
	Genetic factors (e.g., *APOE-4*, *COMT*, SNPs in inflammation-related genes)
	Older age (?)

type of cancer treatment, particularly in the post-treatment period. Together, these findings strongly suggest that host factors play an important role in the development and persistence of cancer-related fatigue.

Longitudinal studies have begun to identify predictors of cancer-related fatigue. These include pre-treatment fatigue, pre-treatment sleep disturbance, history of depression, loneliness, early life stress, physical inactivity, and body mass index (Bower 2014). In addition, patients who engage in negative thoughts or "catastroph-ize" about their fatigue (e.g., I tell myself I don't think I can bear the fatigue any more), report elevated fatigue during and after treatment. Thus, psychosocial and behavioral factors may set the stage for more severe and persistent cancer-related fatigue. Importantly, some of these factors are amenable to intervention, including physical inactivity, high BMI, and catastrophizing.

Genetic factors have also been linked to cancer-related fatigue. Most of the stud-ies in this area have taken a candidate gene approach, focusing on single nucleotide polymorphisms (SNPs) in inflammation-related genes including *IL1B*, *IL6*, and *TNF* given evidence linking circulating inflammatory markers and fatigue. We examined whether polymorphisms in these genes were associated with fatigue within 1 month after treatment, using data from breast cancer survivors enrolled in the MBS study. Consistent with hypotheses, we found that women with the "high expression" versions of these genes reported higher levels of fatigue (Bower et al. 2013a). Similarly, in a small sample of breast cancer survivors assessed several years after treatment, polymorphisms in *ILB* and *IL6* were associated with persis-tent post-treatment fatigue (Collado-Hidalgo et al. 2008). There is also preliminary evidence that polymorphisms in inflammation-related genes are associated with fatigue among patients undergoing radiation therapy, including many breast cancer patients (Aouizerat et al. 2009; Miaskowski et al. 2010).

Alterations in the HPA axis may contribute to cancer-related fatigue, either directly or through effects on inflammatory processes. We found that breast cancer survivors with persistent fatigue had a flatter diurnal cortisol slope (with elevated levels of cortisol in the evening) as well as blunted cortisol responses to psycho-social stress that were correlated with alterations in inflammatory activity (Bower et al. 2005a, b, 2007) Further, genome-wide transcriptional profiling of leukocytes from fatigued breast cancer survivors showed a marked down-regulation of genes with response elements for the glucocorticoid receptor, suggesting a state of func-tional GR resistance which may contribute the tonic upregulation of NF-κB observed in fatigued survivors (Bower et al. 2011a). Fatigue is also associated with alterations in the autonomic nervous system in breast cancer survivors, including lower heart rate variability (an indicator of parasympathetic activity) and elevated norepinephrine (an indicator of sympathetic activity) (Crosswell et al. 2014; Fagundes et al. 2011). Importantly, because all of these studies have been cross-sectional investigations of breast cancer survivors, it is impossible to determine whether neuroendocrine alterations play a causal role in the develop-ment and persistence of this symptom, or arise as a consequence of fatigue and inflammatory activity.

Longitudinal studies that examine risk factors for cancer-related fatigue are still quite limited and few have followed patients from pre-treatment in to the post-treatment period; fewer still have examined mechanisms that underlie effects of these risk factors on fatigue. To advance research in this area, longitudinal studies are required that track patients before, during, and after treatment and include comprehensive assessment of biobehavioral risk factors and underlying mechanisms. This approach will facilitate the identification of distinct trajectories of fatigue, risk factors for fatigue onset and persistence, and the mechanisms that underlie their effects, paving the way for targeted interventions.

Host Factors and the Risk for Cognitive Impairment

Less is known about the host factors associated with the risk of cognitive impairment after breast cancer treatments (see Table 5.1). Ahles and Saykin (2007) reviewed potential mechanisms for the development of cognitive changes and these included genetic susceptibility, endocrine factors (reductions in estrogen and testosterone), DNA damage and telomere length, cytokine dysregulation and disruption in the blood brain barrier. Among these mechanisms, genetic susceptibility has been studied by several groups. Ahles has reported on the association of the *APOE-4* allele, found in Alzheimer's disease, with cancer-related cognitive dysfunction in long-term breast and lymphoma survivors treated with chemotherapy (Ahles et al. 2003). In another sample of breast cancer patients followed prospectively, Small et al. (2011) found that patients with the catechol-o-methyltransferase (COMT) genotype Val + allele had greater cognitive difficulties with attention, verbal fluency and motor speed, with an interaction with chemotherapy for attention. COMT-Val + carriers are thought to metabolize dopamine more rapidly and this might be the putative mechanism. In our MBS study, we have found that a genetic risk score of SNPs for *IL1B*, *IL6*, and *TNF* was significantly associated with memory complaints as well as fatigue (Bower et al. 2013b). Other groups have also found similar associations (Merriman et al. 2013, 2014).

Other contributing factors could be those influences associated with age-related cognitive decline and cognitive reserve may be reduced in individuals with lower education or prior comorbid conditions leading to subclinical brain injury (Ahles 2012; Mandelblatt et al. 2014) (see Fig. 5.2). It is likely that the cognitive complaints that patients report after treatment exposure are a manifestation of having to work harder (recruit more areas of the brain) to retrieve information, multi-task, and perform executive tasks. These are similar to what happens with age-related cognitive decline (Maillet and Rajah 2013). In addition to these factors, age-related vascular disease, diabetes, and hormonal changes may contribute to these problems. However, it is most interesting the manifestations of symptomatic cognitive difficulties are most notable in younger women, similar to what is seen with fatigue. It may be that the everyday demands put upon younger women exacerbate these complaints, whereas older women may be less likely to notice subtle changes in function.

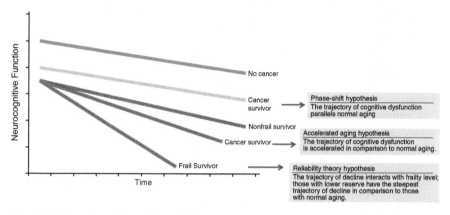

Fig. 5.2 Trajectories of cognitive decline based on theories of aging and frailty phenotype [Adapted from Mandelblatt et al. (2014)]

What Are the Potential Intervention Strategies to Consider for Management of Fatigue or Cognitive Complaints?

Interventions for Cancer-Related Fatigue

A diverse range of treatment approaches have been used to address cancer-related fatigue during and after cancer treatment, including physical activity, psychosocial, mind-body, and pharmacological interventions. Perhaps because the etiology of cancer-related fatigue is multi-factorial and still poorly understood, there is currently no "gold standard" for treatment of this symptom. Still, a number of these approaches have been shown to be beneficial in reducing cancer-related fatigue, as reviewed below. The recently published ASCO Guideline on Fatigue in Cancer Survivors outlines the intervention strategies that should be considered (Bower et al. 2014). A number of randomized controlled trials have examined the effect of exercise on cancer-related fatigue. Overall, meta-analyses of these trials indicate that exercise is effective in reducing fatigue, with effect size estimates ranging from −0.27 to −0.38, indicating a moderate effect (Cramp and Byron-Daniel 2012; Puetz and Herring 2012). Beneficial effects of exercise have been observed in trials conducted with patients during and after treatment, indicating that exercise can be helpful at different stages of the disease trajectory. Aerobic exercise regimens seem to be particularly beneficial. Guidelines from the American College of Sports Medicine (ACSM) recommend that cancer patients and survivors engage in at least 150 min of moderate intensity aerobic activity each week, consistent with recommendations for the general population (Schmitz et al. 2010). ACSM guidelines further recommend that exercise should be tailored to the individual cancer patient to account for exercise tolerance and specific diagnosis, and that patients be closely monitored to safely progress exercise intensity and avoid injury.

Psychosocial interventions are also effective in reducing fatigue, particularly interventions that provide education about fatigue and contributing factors (e.g., physical activity, sleep disturbance) and address dysfunctional fatigue-related thoughts and behaviors. Among women undergoing radiation or chemotherapy for breast cancer, individualized educational and cognitive-behavioral approaches that specifically targeted fatigue buffered the increase in fatigue observed among control patients (Montgomery et al. 2009, 2014; Yates et al. 2005). A brief psychoeducational intervention that provided information about fatigue and modeled adaptive coping strategies (e.g., physical activity) also led to reductions in fatigue among women who had recently completed breast cancer treatment (Stanton et al. 2005). More intensive and targeted treatments have shown benefit for survivors with severe and persistent post-treatment fatigue. These include individual cognitive-behavioral therapy focused on perpetuating factors for persistent fatigue (Gielissen et al. 2006), and a web-based, tailored education program providing information on cancer-related fatigue as well as energy conservation, physical activity, sleep hygiene, distress management, nutrition, and pain control (Yun et al. 2012). Mind-body interventions have also demonstrated efficacy for treating cancer-related fatigue in cancer survivors (see Table 5.2). In particular, specialized programs of acupuncture (Molassiotis et al. 2012), yoga (Bower et al. 2012), and mindfulness (van der Lee and Garssen 2012) led to significant reductions in fatigue among survivors with persistent post-treatment fatigue.

In terms of pharmacologic interventions, there is mixed evidence for the effectiveness of psychostimulants (e.g., methylphenidate) and other wakefulness agents (e.g., modafinil) as treatments for cancer-related fatigue (Minton et al. 2008, 2011). Several large trials of these agents have yielded negative effects, though subgroup analyses suggested that patients with severe fatigue may show some benefit (Jean-Pierre et al. 2010; Moraska et al. 2010). However, there is very limited evidence of their effectiveness in reducing fatigue in patients who are disease free following active treatment. American ginseng may hold promise for treating cancer-related fatigue, particularly among patients undergoing treatment, but more research on this agent is needed (Barton et al. 2013). Of note, very few of the pharmacologic trials have focused specifically on breast cancer patients or survivors.

Interventions for Cognitive Complaints

There have been relatively few studies designed to provide intervention for cognitive dysfunction in cancer survivors, and most of them have been conducted in breast cancer. The first study by Ferguson et al. (2007) was a single arm, individually delivered cognitive behavioral therapy (CBT) approach to memory problems. Due to feasibility and improvements in objective and subjective evaluation, this was expanded to a phase II randomized wait-list controlled trial (Ferguson et al. 2010) that showed trends towards improvement in some aspects of quality of life and memory, but was not definitive. We recently conducted a pilot feasibility trial of a

Table 5.2 Randomized controlled trials of mind-body interventions using cancer-related fatigue as an entry criteria

Author, publication date	Participants	Intervention type	Intervention duration	Control group(s)	Results
Bower (2011)	31 breast cancer survivors with moderate to severe fatigue	Iyengar yoga; group format; focused on postures thought to be effective for reducing cancer-related fatigue (restorative poses, supported back bends, supported inversions)	12 weeks, 2 sessions per week	Health education group	Decrease in fatigue in yoga group vs. controls at post-intervention; group differences maintained over 3 month follow-up
Johns (2014)	35 cancer survivors with moderate to severe fatigue (85.7 % breast)	Mindfulness-based stress reduction; group format; provided training in mindfulness meditation and psycho-education about cancer-related fatigue	7 weeks, 1 session per week	Wait list	Decrease in fatigue in mindfulness group vs. controls at post-intervention; group differences maintained over 1 month follow-up
Molassiotis (2012)	302 breast cancer survivors with moderate to severe fatigue; all post- chemotherapy	Acupuncture; individual sessions; needled 3 standardized points	6 weeks, 1 session per week	Usual care (fatigue information booklet)	Decrease in fatigue in acupuncture group vs. controls at post-intervention
van der Lee (2012)	100 cancer survivors with severe fatigue (58 % breast)	Mindfulness-based cognitive therapy; group format; provided training in mindfulness meditation and using mindfulness to manage automatic negative thoughts about fatigue	9 weeks, 1 session per week	Wait list	Decrease in fatigue in mindfulness group vs. controls at post-intervention; improvement maintained over 6 month follow-up

5 week, group intervention, cognitive rehabilitation program adapted from strategies used in older adults with mild cognitive impairment (Ercoli et al. 2013). This single arm study in 27 breast cancer survivors demonstrated feasibility as well as improvement in self-report and neurocognitive testing up to 6 months post intervention. A small sub-study showed significant normalization of EEG patterns in women who participated in the intervention. Recently, we completed a phase II randomized controlled trial of the same intervention compared to a wait-list control group, and showed highly significant improvements in self-report, neurocognitive tests, and EEG in the intervention group compared to the control group, which was sustained out to 2 months post-intervention, along with improvements in EEG correlating with those who had improved cognitive complaints (Ercoli et al. 2015). These very encouraging findings suggest there is a physiological basis for the improvement in cognitive complaints and test performance.

Other groups have applied computerized technologies to improve cognitive function in breast cancer patients. Kesler et al. (2013a) in a pilot study which randomized 41 breast cancer survivors to a computerized training program focused on executive functioning and memory found significant improvements in those who received the training compared to those who did not. Von Ah et al. (2012) examined a computer-based memory or processing speed training program compared to a wait-list control group of breast cancer survivors. They found that the processing speed training improved that outcome and memory immediately post-intervention and 2 months later. The memory training improved memory performance on neuropsychological testing.

There has also been exploration of psychostimulants to improve fatigue (Jean-Pierre et al. 2010) and secondarily cognitive function, but the findings are not conclusive (Kohli et al. 2009). Other investigators have attempted to examine methylphenidate without success, in terms of adequate recruitment to a treatment trial (Mar Fan et al. 2008). Any such therapy would have to have minimal side effects if it is given chronically, and many breast cancer survivors are averse to continue taking medication long-term if it is not truly necessary or very helpful. Thus behavioral strategies have greater appeal.

What Are the Research Challenges Associated with These Two Common Symptoms?

One of the critical challenges in the area of cancer-related fatigue and cognitive dysfunction is determining the underlying mechanisms for these symptoms. Although cross-sectional research has shown a positive association between inflammatory activity and fatigue in cancer patients and survivors, the causal nature of this association has not been determined. In particular, it is unknown whether inflammation causes fatigue (as observed in experimental models of sickness behavior), or whether inflammation is a consequence of fatigue (perhaps due to reductions in physical activity, alterations in sleep, or other behavioral/physiological changes).

One challenge to advancing research in this area is the lack of animal models of cancer-related fatigue (Dantzer et al. 2012). To directly address the causal role of inflammation in a human model, we conducted a small pilot study to evaluate the acute effects of infliximab, a monoclonal antibody against TNF, in five breast cancer survivors with severe, persistent fatigue. Participants completed daily diaries for 2 weeks before and after receiving a single dose of infliximab to assess changes in the severity and duration of daily fatigue. All five women reported reductions in daily fatigue, including a mean 1.9 point decrease in "worst" fatigue from pre- to post-treatment. These preliminary findings are promising and could be pursued in a larger randomized, placebo-controlled trial to determine the causal role of inflammation in cancer-related fatigue. However, anti-cytokine therapies have well-known side effects that may limit their use among women with breast cancer. In addition, given the multi-factorial nature of fatigue, it is likely that only certain women will respond to these (or other) anti-inflammatory agents. Indeed, a recent trial of infliximab for depression found that only those patients with elevated inflammation at treatment onset showed a positive response to this medication (Raison et al. 2013). Similarly, only patients with elevated inflammation are likely to show reduced cancer-related fatigue (and improvements in cognitive function) following anti-inflammatory therapies. Patients whose fatigue is driven by cognitive processes, such as catastrophizing, may be more responsive to cognitive-behavioral therapies, whereas those fatigue is driven by deconditioning may be responsive to exercise. Of course, these treatments may have multiple targets; for example, in our yoga trial with fatigued breast cancer survivors, women in the intervention group reported higher self-efficacy to manage fatigue symptoms and lower inflammatory activity, both of which may have contributed to their reduced fatigue (Bower et al. 2012, 2014). Identifying appropriate treatments for individual patients is an important challenge for future research. In addition, determining the factors that influence fatigue onset vs. persistence may be helpful in determining which type of interventions may be most helpful during vs. after treatment.

Another topic of considerable interest for research on cancer-related fatigue and cognitive disturbance is the intersection of aging and cancer (Dale et al. 2012). Similar biological processes are involved in aging, fatigue, and cognitive function, including inflammation (Mandelblatt et al. 2013). Indeed, cancer and its treatment may accelerate age-related changes in inflammatory activity and other physiological processes, which may contribute to fatigue and cognitive decline, particularly in vulnerable individuals. Cancer patients and survivors who suffer from fatigue and cognitive problems may look biologically "older" than patients without these problems, which may make them more susceptible to age-related declines in physical and mental function. However, few studies have probed the overlap between age-related processes and cancer-related behavioral disturbances. In addition, potential common and specific mechanisms for fatigue and cognitive function have not been carefully examined.

Clinically, in our practice with breast cancer survivors, persistent fatigue and/or cognitive difficulties often co-occur. In some women, one symptom is more prominent than the other. In our various research studies focused on women with cognitive complaints seeking rehabilitation services, increased fatigue, sleep disturbance and impaired physical function are all self-reported as moderate to severe, even though these complaints are not prominently mentioned. What has been most reassuring to women has been our ability to explain the possible biological factors underlying the development of either persistent fatigue or cognitive complaints, as they frequently feel isolated and rejected by the medical community and even support groups, where other women do not have similar complaints. They are often labeled as being depressed, when they clinically are not, and they are very hard on themselves for not being able to function and work the way they did before their cancer diagnosis and treatment. With the emerging evidence from neuroimaging studies that there are functional cerebral abnormalities associated with breast cancer treatment (especially chemotherapy), it will be critical to develop a better understanding of the natural history of these changes and to determine who is most vulnerable for persistent difficulties that do not resolve or worsen over time. The MBS cohort study is one study, but more are needed. In addition, we need to begin to intervene early in the course of the treatment to try to improve outcomes for women so that they can resume their pre-illness functioning, especially for activities of everyday life which can be compromised in many.

Given the substantial numbers of women who experience persistent fatigue and cognitive difficulties after breast cancer treatment, we can no longer ignore this as a potential toxicity of cancer treatment. Consent forms in clinical trials must address this possibility, and patient reported assessments should be included in clinical trial outcomes. Some of the newer targeted agents, such as everolimus, may have significant impact on fatigue (Baselga et al. 2012) and cognitive difficulties have not been assessed to our knowledge. While we have been successful in reducing the number of women now exposed to adjuvant chemotherapy due to genomic profiles testing, a substantial number will still receive treatments that may cause either fatigue or cognitive difficulties and we need to gather this information to help in management and decision-making regarding treatment.

References

Aggarwal BB, Vijayalekshmi RV, Sung B (2009) Targeting inflammatory pathways for prevention and therapy of cancer: short-term friend, long-term foe. Clin Cancer Res 15:425–430

Ahles TA (2012) Brain vulnerability to chemotherapy toxicities. Psychooncology 21:1141–1148

Ahles TA, Saykin AJ (2007) Candidate mechanisms for chemotherapy-induced cognitive changes. Nat Rev Cancer 7:192–201

Ahles TA, Saykin AJ, Noll WW, Furstenberg CT, Guerin S, Cole B, Mott LA (2003) The relationship of APOE genotype to neuropsychological performance in long-term cancer survivors treated with standard dose chemotherapy. Psychooncology 12:612–619

Ahles TA, Saykin AJ, McDonald BC, Li Y, Furstenberg CT, Hanscom BS, Mulrooney TJ, Schwartz GN, Kaufman PA (2010) Longitudinal assessment of cognitive changes associated with adjuvant treatment for breast cancer: impact of age and cognitive reserve. J Clin Oncol 28:4434–4440

Ahles TA, Root JC, Ryan EL (2012) Cancer- and cancer treatment-associated cognitive change: an update on the state of the science. J Clin Oncol 30:3675–3686

Alexander S, Minton O, Andrews P, Stone P (2009) A comparison of the characteristics of disease-free breast cancer survivors with or without cancer-related fatigue syndrome. Eur J Cancer 45:384–392

Alfano CM, Imayama I, Neuhouser ML, Kiecolt-Glaser JK, Smith AW, Meeske K, McTiernan A, Bernstein L, Baumgartner KB, Ulrich CM, Ballard-Barbash R (2012) Fatigue, inflammation, and omega-3 and omega-6 fatty acid intake among breast cancer survivors. J Clin Oncol 30:1280–1287

Andrykowski MA, Curran SL, Lightner R (1998) Off-treatment fatigue in breast cancer survivors: a controlled comparison. J Behav Med 21:1–18

Aouizerat BE, Dodd M, Lee K, West C, Paul SM, Cooper BA, Wara W, Swift P, Dunn LB, Miaskowski C (2009) Preliminary evidence of a genetic association between tumor necrosis factor alpha and the severity of sleep disturbance and morning fatigue. Biol Res Nurs 11:27–41

Barsevick A, Frost M, Zwinderman A, Hall P, Halyard M (2010) I'm so tired: biological and genetic mechanisms of cancer-related fatigue. Qual Life Res 19:1419–1427

Barton DL, Liu H, Dakhil SR, Linquist B, Sloan JA, Nichols CR, McGinn TW, Stella PJ, Seeger GR, Sood A, Loprinzi CL (2013) Wisconsin Ginseng (Panax quinquefolius) to improve cancer-related fatigue: a randomized, double-blind trial, N07C2. J Natl Cancer Inst 105:1230–1238

Baselga J, Campone M, Piccart M, Burris HA III, Rugo HS, Sahmoud T, Noguchi S, Gnant M, Pritchard KI, Lebrun F, Beck JT, Ito Y, Yardley D, Deleu I, Perez A, Bachelot T, Vittori L, Xu Z, Mukhopadhyay P, Lebwohl D, Hortobagyi GN (2012) Everolimus in postmenopausal hormone-receptor-positive advanced breast cancer. N Engl J Med 366:520–529

Bower JE (2005) Prevalence and causes of fatigue after cancer treatment: the next generation of research. J Clin Oncol 23:8280–8282

Bower JE (2014) Cancer-related fatigue-mechanisms, risk factors, and treatments. Nat Rev Clin Oncol 11(10):597–609

Bower JE, Ganz PA, Desmond KA, Rowland JH, Meyerowitz BE, Belin TR (2000) Fatigue in breast cancer survivors: occurrence, correlates, and impact on quality of life. J Clin Oncol 18:743–753

Bower JE, Ganz PA, Aziz N, Fahey JL (2002) Fatigue and proinflammatory cytokine activity in breast cancer survivors. Psychosom Med 64:604–611

Bower JE, Ganz PA, Dickerson SS, Petersen L, Aziz N, Fahey JL (2005a) Diurnal cortisol rhythm and fatigue in breast cancer survivors. Psychoneuroendocrinology 30:92–100

Bower JE, Ganz PA, Aziz N (2005b) Altered cortisol response to psychologic stress in breast cancer survivors with persistent fatigue. Psychosom Med 67:277–280

Bower JE, Ganz PA, Desmond KA, Bernaards C, Rowland JH, Meyerowitz BE, Belin TR (2006) Fatigue in long-term breast carcinoma survivors: a longitudinal investigation. Cancer 106:751–758

Bower JE, Ganz PA, Aziz N, Olmstead R, Irwin MR, Cole SW (2007) Inflammatory responses to psychological stress in fatigued breast cancer survivors: relationship to glucocorticoids. Brain Behav Immun 21:251–258

Bower JE, Ganz PA, Lin Tao M, Hu W, Belin TR, Sepah S, Cole S, Aziz N (2009) Inflammatory biomarkers and fatigue during radiation therapy for breast and prostate cancer. Clin Cancer Res 15(17):5534–5540

Bower JE, Ganz PA, Irwin MR, Arevalo JM, Cole SW (2011a) Fatigue and gene expression in human leukocytes: increased NF-kappaB and decreased glucocorticoid signaling in breast cancer survivors with persistent fatigue. Brain Behav Immun 25:147–150

Bower JE, Ganz PA, Irwin MR, Kwan L, Breen EC, Cole SW (2011b) Inflammation and behavioral symptoms after breast cancer treatment: do fatigue, depression, and sleep disturbance share a common underlying mechanism? J Clin Oncol 29:3517–3522

Bower JE, Garet D, Sternlieb B, Ganz PA, Irwin MR, Olmstead R, Greendale G (2012) Yoga for persistent fatigue in breast cancer survivors. Cancer 118:3766–3775

Bower JE, Ganz PA, Irwin MR, Castellon S, Arevalo J, Cole SW (2013) Cytokine genetic variations and fatigue among patients with breast cancer. J Clin Oncol 31:1656–1661

Bower JE, Greendale G, Crosswell AD, Garet D, Sternlieb B, Ganz PA, Irwin MR, Olmstead R, Arevalo J, Cole SW (2014) Yoga reduces inflammatory signaling in fatigued breast cancer survivors: a randomized controlled trial. Psychoneuroendocrinology 43:20–9

Bower JE, Bak K, Berger A, Breitbart W, Escalante CP, Ganz PA, Schnipper HH, Lacchetti C, Ligibel JA, Lyman GH, Ogaily MS, Pirl WF, Jacobsen PB (2014) Screening, assessment, and management of fatigue in adult survivors of cancer: an American Society of Clinical Oncology Clinical Practice guideline adaptation. J Clin Oncol 32(17):1840–1850

Broeckel JA, Jacobsen PB, Horton J, Balducci L, Lyman GH (1998) Characteristics and correlates of fatigue after adjuvant chemotherapy for breast cancer. J Clin Oncol 16:1689–1696

Capuron L, Ravaud A, Dantzer R (2000) Early depressive symptoms in cancer patients receiving interleukin 2 and/or interferon alfa-2b therapy. J Clin Oncol 18:2143–2151

Castellon SA, Ganz PA, Bower JE, Petersen LA, Abraham L, Greendale GA (2004) Neurocognitive performance in breast cancer survivors exposed to adjuvant chemotherapy and tamoxifen. J Clin Exp Neuropsychol 26:955–969

Castellon SA, Silverman DH, Ganz PA (2005) Breast cancer treatment and cognitive functioning: current status and future challenges in assessment. Breast Cancer Res Treat 92:199–206

Cella D, Davis K, Breitbart W, Curt G (2001) Cancer-related fatigue: prevalence of proposed diagnostic criteria in a United States sample of cancer survivors. J Clin Oncol 19:3385–3391

Cella D, Lai J, Chang C, Peterman A, Slavin M (2002) Fatigue in cancer patients compared with fatigue in the general United States population. Cancer 94:528–538

Cleeland CS, Bennett GJ, Dantzer R, Dougherty PM, Dunn AJ, Meyers CA, Miller AH, Payne R, Reuben JM, Wang XS, Lee BN (2003) Are the symptoms of cancer and cancer treatment due to a shared biologic mechanism? A cytokine-immunologic model of cancer symptoms. Cancer 97:2919–2925

Collado-Hidalgo A, Bower JE, Ganz PA, Cole SW, Irwin MR (2006) Inflammatory biomarkers for persistent fatigue in breast cancer survivors. Clin Cancer Res 12:2759–2766

Collado-Hidalgo A, Bower JE, Ganz PA, Irwin MR, Cole SW (2008) Cytokine gene polymorphisms and fatigue in breast cancer survivors: early findings. Brain Behav Immun 22:1197–1200

Coussens LM, Werb Z (2002) Inflammation and cancer. Nature 420:860–867

Cramp F, Byron-Daniel J (2012) Exercise for the management of cancer-related fatigue in adults. Cochrane Database Syst Rev 11, CD006145

Crosswell AD, Lockwood KG, Ganz PA, Bower JE (2014) Low heart rate variability and cancer-related fatigue in breast cancer survivors. Psychoneuroendocrinology 45:58–66

Curt GA, Breitbart W, Cella D, Groopman JE, Horning SJ, Itri LM, Johnson DH, Miaskowski C, Scherr SL, Portenoy RK, Vogelzang NJ (2000) Impact of cancer-related fatigue on the lives of patients: new findings from the fatigue coalition. Oncologist 5:353–360

Dale W, Mohile SG, Eldadah BA, Trimble EL, Schilsky RL, Cohen HJ, Muss HB, Schmader KE, Ferrell B, Extermann M, Nayfield SG, Hurria A (2012) Biological, clinical, and psychosocial correlates at the interface of cancer and aging research. J Natl Cancer Inst 104:581–589

Dantzer R, Kelley KW (2007) Twenty years of research on cytokine-induced sickness behavior. Brain Behav Immun 21:153–160

Dantzer R, O'Connor JC, Freund GG, Johnson RW, Kelley KW (2008) From inflammation to sickness and depression: when the immune system subjugates the brain. Nat Rev Neurosci 9:46–56

Dantzer R, Meagher MW, Cleeland CS (2012) Translational approaches to treatment-induced symptoms in cancer patients. Nat Rev Clin Oncol 9:414–426

Deprez S, Amant F, Yigit R, Porke K, Verhoeven J, Van den Stock J, Smeets A, Christiaens MR, Leemans A, Hecke WV, Vandenberghe J, Vandenbulcke M, Sunaert S (2011) Chemotherapy-induced structural changes in cerebral white matter and its correlation with impaired cognitive functioning in breast cancer patients. Hum Brain Mapping 32:480–493

Deprez S, Amant F, Smeets A, Peeters R, Leemans A, Van Hecke W, Verhoeven JS, Christiaens MR, Vandenberghe J, Vandenbulcke M, Sunaert S (2012) Longitudinal assessment of chemotherapy-induced structural changes in cerebral white matter and its correlation with impaired cognitive functioning. J Clin Oncol 30:274–281

Deprez S, Vandenbulcke M, Peeters R, Emsell L, Smeets A, Christiaens MR, Amant F, Sunaert S (2014) Longitudinal assessment of chemotherapy-induced alterations in brain activation during multitasking and its relation with cognitive complaints. J Clin Oncol 32:2031–2038

Donovan KA, Small BJ, Andrykowski MA, Munster P, Jacobsen PB (2007) Utility of a cognitive-behavioral model to predict fatigue following breast cancer treatment. Health Psychol 26:464–472

Ercoli LM, Castellon SA, Hunter AM, Kwan L, Kahn-Mills BA, Cernin PA, Leuchter AF, Ganz PA (2013) Assessment of the feasibility of a rehabilitation intervention program for breast cancer survivors with cognitive complaints. Brain Imaging Behav 7:543–553

Ercoli LM, Castellon SA, Petersen L, Kwan L, Kahn-Mills B, Embree LM, Cernin PA, Hunter AM, Leuchter AF, Ganz PA (2015) Cognitive rehabilitation intervention for breast cancer survivors: results of a randomized clinical trial. Psychooncology

Fagundes CP, Murray DM, Hwang BS, Gouin JP, Thayer JF, Sollers JJ III, Shapiro CL, Malarkey WB, Kiecolt-Glaser JK (2011) Sympathetic and parasympathetic activity in cancer-related fatigue: more evidence for a physiological substrate in cancer survivors. Psychoneuroendocrinology 36:1137–1147

Ferguson RJ, Ahles TA, Saykin AJ, McDonald BC, Furstenberg CT, Cole BF, Mott LA (2007) Cognitive-behavioral management of chemotherapy-related cognitive change. Psychooncology 16:772–777

Ferguson RJ, McDonald BC, Rocque MA, Furstenberg CT, Horrigan S, Ahles TA, Saykin AJ (2010) Development of CBT for chemotherapy-related cognitive change: results of a waitlist control trial. Psychooncology 21(2):176–186

Forlenza MJ, Hall P, Lichtenstein P, Evengard B, Sullivan PF (2005) Epidemiology of cancer-related fatigue in the Swedish twin registry. Cancer 104:2022–2031

Ganz PA (1998) Cognitive dysfunction following adjuvant treatment of breast cancer: a new dose-limiting toxic effect? JNCI J Natl Cancer Inst 90:182–183

Ganz PA, Bower JE, Kwan L, Castellon SA, Silverman DHS, Geist C, Breen EC, Irwin MR, Cole SW (2013a) Does tumor necrosis factor-alpha (TNFalpha) play a role in post-chemotherapy cerebral dysfunction? Brain Behav Immun 30(Supplement):S99–S108

Ganz PA, Kwan L, Castellon SA, Oppenheim A, Bower JE, Silverman DHS, Cole SW, Irwin MR, Ancoli-Israel S, Belin TR (2013b) Cognitive complaints after breast cancer treatments: examining the relationship with neuropsychological test performance. J Natl Cancer Inst 105:791–801

Ganz PA, Petersen L, Castellon SA, Bower JE, Silverman DHS, Cole SW, Irwin MR, Belin TR (2014) Cognitive function after the initiation of adjuvant endocrine therapy in early-stage breast cancer: an observational cohort study. J Clin Oncol 32:3559–3567

Gielissen MFM, Verhagen S, Witjes F, Bleijenberg G (2006) Effects of cognitive behavior therapy in severely fatigued disease-free cancer patients compared with patients waiting for cognitive behavior therapy: a randomized controlled trial. J Clin Oncol 24:4882–4887

Groenvold M, Petersen MA, Idler E, Bjorner JB, Fayers PM, Mouridsen HT (2007) Psychological distress and fatigue predicted recurrence and survival in primary breast cancer patients. Breast Cancer Res Treat 105:209–219

Haroon E, Raison CL, Miller AH (2012) Psychoneuroimmunology meets neuropsychopharmacology: translational implications of the impact of inflammation on behavior. Neuropsychopharmacology 37:137–162

Irvine DM, Vincent L, Graydon JE, Bubela N (1998) Fatigue in women with breast cancer receiving radiation therapy. Cancer Nurs 21:127–135

Irwin MR, Cole SW (2011) Reciprocal regulation of the neural and innate immune systems. Nat Rev Immunol 11:625–632

Jacobsen PB, Hann DM, Azzarello LM, Horton J, Balducci L, Lyman GH (1999) Fatigue in women receiving adjuvant chemotherapy for breast cancer: characteristics, course, and correlates. J Pain Symptom Manage 18:233–242

Jean-Pierre P, Morrow GR, Roscoe JA, Heckler C, Mohile S, Janelsins M, Peppone L, Hemstad A, Esparaz BT, Hopkins JO (2010) A phase 3 randomized, placebo-controlled, double-blind, clinical trial of the effect of modafinil on cancer-related fatigue among 631 patients receiving chemotherapy: a University of Rochester Cancer Center Community Clinical Oncology Program Research base study. Cancer 116:3513–3520

Jim HSL, Phillips KM, Chait S, Faul LA, Popa MA, Lee YH, Hussin MG, Jacobsen PB, Small BJ (2012) Meta-analysis of cognitive functioning in breast cancer survivors previously treated with standard-dose chemotherapy. J Clin Oncol 30(29):3578–3587

Johns SA, Brown LF, Beck-Coon K, Monahan PO, Tong Y, Kroenke K (2014) Randomized controlled pilot study of mindfulness-based stress reduction for persistently fatigued cancer survivors. Psychooncology. Epub ahead of print

Kesler SR, Kent JS, O'Hara R (2011) Prefrontal cortex and executive function impairments in primary breast cancer. Arch Neurol 68:1447–1453

Kesler S, Hadi Hosseini SM, Heckler C, Janelsins M, Palesh O, Mustian K, Morrow G (2013a) Cognitive training for improving executive function in chemotherapy-treated breast cancer survivors. Clin Breast Cancer 13:299–306

Kesler S, Janelsins M, Koovakkattu D, Palesh O, Mustian K, Morrow G, Dhabhar FS (2013b) Reduced hippocampal volume and verbal memory performance associated with interleukin-6 and tumor necrosis factor-alpha levels in chemotherapy-treated breast cancer survivors. Brain Behav Immun 30(Suppl):S109–S116

Kirkwood J (2002) Cancer immunotherapy: the interferon-alpha experience. Semin Oncol 29(3 Suppl 7):18–26

Kohli S, Fisher SG, Tra Y, Adams MJ, Mapstone ME, Wesnes KA, Roscoe JA, Morrow GR (2009) The effect of modafinil on cognitive function in breast cancer survivors. Cancer 115:2605–2616

Liu L, Mills PJ, Rissling M, Fiorentino L, Natarajan L, Dimsdale JE, Sadler GR, Parker BA, Ancoli-Israel S (2012) Fatigue and sleep quality are associated with changes in inflammatory markers in breast cancer patients undergoing chemotherapy. Brain Behav Immun 26:706–713

Maillet D, Rajah MN (2013) Association between prefrontal activity and volume change in prefrontal and medial temporal lobes in aging and dementia: a review. Ageing Res Rev 12:479–489

Mandelblatt JS, Hurria A, McDonald BC, Saykin AJ, Stern RA, VanMeter JW, McGuckin M, Traina T, Denduluri N, Turner S, Howard D, Jacobsen PB, Ahles T (2013) Cognitive effects of cancer and its treatments at the intersection of aging: what do we know; what do we need to know? Semin Oncol 40:709–725

Mandelblatt JS, Jacobsen PB, Ahles T (2014) Cognitive effects of cancer systemic therapy: implications for the care of older patients and survivors. J Clin Oncol 32:2617–2626

Mar Fan HG, Clemons M, Xu W, Chemerynsky I, Breunis H, Braganza S, Tannock IF (2008) A randomised, placebo-controlled, double-blind trial of the effects of d-methylphenidate on fatigue and cognitive dysfunction in women undergoing adjuvant chemotherapy for breast cancer. Support Care Cancer 16:577–583

McDonald B, Conroy S, Ahles T, West J, Saykin A (2010) Gray matter reduction associated with systemic chemotherapy for breast cancer: a prospective MRI study. Breast Cancer Res Treat 123:819–828

McDonald BC, Conroy SK, Ahles TA, West JD, Saykin AJ (2012) Alterations in brain activation during working memory processing associated with breast cancer and treatment: a prospective functional magnetic resonance imaging study. J Clin Oncol 30(20):2500–2508

Merriman JD, Von AD, Miaskowski C, Aouizerat BE (2013) Proposed mechanisms for cancer- and treatment-related cognitive changes. Semin Oncol Nurs 29:260–269

Merriman JD, Aouizerat BE, Cataldo JK, Dunn L, Cooper BA, West C, Paul SM, Baggott CR, Dhruva A, Kober K, Langford DJ, Leutwyler H, Ritchie CS, Abrams G, Dodd M, Elboim C, Hamolsky D, Melisko M, Miaskowski C (2014) Association between an interleukin 1 receptor, type I promoter polymorphism and self-reported attentional function in women with breast cancer. Cytokine 65:192–201

Miaskowski C, Dodd M, Lee K, West C, Paul SM, Cooper BA, Wara W, Swift PS, Dunn LB, Aouizerat BE (2010) Preliminary evidence of an association between a functional interleukin-6 polymorphism and fatigue and sleep disturbance in oncology patients and their family caregivers. J Pain Symptom Manage 40:531–544

Miller AH, Ancoli-Israel S, Bower JE, Capuron L, Irwin MR (2008) Neuroendocrine-immune mechanisms of behavioral comorbidities in patients with cancer. J Clin Oncol 26:971–982

Miller AH, Haroon E, Raison CL, Felger JC (2013) Cytokine targets in the brain: impact on neurotransmitters and neurocircuits. Depress Anxiety 30:297–306

Minton O, Richardson A, Sharpe M, Hotopf M, Stone P (2008) A systematic review and meta-analysis of the pharmacological treatment of cancer-related fatigue. J Natl Cancer Inst 100:1155–1166

Minton O, Richardson A, Sharpe M, Hotopf M, Stone PC (2011) Psychostimulants for the management of cancer-related fatigue: a systematic review and meta-analysis. J Pain Symptom Manage 41:761–767

Mitchell SA (2010) Cancer-related fatigue: state of the science. PM&R 2:364–383

Molassiotis A, Bardy J, Finnegan-John J, Mackereth P, Ryder DW, Filshie J, Ream E, Richardson A (2012) Acupuncture for cancer-related fatigue in patients with breast cancer: a pragmatic randomized controlled trial. J Clin Oncol 30:4470–4476

Monk JP, Phillips G, Waite R, Kuhn J, Schaaf LJ, Otterson GA, Guttridge D, Rhoades C, Shah M, Criswell T, Caligiuri MA, Villalona-Calero MA (2006) Assessment of tumor necrosis factor alpha blockade as an intervention to improve tolerability of dose-intensive chemotherapy in cancer patients. J Clin Oncol 24:1852–1859

Montgomery GH, Kangas M, David D, Hallquist MN, Green S, Bovbjerg DH, Schnur JB (2009) Fatigue during breast cancer radiotherapy: an initial randomized study of cognitive-behavioral therapy plus hypnosis. Health Psychol 28:317–322

Montgomery GH, David D, Kangas M, Green S, Sucala M, Bovbjerg DH, Hallquist MN, Schnur JB (2014) Randomized controlled trial of a cognitive-behavioral therapy plus hypnosis intervention to control fatigue in patients undergoing radiotherapy for breast cancer. J Clin Oncol 32:557–563

Moraska AR, Sood A, Dakhil SR, Sloan JA, Barton D, Atherton PJ, Suh JJ, Griffin PC, Johnson DB, Ali A, Silberstein PT, Duane SF, Loprinzi CL (2010) Phase III, randomized, double-blind, placebo-controlled study of long-acting methylphenidate for cancer-related fatigue: North Central Cancer Treatment Group NCCTG-N05C7 trial. J Clin Oncol 28:3673–3679

Morrow GR, Andrews PL, Hickok JT, Roscoe JA, Matteson S (2002) Fatigue associated with cancer and its treatment. Support Care Cancer 10:389–398

Orre IJ, Reinertsen KV, Aukrust P, Dahl AA, Fossa SD, Ueland T, Murison R (2011) Higher levels of fatigue are associated with higher CRP levels in disease-free breast cancer survivors. J Psychosom Res 71:136–141

Pertl MM, Hevey D, Boyle NT, Hughes MM, Collier S, O'Dwyer AM, Harkin A, Kennedy MJ, Connor TJ (2013) C-reactive protein predicts fatigue independently of depression in breast cancer patients prior to chemotherapy. Brain Behav Immun 34:108–119

Phillips KA, Bernhard J (2003) Adjuvant breast cancer treatment and cognitive function: current knowledge and research directions. J Natl Cancer Inst 95:190–197

Pomykala KL, Ganz PA, Bower JE, Kwan L, Castellon SA, Mallam S, Cheng I, Ahn R, Breen EC, Irwin MR, Silverman DHS (2013) The association between pro-inflammatory cytokines, regional cerebral metabolism, and cognitive complaints following adjuvant chemotherapy for breast cancer. Brain Imaging Behav 1–13

Poulson MJ (2001) Not just tired. J Clin Oncol 19:4180–4181

Puetz TW, Herring MP (2012) Differential effects of exercise on cancer-related fatigue during and following treatment: a meta-analysis. Am J Prev Med 43:e1–24

Raison CL, Rutherford RE, Woolwine BJ, Shuo C, Schettler P, Drake DF, Haroon E, Miller AH (2013) A randomized controlled trial of the tumor necrosis factor antagonist infliximab for treatment-resistant depression: the role of baseline inflammatory biomarkers. JAMA Psychiatry 70:31–41

Reichenberg A, Yirmiya R, Schuld A, Kraus T, Haack M, Morag A, Pollmacher T (2001) Cytokine-associated emotional and cognitive disturbances in humans. Arch Gen Psychiatry 58:445–452

Schagen SB, Hamburger HL, Muller MJ, Boogerd W, van Dam FS (2001) Neurophysiological evaluation of late effects of adjuvant high-dose chemotherapy on cognitive function. J Neurooncol 51:159–165

Schmitz KH, Courneya KS, Matthews C, Demark-Wahnefried W, Galvão DA, Pinto BM, Irwin ML, Wolin KY, Segal RJ, Lucia ALEJ, Schneider CM, von Gruenigen VE, Schwartz AL (2010) American college of sports medicine roundtable on exercise guidelines for cancer survivors. Med Sci Sports Exerc 42:1409–1426

Seigers R, Fardell JE (2011) Neurobiological basis of chemotherapy-induced cognitive impairment: a review of rodent research. Neurosci Biobehav Rev 35:729–741

Seigers R, Schagen SB, Van TO, Dietrich J (2013) Chemotherapy-related cognitive dysfunction: current animal studies and future directions. Brain Imaging Behav 7:453–459

Seruga B, Zhang H, Bernstein LJ, Tannock IF (2008) Cytokines and their relationship to the symptoms and outcome of cancer. Nat Rev Cancer 8:887–899

Small BJ, Rawson KS, Walsh E, Jim HSL, Hughes TF, Iser L, Andrykowski MA, Jacobsen PB (2011) Catechol-O-methyltransferase genotype modulates cancer treatment-related cognitive deficits in breast cancer survivors. Cancer 117:1369–1376

Spath-Schwalbe E, Hansen K, Schmidt F, Schrezenmeier H, Marshall L, Burger K, Fehm HL, Born J (1998) Acute effects of recombinant human interleukin-6 on endocrine and central nervous sleep functions in healthy men. J Clin Endocrinol Metab 83:1573–1579

Stanton AL, Ganz PA, Kwan L, Meyerowitz BE, Bower JE, Krupnick JL, Rowland JH, Leedham B, Belin TR (2005) Outcomes from the moving beyond cancer psychoeducational, randomized, controlled trial with breast cancer patients. J Clin Oncol 23:6009–6018

Stone HB, Coleman CN, Anscher MS, McBride WH (2003) Effects of radiation on normal tissue: consequences and mechanisms. Lancet Oncol 4:529–536

Tannock IF, Ahles TA, Ganz PA, van Dam FS (2004) Cognitive impairment associated with chemotherapy for cancer: report of a workshop. J Clin Oncol 22:2233–2239

Tyring S, Gottlieb A, Papp K, Gordon K, Leonardi C, Wang A, Lalla D, Woolley M, Jahreis A, Zitnik R, Cella D, Krishnan R (2006) Etanercept and clinical outcomes, fatigue, and depression in psoriasis: double-blind placebo-controlled randomised phase III trial. Lancet 367:29–35

Valentine AD, Meyers CA, Kling MA, Richelson E, Hauser P (1998) Mood and cognitive side effects of interferon-alpha therapy. Semin Oncol 25:39–47

van Dam FS, Schagen SB, Muller MJ, Boogerd W, Wall E, Droogleever Fortuyn ME, Rodenhuis S (1998) Impairment of cognitive function in women receiving adjuvant treatment for high-risk breast cancer: high-dose versus standard-dose chemotherapy [see comments]. JNCI J Natl Cancer Inst 90:210–218

van der Lee ML, Garssen B (2012) Mindfulness-based cognitive therapy reduces chronic cancer-related fatigue: a treatment study. Psychooncology 21:264–272

Vardy J, Wefel JS, Ahles T, Tannock IF, Schagen SB (2008) Cancer and cancer-therapy related cognitive dysfunction: an international perspective from the Venice cognitive workshop. Ann Oncol 19:623–629

Von Ah D, Carpenter JS, Saykin A, Monahan P, Wu J, Yu M, Rebok G, Ball K, Schneider B, Weaver M, Tallman E, Unverzagt F (2012) Advanced cognitive training for breast cancer survivors: a randomized controlled trial. Breast Cancer Res Treat 135:799–809

Wefel JS, Vardy J, Ahles T, Schagen SB (2011) International Cognition and Cancer Task Force recommendations to harmonise studies of cognitive function in patients with cancer. Lancet Oncol 12:703–708

Yates P, Aranda S, Hargraves M, Mirolo B, Clavarino A, McLachlan S, Skerman H (2005) Randomized controlled trial of an educational intervention for managing fatigue in women receiving adjuvant chemotherapy for early-stage breast cancer. J Clin Oncol 23:6027–6036

Yun YH, Lee KS, Kim YW, Park SY, Lee ES, Noh DY, Kim S, Oh JH, Jung SY, Chung KW, Lee YJ, Jeong SY, Park KJ, Shim YM, Zo JI, Park JW, Kim YA, Shon EJ, Park S (2012) Web-based tailored education program for disease-free cancer survivors with cancer-related fatigue: a randomized controlled trial. J Clin Oncol 30:1296–1303

Chapter 6
Symptoms: Chemotherapy-Induced Peripheral Neuropathy

Bryan P. Schneider, Dawn L. Hershman, and Charles Loprinzi

Abstract Chemotherapy-induced peripheral neuropathy (CIPN) is a problematic, treatment-induced toxicity that has the potential to impact quality of life and limit the doses of curative intent therapy. This therapy-induced side effect is one of the most troublesome in oncology clinical practices, considering the morbidity, the frequency, and the potential irreversibility of this problem. Patients with breast cancer are particularly impacted by this side effect as multiple agents commonly used for this disease can cause neuropathy. In this chapter, we provide an overview of CIPN, including: clinical predictors, frequency, and its impact on quality of life. Further, we highlight the pathophysiology and review the literature to date for agents designed to prevent or treat CIPN. We also highlight the most important ongoing clinical and translational research questions that hope to help better predict and prevent this toxicity. This includes optimizing the methods of assessment, using host specific factors (Race and genetics) to predict those more likely to experience CIPN, and determining how CIPN might impact clinical decisions toward therapy.

Keywords Neuropathy • CIPN (Chemotherapy-induced peripheral neuropathy) • Taxanes • Breast cancer • Toxicity • Pharmacogenetics • PRO (Patient reported outcomes)

B.P. Schneider (✉)
Associate Professor of Medicine & Medical/Molecular Genetics, Indiana University Simon Cancer Center, Indianapolis, IN, USA
e-mail: bpschnei@iupui.edu

D.L. Hershman
Associate Professor of Medicine and Epidemiology, Herbert Irving Comprehensive Cancer Center, Columbia University, 161 Fort Washington, 1068, New York, NY 10032, USA
e-mail: dlh23@cumc.columbia.edu

C. Loprinzi
Regis Professor of Breast Cancer Research, Division of Medical Oncology, Rochester, MN, USA
e-mail: cloprinzi@mayo.edu

© Breast Cancer Research Foundation 2015
P.A. Ganz (ed.), *Improving Outcomes for Breast Cancer Survivors*,
Advances in Experimental Medicine and Biology 862,
DOI 10.1007/978-3-319-16366-6_6

Overview

Chemotherapy-induced peripheral neuropathy (CIPN) is a problematic, treatment-induced toxicity that has the potential to impact quality of life and limit the doses of curative intent therapy (Cavaletti and Zanna 2002; Hershman et al. 2011). This therapy-induced side effect is one of the most troublesome in oncology clinical practices, considering the morbidity, the frequency, and the potential irreversibility of this problem. Patients with breast cancer are particularly impacted by this side effect as multiple agents commonly used for this disease can cause neuropathy. Breast cancer-related drugs that often cause neuropathy include those used in the metastatic setting such as: platinating agents, vinca alkaloids, eribulin, and ixabepilone. Perhaps the most important class, however, are the taxanes which are commonly employed in both the curative setting and the metastatic setting (Ghersi et al. 2005; Nowak et al. 2004); a class of drugs with potential for serious and, at times, long-lasting neuropathy (Hershman et al. 2011).

CIPN typically induces a sensory neuropathy with symptoms that reflect either a gain in sensory neuronal function, a loss of function or a combination of both. The most common symptoms that likely result from an increase function of a subset of sensory neurons are paresthesias, tingling, pain/allodynia; whereas the most common symptoms that likely reflect loss of function are numbness and dulled sensation, a loss of position and/or vibratory sense (Stubblefield et al. 2009; Cavaletti et al. 2013), and diminished reflexes. Motor neuropathy symptoms also occur, although they are markedly less common (Argyriou et al. 2012). It is not clear whether motor neuropathy is simply a severe variant of the same process or whether the mechanism is completely different. Further, it is not clear why some patients experience predominantly symptoms of loss of function and others symptoms of enhanced excitability or whether this matters when considering future preventive therapeutics.

Specific to the taxanes, the frequency and severity of peripheral neuropathy is related to the specific drug, dose, schedule, and duration of therapy. From the large adjuvant trials, the rates of taxane-induced neuropathy range from 15 to 23 % grade 2–4, as graded by the Common Terminology Criteria Adverse Event (CTCAE) system (Hershman et al. 2011; Lee and Swain 2006). Patients with grade 2 neuropathy have interference with function (e.g. difficulty buttoning a shirt), those with grade 3 have interference with activities of daily living (e.g. brushing teeth or bathing), and those with grade 4 have permanent and disabling symptoms. In general the rates are higher for paclitaxel, compared with docetaxel (while acute and hematologic toxicities are more prevalent in the latter) (Sparano et al. 2008). The frequency and severity of neuropathy increases with increasing dose for both agents. The frequency of neuropathy is also schedule dependent with the weekly dosing for paclitaxel having more neuropathy when compared with every 3-week dosing; although the former also has more anti-tumor efficacy against breast cancer (Sparano et al. 2008). The likelihood of neuropathy may be higher in patients who have other contributing predispositions to neuropathy, such as diabetes mellitus (Gogas et al. 1996). Additionally, those patients who are obese and older age are at greater risk (Rowinsky et al. 1993a, b). Finally, recent data suggest that African American patients might also be at a markedly higher risk for paclitaxel induced CIPN (Schneider et al. 2011). Thus, special attention must be paid to these patient populations when preparing to treat them with a potentially neurotoxic agent.

In addition to the classic chronic CIPN caused by paclitaxel, usually presenting in a stocking/glove distribution (Cavaletti and Zanna 2002; Stubblefield et al. 2009), there are data to strongly support that the acute pain syndrome (which, for a long time had been labeled as being from arthralgias/myalgias) is actually an acute form of neuropathy (Loprinzi et al. 2011). This is similar to oxaliplatin causing an acute neuropathy along with a more chronic neuropathy (Argyriou et al. 2012; Velasco et al. 2014).

There are two major clinical tensions that relate to CIPN. One is the direct impact on quality of life and functionality (Hershman et al. 2011). The second is the potential to limit the use of an effective agent. For the latter, this can mean the permanent discontinuation of an effective drug when treating metastatic breast cancer and less than desired dose-intensity in the curative setting. Specifically, a highly effective adjuvant regimen for high-risk patients includes weekly paclitaxel, which unfortunately also has one of the highest incidences of CIPN (Sparano et al. 2008). Thus, for those at high risk for disease recurrence, a major concern is the patient's inability to tolerate the full dose/duration of therapy when the treatment is likely to be life-saving. An equally problematic situation occurs when deciding on adjuvant treatment in patients at very low risk for recurrence, but deemed eligible for chemotherapy. The use of taxane-based regimens in this setting has become commonplace in order to avoid anthracyclines (Jones et al. 2006). While this approach has removed the rare, but serious risks of congestive heart failure and myelodysplasia/leukemia, it has highlighted the marginal risk-benefit ratio for this patient population in whom the incremental gain in curability may be quite small and the potential for a devastating, permanent neurotoxicity may be larger. This problem is exacerbated by the inability to predict, a priori, which patients might be preferentially affected by CIPN.

Understanding the mechanism for CIPN is critical toward identifying potential targets for preventive and therapeutic interventions. The current understanding of what causes CIPN is incomplete (Cavaletti et al. 1995; Flatters and Bennett 2006; Jimenez-Andrade et al. 2006; Nakata and Yorifuji 1999; Pachman et al. 2011; Persohn et al. 2005; Peters et al. 2007; Raine et al. 1987; Theiss and Meller 2000; Witte et al. 2008). Taxanes promote microtubule stabilization, which causes cell death by interfering with normal cell division. Similar aggregation of the microtubules in the neuronal cell bodies may also lead to the disturbances in neuronal function by impacting microtubule based axonal transport, mitochondrial dysfunction, or through direct damage to DNA. In pain models, damage to peripheral nerves leads to spontaneous activation of afferent pain nerve fibers with an increase in voltage gated sodium and calcium channels as well as an up-regulation of a variety of receptor proteins. The activation of the nerve fibers also causes hyper-excitability of the dorsal column of the spinal cord and the dorsal horn (Baron et al. 2010). Additionally, there is loss of GABA releasing neurons and descending inhibitory pathways involving serotonin and norepinephrine, which further amplifies the central sensitization. After central sensitization, input from even non-nociceptive nerve fibers can be interpreted as painful (Baron et al. 2010). Much of the work to date has been carried out in mouse or rat models. A limitation of this work has been the inability to recapitulate some of the varied phenotypes. Thus, although models of pain are robust, excellent models for paresthesias and numbness are lacking.

Clinical Research Questions

Prevention and Treatment Strategies

The major research questions to date have placed great emphasis on identifying agents that might either treat or prevent neuropathy without adversely impact the efficacy of the drugs. To date there have been 42 randomized controlled clinical trials of agents to prevent CIPN (Hershman et al. 2014). Unfortunately, none of these trials have provided any convincing evidence for a beneficial agent. The inability to identify a successful protective agent is, in part, a reflection of our inability to fully understand the mechanism of this toxicity.

There have also been multiple randomized trials, which have attempted to identify therapies that might treat the problem after it has occurred. Similar to the trials designed to prevent CIPN, most of the trials for treatment of the toxicity have been negative (Table 6.1) (Hershman et al. 2014). One of the most compelling studies, however, was a trial that demonstrated superiority of duloxetine over placebo (Smith et al. 2013a). This trial demonstrated a significant reduction in pain ($p = 0.003$) as well as a suggestion of benefit on numbness and tingling. In an exploratory subgroup analysis, however, the benefit was less clear for the taxanes compared with oxaliplatin. Another relatively-positive result was seen with the use of a topical cream composed of baclofen, amitriptyline, and ketamine (BAK) in a small randomized trial (Barton et al. 2011). Based on the existing data, the American Society of Clinical Oncology CIPN guideline committee (Table 6.2) recommended that clinicians should consider duloxetine for CIPN (Hershman et al. 2014). Additionally, this committee suggested that, although there were not as convincing data with other agents, the following agents could be considered for a trial treatment in selected patients: gabapentin/pregabalin, tricyclic antidepressants, and the above-noted BAK cream (Hershman et al. 2014). Despite the relatively sparse data

Table 6.1 Summary of randomized controlled trials for the treatment of established chemotherapy induced peripheral neuropathy Hershman et al. (2014)

Pharmacologic intervention	Neurotoxic agent	Reference
Duloxetine	Taxane or platinum	Smith et al. (2013a)
Gabapentin	Vinca or platinum or taxane	Rao et al. (2007)
Lamotrigine	Vinca or platinum or taxane	Rao et al. (2008)
Nortriptyline	Cisplatin	Hammack et al. (2002)
	Vinca or platinum or taxane	Kautio et al. (2008)
Topical amitriptyline, ketamine ± baclofen (BAK)	Vinca or platinum or taxane or thalidomide	Barton et al. (2011)

Table 6.2 ASCO practice guidelines for chemotherapy induced peripheral neuropathy Hershman et al. (2014)

Prevention of CIPN

There are no established agents recommended for the prevention of CIPN in patients with cancer undergoing treatment with neurotoxic agents. This is based on the paucity of high-quality, consistent evidence and a balance of benefits versus harms

- Clinicians should **not** offer the following agents for the prevention of CIPN to patients with cancer undergoing treatment with neurotoxic agents:
    - Acetyl-L-carnitine (ALC)
    - Amifostine
    - Amitriptyline
    - CaMg for patients receiving oxaliplatin-based chemotherapy
    - Diethyldithio-carbamate (DDTC)
    - Glutathione (GSH) for patients receiving paclitaxel/carboplatin chemotherapy
    - Nimodipine
    - Org 2766
    - All-*trans*-retinoic acid
    - rhuLIF
    - Vitamin E
    - Venlafaxine is not recommended for routine use in clinical practice. Although the venlafaxine data support its potential utility, the data were not strong enough to recommend its use in clinical practice, until additional supporting data become available
    - No recommendations can be made on the use of N-acetylcysteine, carbamazepine, glutamate, GSH for patients receiving cisplatin or oxaliplatin-based chemotherapy, goshajinkigan (GJG), omega-3 fatty acids, or oxycarbazepine for the prevention of CIPN at this time

Treatment of CIPN

For patients with cancer experiencing CIPN, clinicians may offer duloxetine

No recommendations can be made on the use of:

- ALC, noting that a positive phase III abstract supported its value, but this work has not yet been published in a peer-reviewed journal, and a prevention trial suggested that this agent was associated with worse outcomes
- Tricyclic antidepressants; however, based on the limited options that are available for this prominent clinical problem and the demonstrated efficacy of these drugs for other neuropathic pain conditions, it is reasonable to try a tricyclic antidepressant (e.g. nortriptyline or desipramine) in patients suffering from CIPN after a discussion with the patients about the limited scientific evidence for CIPN, potential harms, benefits, cost, and patient preferences
- Gabapentin, noting that the available data were limited regarding its efficacy for treating CIPN. However, the panel felt that this agent is reasonable to try for selected patients with CIPN pain given that only a single negative randomized trial for this agent was completed, the established efficacy of gabapentin and pregabalin for other forms of neuropathic pain, and the limited CIPN treatment options. Patients should be informed about the limited scientific evidence for CIPN, potential harms, benefits, and costs
- A topical gel treatment containing baclofen (10 mg), amitriptyline HCl (40 mg), and ketamine (20 mg), noting that a single trial indicated that this product did decrease CIPN symptoms. Given the available data, the panel felt that this agent is reasonable to try for selected patients with CIPN pain. Patients should be informed about the limited scientific evidence for the treatment of CIPN, potential harms, benefits, and costs

supporting these therapies, data regarding some of them on other forms of neuropathy (i.e. diabetic neuropathy and acute post-herpetic neuralgia) influenced this recommendation. Opiates are also used for painful neuropathy without a good feeling for the benefit/risk ratio regarding them.

A major limitation for the intervention trials to date is a limited understanding of the underlying pathophysiology. If the goal of therapy is to repair an underlying problem then lumping patients with different types of sensory or motor neuropathy may be as inefficient as studying anti-HER2 therapies for all tumors regardless of HER2 status.

Assessment of Neurotoxicity and Relationship to Mechanisms

As stated above, much of what we know about the frequency and severity of CIPN is derived from the CTCAE as this has been widely employed in many of the large clinical trials that have studied these agents. There are multiple limitations to this reporting methodology (Hershman et al. 2011). This criterion is largely based on the degree of impact on functionality. This is a practical criterion when considering the need to dose reduce but is not overly helpful in distinguishing the various types/manifestations of the process. This limits the ability to fully characterize the true diversity and frequency of the toxicity. Importantly, it hinders correlative work aimed at predicting the toxicity and unveiling the mechanistic underpinnings. If, indeed, the various types of neuropathy symptoms reflect differences in unique pathophysiologies between the different neurotoxic chemotherapy agents, then correlative biomarker work requiring large sample sizes where CTCAE was used will suffer from dilution of the true associations. Additionally, recent data suggest poor concordance among raters for cancer therapy-induced toxicities (Cella et al. 2003, Cancer Therapy Evaluation Program, August 9, 2006). Further, there is discordance in agreement between clinician raters and the patients who experience these toxicities. Specific to taxane-induced peripheral neuropathy, the use of patient reported outcomes (PROs) correlate well with vibration threshold testing and are effective for both acute symptoms and over long-term follow-up (Hershman et al. 2011). With the recognition that the toxicity profile is an important piece to optimize the therapeutic index, many of the large studies have begun to incorporate PROs as a superior endpoint/phenotype. Finally, and perhaps most importantly, many trials do not capture the long-term frequency of CIPN. This is a big limitation as enduring or irreversible neuropathy may be the most clinically important phenotype to identify and study.

Newer Research Strategies

There are a number of ongoing clinical trials to further identify agents that might prevent or treat CIPN. In addition, other modalities are currently undergoing testing such as acupuncture, topical menthol and cutaneous electro-stimulation devices. With anticipated new insights into the mechanism of CIPN, additional advances can be made with rational selection of drugs. The identification of common mechanisms of neuropathy caused across drug classes will be important for the development of drugs that can be implemented broadly. Additionally, understanding the pathophysiology for the spectrum of CIPN symptoms will be critical to optimal drug development.

Identifying Host Factors Related to Risk for CIPN

Another evolving area of research is the use of germline genetic variability (i.e. SNPs, copy number variations, etc.) to predict drug-induced toxicity. This has become a provocative area of research as variants can impact the metabolism, transport, and excretion of drugs, but can also impact the target tissue (i.e., neurons). A candidate study from an institutional series demonstrated an association between a variant in a paclitaxel metabolizing enzyme, CYP2C8*3 and neuropathy (Hertz et al. 2013). Another candidate approach from the adjuvant breast cancer trial SWOG-0221, demonstrated an association between a SNP in *FANCD2* and taxane induced neuropathy (Sucheston et al. 2011). Recently, several large genome wide association studies (GWAS) have been conducted from large clinical trials involving taxanes. The CALGB-40101 investigators identified a SNP in *FDG4* that correlated with increased likelihood of paclitaxel-induced neuropathy (Baldwin et al. 2012). *FDG4* is associated with the hereditary neuropathy condition of Charcot-Marie-Tooth disease. Subsequent pathway and modeling work with this data set have suggested that a hereditable predisposition to this toxicity may lie in genes involved in axon outgrowth (Chhibber et al. 2014). Another trial specifically focused on more rare variants using massively parallel sequencing of 20,794 genes associated with heredity neuropathy from patients who had received paclitaxel-based chemotherapy (Beutler et al. 2013). The investigators reported an association between EPHA5, ARHGEF10, and PRX and paclitaxel-induced neuropathy. It is hopeful that the identification of genomic predictors might not only play a useful role in predicting who will be at high or low risk of this toxicity but may also shed insight into the biological underpinnings to help with future drug development. Further, the integration of these genetic factors with other predictors such as race, weight, or co-morbid states might allow for a truly personalized and successful predictor for likelihood of this toxicity.

Future Directions

There are multiple areas of research progress to improve our approach to those who might be at risk for CIPN and here we outline three immediate areas of need: education, drug development, and predictive biomarkers.

For any toxicity, patient and physician education are paramount to successful management. Physicians who fail to prioritize toxicities cannot adequately counsel the true risk to benefit ratio of the therapies they plan to deliver. This is particularly true in the case of adjuvant chemotherapy, where the vast majority of women can expect to be long-term survivors. Additionally, this makes it difficult for patients to prepare themselves mentally for potential challenges and hurdles that await them. Recent data demonstrated that the counseled frequency and severity of neuropathy could impact the specific regimen a patient might choose (Smith et al. 2013b). Further, patients who had previously experienced neuropathy were actually more likely to choose (less worried about) a regimen that would cause mild neuropathy and markedly less likely to choose (more worried about) a regimen that would cause severe neuropathy (Smith et al. 2013b). These data demonstrate that those patients who experienced the toxicity are more nuanced in their decision-making based on their personal understanding of the toxicity. This implies that physicians must strive to educate patients in a more detailed fashion so that they might make the best possible decision for their therapy.

Improved drug development is also drastically needed. The bar is high, however, for drugs that prevent or treat a specific side effect. The first hurdle is to identify drugs that are highly effective. As outlined above this has not been an easy task, to date, in part because the underlying pathophysiology is poorly understood. Second, the preventive drug must not have significant toxicity. Many patients are willing to accept substantial drug-induced toxicity for the payoff of increased cure rate, but few like the idea of trading one drug side effect for another. Finally, the preventive drug, ideally, will be affordable. In our current healthcare economic environment, extremely expensive supportive care drugs will be less likely to be paid for by insurance without substantial evidence of benefit and this may leave many patients unable to afford the option.

Finally, genetic biomarkers to predict which patients are at highest risk or those preferentially protected would be clinically valuable. As outlined above, there are provocative genomic data from large clinical trials implementing taxanes that may lead to such decision-making information in the future. However, there are several hurdles that must be overcome before clinical implementation is possible.

Regarding this, it is clear that the findings from the studies done to date have identified non-overlapping associations. This is not surprising as often the true-positive associations aren't necessary those with the top p-values. This makes overlapping of other rich data sets extremely important to identify the true positive associations. Attempts at additional confirmation of these data may soon be on the way. Several other GWAS have been completed across the Cooperative group system that might allow for validation of the existing findings, including that from the SWOG-0221 trial and ECOG-5103 trial (Schneider et al. 2011). This could provide an amazing opportunity to perform a meta-analysis across these trials; and this has been proposed. Another layer of complexity is that for complex pathophysiological processes, the underlying predispositions might be multigenic. This requires sophisticated pathway and modeling approaches. While much of the work to date has focused on common variants (which likely will have modest effect sizes), it is also very likely that rare variants (with large effect sizes) might also be important.

Unfortunately, many of the standard GWAS platforms do not cover rare variants and thus this exploration requires more deep sequencing approaches, as demonstrated above.

Additionally, the ability to identify a true association depends not only on adequate power and meticulous adherence to genomic quality control, but also consistent and accurate phenotyping. As outlined above, many of the correlative studies have been performed on trials where the CTCAE was the only methodology for case definitions. The more recent integration of PROs, however, might provide a new level of insight and biomarker discovery.

It will be important to develop a user-friendly decision-making tool to help guide physicians regarding how to understand and react to these genomic markers. Unlike many of the current genomic tests being used in breast cancer (i.e. Oncotype Dx), the decision to react to a toxicity marker must also consider the patient's risk of disease and the alternative approaches available.

In conclusion, CIPN is a major problem for patients with breast cancer. Much work is ongoing to identify predictive biomarkers, improve education, understand the underlying pathophysiology, and to identify drugs to treat or prevent this undesirable side effect.

References

Argyriou AA, Bruna J, Marmiroli P, Cavaletti G (2012) Chemotherapy-induced peripheral neurotoxicity (CIPN): an update. Crit Rev Oncol Hematol 82:51–77

Baldwin RM, Owzar K, Zembutsu H, Chhibber A, Kubo M, Jiang C, Watson D, Eclov RJ, Mefford J, McLeod HL, Friedman PN, Hudis CA, Winer EP, Jorgenson EM, Witte JS, Shulman LN, Nakamura Y, Ratain MJ, Kroetz DL (2012) A genome-wide association study identifies novel loci for paclitaxel-induced sensory peripheral neuropathy in CALGB 40101. Clin Cancer Res 18:5099–5109

Baron R, Binder A, Wasner G (2010) Neuropathic pain: diagnosis, pathophysiological mechanisms, and treatment. Lancet Neurol 9:807–819

Barton DL, Wos EJ, Qin R, Mattar BI, Green NB, Lanier KS, Bearden JD 3rd, Kugler JW, Hoff KL, Reddy PS, Rowland KM Jr, Riepl M, Christensen B, Loprinzi CL (2011) A double-blind, placebo-controlled trial of a topical treatment for chemotherapy-induced peripheral neuropathy: NCCTG trial N06CA. Support Care Cancer 19:833–841

Beutler AS, Kulkarni A, Kanwar R, Qin R, Cunningham JM, Therneau TM, Loprinzi CL (2013) Abstract LB-196: sequencing symptom control: results from the alliance N08C1 and N08CA genetics of chemotherapy neuropathy trials. Cancer Res 73(1)

Cancer Therapy Evaluation Program (2006) Common terminology criteria for adverse events, version 3.0, DCTD, NCI, NIH, DHHS. Accessed 31 Mar 2003

Cavaletti G, Zanna C (2002) Current status and future prospects for the treatment of chemotherapy-induced peripheral neurotoxicity. Eur J Cancer 38:1832–1837

Cavaletti G, Tredici G, Braga M, Tazzari S (1995) Experimental peripheral neuropathy induced in adult rats by repeated intraperitoneal administration of taxol. Exp Neurol 133:64–72

Cavaletti G, Cornblath DR, Merkies IS, Postma TJ, Rossi E, Frigeni B, Alberti P, Bruna J, Velasco R, Argyriou AA, Kalofonos HP, Psimaras D, Ricard D, Pace A, Galie E, Briani C, Dalla Torre C, Faber CG, Lalisang RI, Boogerd W, Brandsma D, Koeppen S, Hense J, Storey D, Kerrigan S, Schenone A, Fabbri S, Valsecchi MG, CI-PeriNomS Group (2013) The chemotherapy-induced peripheral neuropathy outcome measures standardization study: from consensus to the first validity and reliability findings. Ann Oncol 24:454–462

Cella D, Peterman A, Hudgens S, Webster K, Socinski MA (2003) Measuring the side effects of taxane therapy in oncology: the functional assessment of cancer therapy-taxane (FACT-taxane). Cancer 98:822–831

Chhibber A, Mefford J, Stahl EA, Pendergrass SA, Baldwin RM, Owzar K, Li M, Winer EP, Hudis CA, Zembutsu H, Kubo M, Nakamura Y, Mcleod HL, Ratain MJ, Shulman LN, Ritchie MD, Plenge RM, Witte JS, Kroetz DL (2014) Polygenic inheritance of paclitaxel-induced sensory peripheral neuropathy driven by axon outgrowth gene sets in CALGB 40101 (Alliance). Pharmacogenomics J 14(4):336–342

Flatters SJ, Bennett GJ (2006) Studies of peripheral sensory nerves in paclitaxel-induced painful peripheral neuropathy: evidence for mitochondrial dysfunction. Pain 122:245–257

Ghersi D, Wilcken N, Simes RJ (2005) A systematic review of taxane-containing regimens for metastatic breast cancer. Br J Cancer 93:293–301

Gogas H, Shapiro F, Aghajanian C, Fennelly D, Almadrones L, Hoskins WJ, Spriggs DR (1996) The impact of diabetes mellitus on the toxicity of therapy for advanced ovarian cancer. Gynecol Oncol 61:22–26

Hammack JE, Michalak JC, Loprinzi CL, Sloan JA, Novotny PJ, Soori GS, Tirona MT, Rowland KM, Stella PJ JR, Johnson JA (2002) Phase III evaluation of nortriptyline for alleviation of symptoms of cis-platinum-induced peripheral neuropathy. Pain 98:195–203

Hershman DL, Weimer LH, Wang A, Kranwinkel G, Brafman L, Fuentes D, Awad D, Crew KD (2011) Association between patient reported outcomes and quantitative sensory tests for measuring long-term neurotoxicity in breast cancer survivors treated with adjuvant paclitaxel chemotherapy. Breast Cancer Res Treat 125:767–774

Hershman DL, Lacchetti C, Dworkin RH, Lavoie Smith EM, Bleeker J, Cavaletti G, Chauhan C, Gavin P, Lavino A, Lustberg MB, Paice J, Schneider B, Smith ML, Smith T, Terstriep S, Wagner-Johnston N, Bak K, Loprinzi CL (2014) Prevention and management of chemotherapy-induced peripheral neuropathy in survivors of adult cancers: American society of clinical oncology clinical practice guideline. J Clin Oncol 32:1941–1967

Hertz DL, Roy S, Motsinger-Reif AA, Drobish A, Clark LS, Mcleod HL, Carey LA, Dees EC (2013) CYP2C8*3 increases risk of neuropathy in breast cancer patients treated with paclitaxel. Ann Oncol 24:1472–1478

Jimenez-Andrade JM, Peters CM, Mejia NA, Ghilardi JR, Kuskowski MA, Mantyh PW (2006) Sensory neurons and their supporting cells located in the trigeminal, thoracic and lumbar ganglia differentially express markers of injury following intravenous administration of paclitaxel in the rat. Neurosci Lett 405:62–67

Jones SE, Savin MA, Holmes FA, O'Shaughnessy JA, Blum JL, Vukelja S, McIntyre KJ, Pippen JE, Bordelon JH, Kirby R, Sandbach J, Hyman WJ, Khandelwal P, Negron AG, Richards DA, Anthony SP, Mennel RG, Boehm KA, Meyer WG, Asmar L (2006) Phase III trial comparing doxorubicin plus cyclophosphamide with docetaxel plus cyclophosphamide as adjuvant therapy for operable breast cancer. J Clin Oncol 24:5381–5387

Kautio AL, Haanpaa M, Saarto T, Kalso E (2008) Amitriptyline in the treatment of chemotherapy-induced neuropathic symptoms. J Pain Symptom Manage 35:31–39

Lee JJ, Swain SM (2006) Peripheral neuropathy induced by microtubule-stabilizing agents. J Clin Oncol 24:1633–1642

Loprinzi CL, Reeves BN, Dakhil SR, Sloan JA, Wolf SL, Burger KN, Kamal A, Le-Lindqwister NA, Soori GS, Jaslowski AJ, Novotny PJ, Lachance DH (2011) Natural history of paclitaxel-associated acute pain syndrome: prospective cohort study NCCTG N08C1. J Clin Oncol 29:1472–1478

Nakata T, Yorifuji H (1999) Morphological evidence of the inhibitory effect of taxol on the fast axonal transport. Neurosci Res 35:113–122

Nowak AK, Wilcken NR, Stockler MR, Hamilton A, Ghersi D (2004) Systematic review of taxane-containing versus non-taxane-containing regimens for adjuvant and neoadjuvant treatment of early breast cancer. Lancet Oncol 5:372–380

Pachman DR, Barton DL, Watson JC, Loprinzi CL (2011) Chemotherapy-induced peripheral neuropathy: prevention and treatment. Clin Pharmacol Ther 90:377–387

Persohn E, Canta A, Schoepfer S, Traebert M, Mueller L, Gilardini A, Galbiati S, Nicolini G, Scuteri A, Lanzani F, Giussani G, Cavaletti G (2005) Morphological and morphometric analysis of paclitaxel and docetaxel-induced peripheral neuropathy in rats. Eur J Cancer 41:1460–1466

Peters CM, Jimenez-Andrade JM, Kuskowski MA, Ghilardi JR, Mantyh PW (2007) An evolving cellular pathology occurs in dorsal root ganglia, peripheral nerve and spinal cord following intravenous administration of paclitaxel in the rat. Brain Res 1168:46–59

Raine CS, Roytta M, Dolich M (1987) Microtubule-mitochondrial associations in regenerating axons after taxol intoxication. J Neurocytol 16:461–468

Rao RD, Michalak JC, Sloan JA, Loprinzi CL, Soori GS, Nikcevich DA, Warner DO, Novotny P, Kutteh LA, Wong GY, North Central Cancer Treatment Group (2007) Efficacy of gabapentin in the management of chemotherapy-induced peripheral neuropathy: a phase 3 randomized, double-blind, placebo-controlled, crossover trial (N00C3). Cancer 110:2110–2118

Rao RD, Flynn PJ, Sloan JA, Wong GY, Novotny P, Johnson DB, Gross HM, Renno SI, Nashawaty M, Loprinzi CL (2008) Efficacy of lamotrigine in the management of chemotherapy-induced peripheral neuropathy: a phase 3 randomized, double-blind, placebo-controlled trial, N01C3. Cancer 112:2802–2808

Rowinsky EK, Chaudhry V, Cornblath DR, Donehower RC (1993) Neurotoxicity of taxol. J Natl Cancer Inst Monogr (15):107–115

Rowinsky EK, Eisenhauer EA, Chaudhry V, Arbuck SG, Donehower RC (1993b) Clinical toxicities encountered with paclitaxel (Taxol). Semin Oncol 20:1–15

Schneider BP, Li L, Miller K, Flockhart D, Radovich M, Hancock BA, Kassem N, Foroud T, Koller DL, Badve SS, Li Z, Partridge AH, O'Neill AM, Sparano JA, Dang CT, Northfelt DW, Smith ML, Railey E, Sledge GW (2011) Genetic associations with taxane-induced neuropathy by a genome-wide association study (GWAS) in E5103. J Clin Oncol 29(suppl; abstr 1000):80s

Smith EM, Pang H, Cirrincione C, Fleishman S, Paskett ED, Ahles T, Bressler LR, Fadul CE, Knox C, Le-Lindqwister N, Gilman PB, Shapiro CL, Alliance for Clinical Trials In Oncology (2013a) Effect of duloxetine on pain, function, and quality of life among patients with chemotherapy-induced painful peripheral neuropathy: a randomized clinical trial. JAMA 309:1359–1367

Smith ML, Railey E, White CB, Schneider BP (2013b) Discerning clinical relevance of biomarkers in early stage breast cancer. The San Antonio breast cancer symposium, abstract P6-08-05

Sparano JA, Wang M, Martino S, Jones V, Perez EA, Saphner T, Wolff AC, Sledge GW, Wood WC JR, Davidson NE (2008) Weekly paclitaxel in the adjuvant treatment of breast cancer. N Engl J Med 358:1663–1671

Stubblefield MD, Burstein HJ, Burton AW, Custodio CM, Deng GE, Ho M, Junck L, Morris GS, Paice JA, Tummala S, Von Roenn JH (2009) NCCN task force report: management of neuropathy in cancer. J Natl Compr Canc Netw 7(5):S1–S26, quiz S27–8

Sucheston LE, Zhao H, Yao S, Zirpoli G, Liu S, Barlow WE, Moore HC, Thomas Budd G, Hershman DL, Davis W, Ciupak GL, Stewart JA, Isaacs C, Hobday TJ, Salim M, Hortobagyi GN, Gralow JR, Livingston RB, Albain KS, Hayes DF, Ambrosone CB (2011) Genetic predictors of taxane-induced neurotoxicity in a SWOG phase III intergroup adjuvant breast cancer treatment trial (S0221). Breast Cancer Res Treat 130:993–1002

Theiss C, Meller K (2000) Taxol impairs anterograde axonal transport of microinjected horseradish peroxidase in dorsal root ganglia neurons in vitro. Cell Tissue Res 299:213–224

Velasco R, Bruna J, Briani C, Argyriou AA, Cavaletti G, Alberti P, Frigeni B, Cacciavillani M, Lonardi S, Cortinovis D, Cazzaniga M, Santos C, Kalofonos HP (2014) Early predictors of oxaliplatin-induced cumulative neuropathy in colorectal cancer patients. J Neurol Neurosurg Psychiatry 85:392–398

Witte H, Neukirchen D, Bradke F (2008) Microtubule stabilization specifies initial neuronal polarization. J Cell Biol 180:619–632

Chapter 7
Symptoms: Aromatase Inhibitor Induced Arthralgias

Dawn L. Hershman, Charles Loprinzi, and Bryan P. Schneider

Abstract Recent clinical trials have demonstrated that aromatase inhibitors (AIs) are slightly more effective than tamoxifen at reducing breast cancer recurrences. However, breast cancer patients receiving AIs have a higher incidence of musculoskeletal symptoms, particularly joint pain and stiffness. Musculoskeletal pain and stiffness can lead to noncompliance and increased utilization of health care resources. There is a suggestion that the syndrome is the result of estrogen deprivation and may share components with autoimmune diseases such as Sjögren's syndrome. Several factors may increase the likelihood of developing AI arthralgia, such as prior chemotherapy, prior hormone replacement therapy, and increased weight; there are inconsistencies with regard to the data on genetic predispositions to this syndrome. While several studies have been done to evaluate interventions to treat or prevent AI arthralgia, no clear treatment has emerged as being particularly beneficial. Much of the research has been limited by small sample size, difficulty blinding patients to placebo, inconsistent definitions of the syndrome, multiple patient reported outcomes, lack of objective outcome measures and heterogeneous patient populations. We are at the early stages of research in characterizing, understanding etiology, preventing and treating AI arthralgias; however much work is being done in this area which, hopefully, will ultimately improve the lives of women with breast cancer.

Keywords Breast cancer • Aromatase inhibitors • Arthralgias

D.L. Hershman (✉)
Associate Professor of Medicine and Epidemiology, Herbert Irving Comprehensive
Cancer Center, Columbia University, 161 Fort Washington, 1068,
New York, NY 10032, USA
e-mail: dlh23@cumc.columbia.edu

C. Loprinzi
Regis Professor of Breast Cancer Research, Division of Medical Oncology,
Rochester, MN, USA
e-mail: cloprinzi@mayo.edu

B.P. Schneider
Associate Professor of Medicine & Medical/Molecular Genetics,
Indiana University Simon Cancer Center, Indianapolis, IN, USA
e-mail: bpschnei@iupui.edu

© Breast Cancer Research Foundation 2015   89
P.A. Ganz (ed.), *Improving Outcomes for Breast Cancer Survivors*,
Advances in Experimental Medicine and Biology 862,
DOI 10.1007/978-3-319-16366-6_7

Overview

Due to early detection and improved treatments, there has been a 30 % reduction in breast cancer (BC) mortality over the past two decades (DeSantis et al. 2014). The increase in BC survival is largely due to the benefits of hormonal therapy in women with hormone receptor (HR) positive breast cancer. Recent clinical trials have demonstrated that aromatase inhibitors (AIs) are more effective than tamoxifen at reducing BC recurrences (Baum et al. 2002; Goss et al. 2003, 2005; Howell et al. 2005; Thurlimann et al. 2005; Coombes et al. 2004). However, BC patients receiving AIs have a higher incidence of musculoskeletal symptoms, particularly joint pain and stiffness. Musculoskeletal pain and stiffness leads to noncompliance and increased utilization of health care resources (Henry et al. 2012.; Scudds and Mc 1998; Kewman et al. 1991; Carey et al. 1995). In a prospective study of 1,976 patients, a 10 % increase in arthralgia was associated with a 20 % increase risk of non-compliance to AI therapy (Hadji et al. 2014). Since women with HR-positive BC benefit from long-term hormonal therapy for 5–10 years, it is important to try to minimize side effects, to enhance patient adherence and to improve quality of life (QOL). Therefore, safe and effective treatments that alleviate these symptoms are needed. There is no standard definition, consistent terminology or agreed upon outcome measures for this condition. Some refer to it as AI Arthralgia (AIA) or AI Musculoskeletal Syndrome (AIMSS) (Niravath 2013) (Fig. 7.1).

In large adjuvant trials involving AIs, the incidence of musculoskeletal disorders was reported in 19–35 % of patients on AI's and 12–29 % of patients on tamoxifen (Baum et al. 2002; Goss et al. 2003). However, prospective cohort studies assessing symptoms with patient reported outcome measures suggest that 40–50 % of women have either

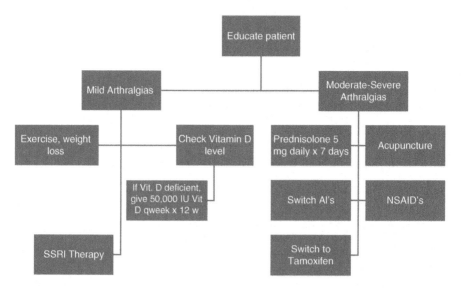

Fig. 7.1 Possible management algorithm from Niravath (2013)

new onset or worsening AI-related arthralgias (Crew et al. 2007; Henry et al. 2008, 2012). In a small prospective study of patients initiating AI therapy, the median time to development of AI arthralgias was 7 weeks, and by 12 weeks 55 % of patients had at least one complaint, and the incidence increased steadily over time (Shi et al. 2013). Other prospective cohort studies have found a similar incidence (Laroche et al. 2014).

Several studies have suggested an association between the development of AI arthralgias and improved disease free survival outcomes; however other studies have not shown this association. For example, a retrospective analysis of the ATAC data shows that women who developed arthralgia had a breast cancer recurrence HR of 0.65 ($P=0.001$) when compared with women with no arthralgia (Cuzick et al. 2008). Similarly, analysis of the TEAM trial showed improvements in disease-free survival in patients who had arthralgia while on endocrine therapy (Hadji et al. 2012). This is in contrast to the Intergroup Exemestane study that did not find this association (Mieog et al. 2012). Measurement error is a real problem with these studies, as they primarily rely on CTCAE reporting, and not patient reported outcomes.

Etiology

Estrogen deficiency after menopause has been linked to an increase in several chronic inflammatory conditions, including osteoporosis and osteoarthritis (OA) (Riggs and Melton 1992; Sherwin 1996). Estrogen can influence chondrocyte formation on multiple levels by interacting with cellular growth factors, adhesion molecules, and cytokines (Ushiyama et al. 1995; Rosner et al. 1982; Dayani et al. 1988). A dose-dependent change in matrix protein turnover occurs when cultured chondrocytes are exposed to estradiol (Richmond et al. 2000; Dayani et al. 1988; Blanchard et al. 1991; Rosner et al. 1982). Production of interleukin-6 (IL-6) and type II collagen in articular chondrocytes is also affected by estradiol, suggesting it may affect cartilage metabolism (Guerne et al. 1990; Claassen et al. 2006; Richette et al. 2003). Additional support that estrogen deprivation results in this syndrome comes from studies showing that hormone replacement with conjugated equine estrogens result in decreased joint pain, pain severity and joint swelling in postmenopausal women (Chlebowski et al. 2013).

In addition, there may be an autoimmune component to the syndrome. Animal models, where aromatase is knocked out, manifest symptoms similar to Sjögren's syndrome. In a study of patients referred to a rheumatologist, 50 % met the criteria for sicca syndrome (Laroche et al. 2007). Several small studies have also evaluated the influence AI therapy on inflammatory serum markers but results evaluating CRP, IL-6, and TNFα have been inconsistent (Dougherty et al. 2005; Azria et al. 2007; Harputluoglu et al. 2008). Even in studies showing AI-related changes to inflammatory markers, these changes were not correlated with the development of AI arthralgia (Azria et al. 2007).

Studies assessing AI-induced arthralgias have shown a correlation between PROs and objective findings. Morales et al. demonstrated that the subjective symptoms of AI-induced arthralgias in the hands are associated with physiologic changes to joints and functional impairments (Morales et al. 2008). Women taking AIs are more likely to have an increase in tenosynovial changes as seen on MRI, a decrease in grip strength as measured by a sphygmomanometer, as well as increased pain and stiffness as measured by self-administered questionnaires (Morales et al. 2008). In a study conducted by Dizdar et al., women taking AIs had increased tendon thickness and higher rates of effusions in hand joints/tendons on musculoskeletal sonography, compared to women who never received AIs (Dizdar et al. 2009; Lintermans et al. 2011). AI use is also associated with a greater incidence of carpal tunnel syndrome of moderate intensity and short duration (Sestak et al. 2009). With regard to pain sensitivity, the syndrome does not appear to result in impairment of descending pain inhibitory pathways as measured by pressure pain testing or conditioned pain modulation testing (Henry et al. 2014).

Risk Factors

The risk factors for developing AI-associated arthralgia are unclear. In some studies high BMI, prior chemotherapy, and a history of hormone replacement therapy are major risk factors for developing joint symptoms (Sestak et al. 2008). Other studies show prior taxane chemotherapy, symptoms at the time of treatment initiation and time from menopause are also associated with severity of AI arthralgias (Shi et al. 2013; Crew et al. 2007; Mao et al. 2011). One prospective cohort study found that additional risk factors for the development of pain included higher levels of anxiety and impaired quality of life at the time of initiation of therapy (Laroche et al. 2014).

The question of genetic susceptibility to toxicity has been addressed as well. In a prospective cohort study of 343 post-menopausal women starting AI therapy, single nucleotide polymorphisms (SNPs) in genes encoding for the metabolism of estrogens (CYP17A1) and vitamin D (VDR, CYP27B1) were associated with self-reported arthralgia (Garcia-Giralt et al. 2013). In addition, patients who had SNP's for multiple genes had the highest risk for AI arthralgia. A cross-sectional study in 390 patients also found that repeats in the CYP19A1 gene were associated with AI arthralgias (Mao et al. 2011). A better understanding of genomic and clinical risk factors can help identify patients who can be targeted for specific interventions to prevent this syndrome. An ongoing ECOG prospective cohort study in 1,000 women evaluating genomic predictors of AI arthralgias and early AI discontinuation should further clarify this issue.

Treatment

The use of a non-steroidal anti-inflammatory agent, or simply switching to an alternative AI, are common clinical approaches for patients experiencing significant arthralgias. Interestingly, approximately a third of patients will experience some improvement in symptoms by simply switching to another AI (Henry et al. 2012).

Table 7.1 Summary of trials for treatment or prevention of AI arthralgia

Therapy	N	Blinded	Randomized	Outcome
Supplements				
Vitamin D (Khan et al. 2012)	160	Y	Y	In this prevention trial, increased pain was observed in 38 % of patients receiving vitamin D, versus 61 % on placebo ($p = 0.008$)
Glucosamine (Greenlee et al. 2013)	53	N	N	50 % of patients with ≥20 % reduction in pain
Omega 3 fatty acid (Hershman et al. 2014)	240	Y	Y	50 % reduction in pain/stiffness in both arms
Drugs				
Duloxetine[a] (Henry et al. 2011)	29	N	N	74 % of patients had at least a 30 % decrease in average pain
Testosterone[a] (Birrell and Tilley 2009)	90	Y	Y	The higher dose of tested testosterone dose decreased pain more than did the placebo ($p = 0.04$)
Prednisolone (Kubo et al. 2012)	29	N	N	67 % of patients reported symptom improvement
Other				
Acupuncture[a, b] (Crew et al. 2010)	40	Y	Y	50 % decreased pain in the active acupuncture arm, as opposed to no change in the sham arm
Exercise[b] (Irwin et al. 2013)	121	N	Y	24 % decrease in pain scores with exercise versus virtually no change in the usual care group ($p = 0.013$)

[a]Large randomized controlled trial ongoing
[b]Additional studies also published; see text

There are, however, currently no proven treatments for AI-related arthralgias. Researchers have investigated interventions that have been studied in patients with chronic pain conditions, osteoarthritis and rheumatologic arthritis. Patients are often not willing to take medications to treat side effects, that have the potential for additional side effects, so many have gravitated to natural products, mind-body interventions and exercise. Many prospective trials are collecting blood and DNA to perform analysis that will be critical in elucidating the mechanism of this side effect as well as genetic susceptibility (Table 7.1).

Vitamin D

Vitamin D deficiency and insufficiency may contribute to musculoskeletal symptoms. In a prospective study, 60 women who were beginning adjuvant AI therapy had baseline vitamin D (25OHD) levels measured. At the conclusion of 16 weeks of letrozole, 52 % of women with baseline 25OHD levels >66 ng/ml reported no disability from joint pain, whereas only 19 % of those with levels <66 ng/ml had no disabling joint pain (Khan et al. 2010). In a subsequent randomized VITAL trial (Vitamin D for Arthralgias From Letrozole), 160 postmenopausal women with a serum vitamin D level of <40 ng/mL were randomized to receive 30,000 IU of oral vitamin D3 weekly for 24 weeks; the other was given a placebo. About 61 % of controls and 38 % of those on vitamin D reported an increase in pain ($P = .008$) (Khan et al. 2012).

Glucosamine Chondroitin

Glucosamine and chondroitin are popular dietary supplements frequently used with the goal of treating arthritic pain. In a non-randomized phase II trial of glucosamine and chondroitin to treat moderate-to-severe aromatase inhibitor induced joint pain, approximately 50 % of participants self-reported a ≥20 % improvement in pain, stiffness and function. The intervention was well-tolerated with minimal toxicities and no changes in estradiol levels were observed (Greenlee et al. 2013). Nonetheless, a placebo effect may be largely responsible for this finding.

Omega-3

Omega-3-fatty acids have anti-inflammatory effects and can be effective in decreasing arthralgias from rheumatologic conditions. A placebo-controlled trial of 3.3 g of Omega-3-fatty acids was conducted among 249 women on AIs with severe (≥5 of 10) pain and or stiffness. Interestingly a 60 % improvement was observed in the group randomized to Omega-3. However, a similar reduction was seen in the placebo arm. At 24 weeks, both groups had about a 2-point improvement from baseline on a 10 point scale (Hershman et al. 2014). This study demonstrates the difficulty in relying on patient-reported outcomes and the strength of the placebo effect. It also raises questions about the results of other trials where the intervention could not be truly blinded.

Duloxetine

Duloxetine is a selective serotonin and norepinephrine reuptake inhibitor used for treating pain. A single-arm, open-label phase 2 study of duloxetine was studied in women with breast cancer who developed new or worsening pain after treatment with an AI. Twenty-one of twenty-nine evaluable patients (72.4 %) achieved at least a 30 % decrease in average pain. The mean percentage reduction in average pain severity was 60.9 % (Henry et al. 2011). Based on the results of this study, a randomized placebo-controlled trial is being conducted in SWOG.

Testosterone

A double blind placebo-controlled, randomized pilot study of a transdermal testosterone preparation supported that this approach was helpful for alleviating aromatase inhibitor-induced arthralgias (Birrell and Tilley 2009). This trial involved 90 patients with baseline AI arthralgia pain and/or stiffness be greater than 50 on a 0–100 point pain scale. Patients were randomized into one of three study arms to receive a low testosterone dose versus an intermediate testosterone dose versus a placebo. After 3 months, the pain scores decreased more in the intermediate dose testosterone arm compared to the placebo arm ($P=0.04$). Likewise, stiffness scores decreased more in the intermediate dose testosterone arm, compared to the placebo arm ($P=0.06$). While serum testosterone concentrations increased in the groups getting testosterone, there was no suggestion that estrogen concentrations were any higher with testosterone, compared to the placebo arm. Based on these promising findings a phase III randomized placebo-controlled trial, using intradermal testosterone pellets, is being conducted in women with AI arthralgias, through the Alliance cooperative group.

Prednisolone

Autoimmune diseases are often treated with low dose steroids, and as mentioned above, there is some similarities between the arthralgia syndrome from AI's and Sjögren's syndrome. To test this approach, patients with AI arthralgia were administered 5 mg of oral prednisolone once a day in the morning for only 1 week. Patients were then asked to answer a questionnaire about joint pain symptoms at 1 week, 1 month and 2 months after the beginning of prednisolone use. Joint pain symptoms improved in 67 % of patients immediately after prednisolone use, with 63 % still reporting analgesic effect at 1 month, and 52 % at 2 months after beginning the short-term use of prednisolone (Kubo et al. 2012).

Acupuncture

Acupuncture is a popular non-pharmacologic modality that has been shown to be a useful adjunct in a range of painful conditions, including musculoskeletal pain (Anonymous 1998). Small pilot trials for AI arthralgias have reported conflicting results. A randomized, sham-controlled, blinded trial to assess the effect of a 6-week intervention of acupuncture in 38 women with AI-associated joint symptoms reported that true acupuncture group had a 50 % decrease pain compared to no change in the sham acupuncture group (Crew et al. 2010). Other smaller studies have suggested a benefit of both standard and electroacupuncture (Oh et al. 2013; Mao et al. 2014). A larger multicenter randomized trial with a waitlist control, sham, and true acupuncture is being conducted in SWOG.

Exercise

Several studies have suggested that exercise can reduce treatment-related adverse effects. A randomized trial of 121 women with AI arthralgia reported that pain scores decreased by 24 % at 12 months among women randomized to exercise vs. no change among women randomized to usual care (mean baseline to 12-month change: $-1.27+0.34$ vs. $-0.01+0.35$, respectively; $P=.013$). A dose–response effect was also observed with greater exercise leading to less pain severity (Irwin et al. 2013). In addition, a small pilot study of tai chi in 12 women with self reported AI arthralgia demonstrated a reduction in pain (Galantino et al. 2013). Additional work in this area is warranted, however, these studies are limited by the inability to blind participants.

Switching

Two studies have been done suggesting switching AI's can result in improvement of symptoms. In one study, 60 % of patients that switched remained on the alternate AI at 6 months, and 15 % had no complaints of joint symptoms (Briot et al. 2010). Another study showed that 39 % of patients were able to tolerate the second AI (Henry et al. 2012). Given the strong placebo effect, these results should be interpreted with caution with regard to the biologic effect of switching treatments. Another approach is to switch to tamoxifen, a therapy with similar long-term benefits.

Future Directions

There is enormous discrepancy between studies evaluating AI arthralgia due to lack of uniformity in both subjective and objective outcome measures and inconsistency in reporting. As a result priorities going forward might focus on uniform definitions, a better understanding of the natural history, defining mechanisms and determining effective treatment and prevention strategies. While there has been some work evaluating the syndrome, the heterogeneity in terminology and definitions can make interpreting the findings difficult. A consensus on consistent terminology and definition might help with future studies.

The original large phase III clinical trials resulting in drug approval did not capture patient reported outcomes, which was a missed opportunity for understanding this syndrome in a large number of women. Because the symptoms were often not attributed to the drug, these trials underestimated the degree to which these side effects interfere with quality of life, adherence and function. Cohort studies have used a variety of patient reported outcomes such as the Brief Pain Inventory (BPI), the Health Assessment Questionnaire (HAQ), the Western Ontario and McMaster Universities Arthritis Index (WOMAC) and the Score for Assessment and Quantification of Chronic Rheumatic Affections of the Hands (SACRAH). Consistent outcome measures would allow for better consistency of interpreting the results of interventional trials.

There are ongoing cohort studies, as the one being done through ECOG, where 1,000 patients are being followed at initiation of AI therapy and evaluated over the course of a year. In addition DNA and serum are being collected to clarify if there are genetic determinants of risk. This study should help clarify the short-term natural history. However the 1 year follow-up will limit the understanding of delayed symptoms and poor adherence. Another shortcoming of this trial, as opposed to the missed opportunity in the early randomized trials is that there is no placebo arm with which to better understand any nocebo effect. In addition, understanding the factors that contribute to improvement of symptoms in some patients, as opposed to others, may help physicians make better therapeutic recommendations.

A clearer understanding of the mechanism behind AI arthralgia may result in more targeted interventions or drug modifications that could reduce the development of this secondary effect. However, it may be that the exact mechanism that results in the drug effectiveness, i.e., the lowering of estradiol, may be the inciting factor. Careful attention will need to be paid to the fact that improvements in symptoms could affect the efficacy of the therapy if directed to the mechanism of action. As a result pure management of symptoms with interventions known to improve pain or treat other forms of arthritis have been studied.

Understanding risk factors may help risk stratify patients for treatment with tamoxifen or AI therapy, and may help target preventive interventions. Early suggestions from a biologic perspective have focused on estrogen-related pathways and polymorphisms in the aromatase pathway. It is clear that prior chemotherapy, prior hormone replacement therapy and baseline psychological state may influence the development of symptoms and adherence. These factors as well as genetic factors may help determine which patients should avoid AIs upfront and be treated with tamoxifen from the start. It will be crucial to understand if these individuals have a different prognosis.

The optimal outcome measure and timing of assessments is unclear, therefore clinical trials often vary from each other in primary outcome, duration and patient populations. The issue of placebo effect, as demonstrated by the SWOG Omega-3 study makes clinical trials challenging, and should push the field to try to better define objective as well as subjective definitions of this syndrome. Furthermore, many clinical trials cannot be truly blinded and may result in inaccurate conclusions. Interventional studies are subject to biases resulting from a very strong placebo effect and a waxing and waning symptom course.

The ultimate goal of treating or preventing AI arthralgias is to improve quality of life and increase adherence while maintaining efficacy, so these outcomes need to be considered in prevention and treatment studies.

References

Anonymous (1998) NIH consensus conference. Acupuncture. JAMA 280:1518–1524

Azria D, Lamy Y, Belkacemi G et al (2007) Letrozole-induced arthralgia: results of a multicenteric prospective trial exploring clinical parameters and plasma biomarkers. ASCO Breast Cancer Symposium

Baum M, Budzar AU, Cuzick J (2002) Anastrozole alone or in combination with tamoxifen versus tamoxifen alone for adjuvant treatment of postmenopausal women with early breast cancer: first results of the ATAC randomised trial. Lancet 359:2131–2139 [see comment][erratum appears in Lancet 2002 Nov 9;360(9344):1520]

Birrell S, Tilley W (2009) Testosterone undecanoate treatment reduces joint morbidities induced by anastrozole therapy in postmenopausal women with breast cancer: results of a double-blind, randomized phase II trial. San Antonio breast cancer symposium

Blanchard O, Tsagris L, Rappaport R et al (1991) Age-dependent responsiveness of rabbit and human cartilage cells to sex steroids in vitro. J Steroid Biochem Mol Biol 40:711–716

Briot K, Tubiana-Hulin M, Bastit L et al (2010) Effect of a switch of aromatase inhibitors on musculoskeletal symptoms in postmenopausal women with hormone-receptor-positive breast cancer: the ATOLL (articular tolerance of letrozole) study. Breast Cancer Res Treat 120:127–134

Carey TS, Evans A, Hadler N et al (1995) Care-seeking among individuals with chronic low back pain. Spine 20:312–317

Chlebowski RT, Cirillo DJ, Eaton CB et al (2013) Estrogen alone and joint symptoms in the women's health initiative randomized trial. Menopause 20:600–608

Claassen H, Schluter M, Schunke M et al (2006) Influence of 17beta-estradiol and insulin on type II collagen and protein synthesis of articular chondrocytes. Bone 39:310–317

Coombes RC, Hall E, Gibson LJ et al (2004) A randomized trial of exemestane after two to three years of tamoxifen therapy in postmenopausal women with primary breast cancer. N Engl J Med 350:1081–1092

Crew KD, Greenlee H, Capodice J et al (2007) Prevalence of joint symptoms in postmenopausal women taking aromatase inhibitors for early-stage breast cancer. J Clin Oncol 25:3877–3883

Crew KD, Capodice J, Greenlee H et al (2010) Randomized, blinded, sham-controlled trial of acupuncture for the management of aromatase inhibitor-associated joint symptoms in women with early stage breast cancer. J Clin Oncol 28:1154–1160

Cuzick J, Sestak I, Cella D et al (2008) Treatment-emergent endocrine symptoms and the risk of breast cancer recurrence: a retrospective analysis of the ATAC trial. Lancet Oncol 9:1143–1148

Dayani N, Corvol MT, Robel P et al (1988) Estrogen receptors in cultured rabbit articular chondrocytes: influence of age. J Steroid Biochem 31:351–356

DeSantis C, Ma J, Bryan L et al (2014) Breast cancer statistics, 2013. CA Cancer J Clin 64:52–62

Dizdar O, Ozcakar L, Malas FU et al (2009) Sonographic and electrodiagnostic evaluations in patients with aromatase inhibitor-related arthralgia. J Clin Oncol 27:4955–4960

Dougherty RH, Rohrer JL, Hayden D et al (2005) Effect of aromatase inhibition on lipids and inflammatory markers of cardiovascular disease in elderly men with low testosterone levels. Clin Endocrinol (Oxf) 62:228–235

Galantino ML, Callens ML, Cardena GJ et al (2013) Tai chi for well-being of breast cancer survivors with aromatase inhibitor-associated arthralgias: a feasibility study. Altern Ther Health Med 19:38–44

Garcia-Giralt N, Rodriguez-Sanz M, Prieto-Alhambra D et al (2013) Genetic determinants of aromatase inhibitor-related arthralgia: the B-ABLE cohort study. Breast Cancer Res Treat 140:385–395

Goss PE, Ingle JN, Martino S et al (2003) A randomized trial of letrozole in postmenopausal women after five years of tamoxifen therapy for early-stage breast cancer. N Engl J Med 349:1793–1802 [see comment]

Goss PE, Ingle JN, Martino S et al (2005) Randomized trial of letrozole following tamoxifen as extended adjuvant therapy in receptor-positive breast cancer: updated findings from NCIC CTG MA.17. J Natl Cancer Inst 97:1262–1271

Greenlee H, Crew KD, Shao T et al (2013) Phase II study of glucosamine with chondroitin on aromatase inhibitor-associated joint symptoms in women with breast cancer. Support Care Cancer 21:1077–1087

Guerne PA, Carson DA, Lotz M (1990) IL-6 production by human articular chondrocytes. Modulation of its synthesis by cytokines, growth factors, and hormones in vitro. J Immunol 144:499–505

Hadji P, Kieback DG, Tams J et al (2012) Correlation of treatment-emergent adverse events and clinical response to endocrine therapy in early breast cancer: a retrospective analysis of the German cohort of TEAM. Ann Oncol 23:2566–2572

Hadji P, Jackisch C, Bolten W et al (2014) COMPliance and arthralgia in clinical therapy: the COMPACT trial, assessing the incidence of arthralgia, and compliance within the first year of adjuvant anastrozole therapy. Ann Oncol 25:372–377

Harputluoglu H, Dizdar O, Malas U et al (2008) Aromatase inhibitor-associated arthralgia: prevalence, clinical and serum parameters among Turkish postmenopausal breast cancer patients. ASCO Annual Meeting. J Clin Oncol (May 20 supplement)

Henry NL, Giles JT, Ang D et al (2008) Prospective characterization of musculoskeletal symptoms in early stage breast cancer patients treated with aromatase inhibitors. Breast Cancer Res Treat 111:365–372

Henry NL, Banerjee M, Wicha M et al (2011) Pilot study of duloxetine for treatment of aromatase inhibitor-associated musculoskeletal symptoms. Cancer 117:5469–5475

Henry NL, Azzouz F, Desta Z et al (2012) Predictors of aromatase inhibitor discontinuation as a result of treatment-emergent symptoms in early-stage breast cancer. J Clin Oncol 30:936–942

Henry NL, Conlon A, Kidwell KM et al (2014) Effect of estrogen depletion on pain sensitivity in aromatase inhibitor-treated women with early-stage breast cancer. J Pain 15:468–475

Hershman D, Unger J, Crew K et al (2014) Omega-3 fatty acids for aromatase inhibitor–induced musculoskeletal symptoms in women with early-stage breast cancer (SWOG S0927)

Howell A, Cuzick J, Baum M et al (2005) Results of the ATAC (Arimidex, Tamoxifen, Alone or in Combination) trial after completion of 5 years' adjuvant treatment for breast cancer. Lancet 365:60–62

Irwin M, Cartmel B, Gross C et al (2013) Effect of exercise vs. usual care on aromatase inhibitor-associated arthralgias in women with early stage breast cancer: the hormones and physical exercise (HOPE) Study. SABCS

Kewman DG, Vaishampayan N, Zald D et al (1991) Cognitive impairment in musculoskeletal pain patients. Int J Psychiatry Med 21:253–262

Khan QJ, Reddy PS, Kimler BF et al (2010) Effect of vitamin D supplementation on serum 25-hydroxy vitamin D levels, joint pain, and fatigue in women starting adjuvant letrozole treatment for breast cancer. Breast Cancer Res Treat 119(1):111–118

Khan Q, Kimler B, Reddy P et al (2012) Randomized trial of vitamin D3 to prevent worsening of musculoskeletal symptoms and fatigue in women with breast cancer starting adjuvant letrozole: the VITAL trial. J Clin Oncol 30(suppl; abstr 9000)

Kubo M, Onishi H, Kuroki S et al (2012) Short-term and low-dose prednisolone administration reduces aromatase inhibitor-induced arthralgia in patients with breast cancer. Anticancer Res 32:2331–2336

Laroche M, Borg S, Lassoued S et al (2007) Joint pain with aromatase inhibitors: abnormal frequency of Sjogren's syndrome. J Rheumatol 34:2259–2263

Laroche F, Coste J, Medkour T et al (2014) Classification of and risk factors for estrogen deprivation pain syndromes related to aromatase inhibitor treatments in women with breast cancer: a prospective multicenter cohort study. J Pain 15:293–303

Lintermans A, Van Calster B, Van Hoydonck M et al (2011) Aromatase inhibitor-induced loss of grip strength is body mass index dependent: hypothesis-generating findings for its pathogenesis. Ann Oncol 22:1763–1769

Mao JJ, Su HI, Feng R et al (2011) Association of functional polymorphisms in CYP19A1 with aromatase inhibitor associated arthralgia in breast cancer survivors. Breast Cancer Res 13:R8

Mao JJ, Xie SX, Farrar JT et al (2014) A randomised trial of electro-acupuncture for arthralgia related to aromatase inhibitor use. Eur J Cancer 50:267–276

Mieog JS, Morden JP, Bliss JM et al (2012) Carpal tunnel syndrome and musculoskeletal symptoms in postmenopausal women with early breast cancer treated with exemestane or tamoxifen after 2-3 years of tamoxifen: a retrospective analysis of the intergroup exemestane study. Lancet Oncol 13:420–432

Morales L, Pans S, Verschueren K et al (2008) Prospective study to assess short-term intra-articular and tenosynovial changes in the aromatase inhibitor-associated arthralgia syndrome. J Clin Oncol 26:3147–3152

Niravath P (2013) Aromatase inhibitor-induced arthralgia: a review. Ann Oncol 24:1443–1449

Oh B, Kimble B, Costa DS et al (2013) Acupuncture for treatment of arthralgia secondary to aromatase inhibitor therapy in women with early breast cancer: pilot study. Acupunct Med 31:264–271

Richette P, Corvol M, Bardin T (2003) Estrogens, cartilage, and osteoarthritis. Joint Bone Spine 70:257–262

Richmond RS, Carlson CS, Register TC et al (2000) Functional estrogen receptors in adult articular cartilage: estrogen replacement therapy increases chondrocyte synthesis of proteoglycans and insulin-like growth factor binding protein 2. Arthritis Rheum 43:2081–2090

Riggs BL, Melton LJ 3rd (1992) The prevention and treatment of osteoporosis. N Engl J Med 327:620–627 [see comment][erratum appears in N Engl J Med. 1993 Jan 7;328(1):65; author reply 66; PMID: 8416278]

Rosner IA, Manni A, Malemud CJ et al (1982) Estradiol receptors in articular chondrocytes. Biochem Biophys Res Commun 106:1378–1382

Scudds RJ, Mc DRJ (1998) Empirical evidence of the association between the presence of musculoskeletal pain and physical disability in community-dwelling senior citizens. Pain 75:229–235

Sestak I, Cuzick J, Sapunar F et al (2008) Risk factors for joint symptoms in patients enrolled in the ATAC trial: a retrospective, exploratory analysis. Lancet Oncol 9:866–872

Sestak I, Sapunar F, Cuzick J (2009) Aromatase inhibitor-induced carpal tunnel syndrome: results from the ATAC trial. J Clin Oncol 27:4961–4965

Sherwin BB (1996) Hormones, mood, and cognitive functioning in postmenopausal women. Obstet Gynecol 87

Shi Q, Giordano SH, Lu H et al (2013) Anastrozole-associated joint pain and other symptoms in patients with breast cancer. J Pain 14:290–296

Thurlimann B, Keshaviah A, Coates AS et al (2005) A comparison of letrozole and tamoxifen in postmenopausal women with early breast cancer. N Engl J Med 353:2747–2757

Ushiyama T, Inoue K, Nishioka J (1995) Expression of estrogen receptor related protein (p29) and estradiol binding in human arthritic synovium. J Rheumatol 22:421–426

Chapter 8
Symptoms: Lymphedema

Electra D. Paskett

Abstract Lymphedema is one of the main late effects from breast cancer treatment affecting 3–60 % of breast cancer survivors. Primarily occurring in the hand, arm, and/or affected breast, symptoms of lymphedema include swelling, pain, redness, restriction of arm/hand movement, tightness and feelings of fullness. These symptoms not only may limit physical functioning but also negatively affect quality of life, body image, social functioning, and financial status of breast cancer survivors with lymphedema. Unfortunately, there are no standardized methods for prevention, diagnosis, and treatment of breast cancer-related lymphedema. Despite its prevalence and lack of clinical guidelines, lymphedema is one of the most poorly understood, relatively underestimated, and least researched complications of cancer treatment. This chapter reviews the current problem of breast cancer-related lymphedema by investigating prevention and risk reduction strategies, diagnosis, and treatment. In addition, this chapter identifies future research opportunities focusing on prevention and risk reduction strategies, quality of life and physical function, surveillance, patient education, cost, diagnosis, and treatment. Challenges and recommendations for future research in these areas, particularly among underserved populations, are discussed.

Keywords Breast cancer • Lymphedema • Swelling • Symptoms • Risk reduction • Prevention • Diagnosis • Treatment

Introduction

Due to improved treatments and earlier detection of smaller, treatable tumors, there are more breast cancer survivors living longer. Therefore, these women are at increased risk for a multitude of late effects for a long time after diagnosis and treatment. Lymphedema is one such effect of treatment for which women are at risk during their lifetime. Lymphedema may occur in the hand, arm, and/or affected

E.D. Paskett, Ph.D. (✉)
Department of Internal Medicine, The Ohio State University College of Medicine,
Columbus, OH, USA
e-mail: electra.paskett@osumc.edu

© Breast Cancer Research Foundation 2015   101
P.A. Ganz (ed.), *Improving Outcomes for Breast Cancer Survivors*,
Advances in Experimental Medicine and Biology 862,
DOI 10.1007/978-3-319-16366-6_8

breast due to surgery (node dissection, sampling or mastectomy/lumpectomy), chemotherapy and/or radiation (Mortimer 1998; Rockson 2012). Causes are related to the disruption of lymph flow caused by these treatment modalities.

The most known feature of lymphedema is swelling, however, pain, redness, restriction of arm/hand movement, tightness and feelings of fullness are also reported symptoms (Armer and Fu 2005; Ridner et al. 2012). The resulting impact on women who experience these symptoms includes not only limitations in physical functioning, but also quality of life, body image issues, social functioning, and in some cases, employment disruption (McWayne and Heiney 2005; Shigaki et al. 2013; Cormier et al. 2009; Fu et al. 2013; Park et al. 2012). A better understanding of the magnitude and risk factors for lymphedema are needed, as well as better ways to detect lymphedema early and treat it.

Statement of Current Problem

What we know about lymphedema has been garnered from a variety of studies focused on the prevalence of lymphedema and its risk factors. Previous studies have estimated that anywhere from 3–60 % of breast cancer survivors are at risk for lymphedema; however, these estimates vary by type of population studied, type of axillary node dissection, measurements used, and length of follow-up from treatment. For example, among women with sentinel node biopsy, the prevalence is 3–10 %, whereas among women with full axillary node dissection, reports of lymphedema range from 20–60 %. In addition to treatment factors, obesity at diagnosis (Dominick et al. 2013; Ridner et al. 2011; Clark et al. 2005; Ozaslan and Kuru 2004), infection/injury (Clark et al. 2005), older age (Hayes et al. 2008), excessive use of arm/hand, and hand dominance have been found to be potential risk factors (Ridner et al. 2011; Soran et al. 2006; Mak et al. 2008). Disease-related factors also play a role, such as nodal status and tumor factors (Dominick et al. 2013; McLaughlin et al. 2008). Reported risk factors are presented in Table 8.1.

Health care costs, both to the patient and to society, have been less studied. Breast cancer patients diagnosed with lymphedema incur an estimated $22,153

Table 8.1 Risk factors for lymphedema

Treatment factors	Patient factors	Disease-related factors
Sentinel node biopsy	Older age	Worse pathologic nodal status
Axillary lymph node dissection	Obesity and/or high BMI	Worse T stage
Post-operative axillary radiation	History of infection/soft tissue infection (i.e., recurrent cellulitis) in arm/hand	Advanced stages of disease
	Upper extremity injury	
	Excessive use of arm/hand/hand dominance	

more in total healthcare costs (e.g., cancer treatments, outpatient visits unrelated to cancer treatment, complications of lymphedema, physical therapy, etc.) than their counterparts with no diagnosis of breast cancer-related lymphedema (BCRL) (Shih et al. 2009), and women diagnosed with late-stage BCRL had yearly healthcare costs of $3,124.92, whereas early stage-BCRL patients had yearly costs of $636.19 (Stout et al. 2012). Costs are due to mental health care, diagnostic imaging for BCRL and complex, treatment-related visits. Women with lymphedema also report a greater frequency of infections, such as cellulitis, again increasing costs (economic and other types) (Shih et al. 2009).

Disparities in both diagnosis and treatment of lymphedema have also been noted for minority women. In particular, African American women are more likely than White women to have undiagnosed lymphedema, and if they are diagnosed with lymphedema by a physician, they are more likely to receive only bandaging and compression treatments as opposed to complete decongestive therapy (Sayko et al. 2013). No studies have explored the impact of costs of treatment among low-income and under/uninsured women on receiving prompt and proper treatment.

Areas of Current Investigation

Areas of investigation for lymphedema have included prevention/risk reduction strategies, diagnosis, and treatment.

Prevention and Risk Reduction Strategies Prevention has focused on taking what we know causes lymphedema and developing risk reduction strategies. Most importantly, sentinel lymph node dissection (SLND) has now replaced full axillary lymph node dissection (ALND) where possible, reducing the risk of lymphedema. Infection prevention and education about precautionary guidelines (Armer et al. 2013; Paskett et al. 2012; Bernas 2013; Bernas et al. 2010; Erickson et al. 2001; Golshan and Smith 2006; Shah and Vicini 2011; Shah et al. 2012a; Soran et al. 2012; Stout et al. 2013) have not been tested as risk reducing strategies, although risk and prevention messages have been targeted to both providers—in terms of risk and how to reduce it, minimize risk of infection (i.e., draw blood only from untreated side) (Armer et al. 2013; Bernas 2013; Bernas et al. 2010; Shah and Vicini 2011; Soran et al. 2012; Shah et al. 2012b; Cassileth et al. 2013; O'Toole et al. 2013; Rourke et al. 2010; Schwartz 2012; Stout Gergich et al. 2008; Tam et al. 2012; Fu et al. 2012)— and survivors—to recognize early signs, and understand methods of risk reduction (Soran et al. 2012; Schwartz 2012; McLaughlin et al. 2013; Meneses et al. 2007; Sherman and Koelmeyer 2011). More recently, physical activity (Ahmed et al. 2006; Brennan and Miller 1998; Jammallo et al. 2013; Jonsson and Johansson 2009; Katz et al. 2010; McNeely et al. 2010; Schmitz 2010; Schmitz et al. 2009, 2010) and weight reduction have been explored as prevention options with results still pending; however, some studies show no harm with physical activity (Ahmed et al. 2006; Cormie et al. 2013; Courneya et al. 2007). The use of compression garments for air travel is still controversial (Graham 2002; Kilbreath et al. 2010) and has yet to be evaluated.

Diagnosis Uncertainties about diagnostic measures for lymphedema exist because current methods vary greatly in their validity, reliability and acceptability to both women and providers/clinics. Methods studied include: water displacement (Sagen et al. 2009), lymphoscintigraphy (Moshiri et al. 2002; Szuba et al. 2002), high-frequency ultrasound (Adriaenssens et al. 2012), bioimpedance (Cornish et al. 2001; Ward et al. 1992), arm circumference (Deutsch et al. 2008; Chen et al. 2008), and self-report (Czerniec et al. 2010). Each method has strengths and weaknesses; however, the fact that there are so many tools reduces the ability of common estimates of lymphedema to be valid and reliable. A summary of diagnostic methods are presented in Table 8.2. In addition, because there is no commonly accepted measurement tool, the ability of any tool to be used for early detection, when early treatment can eliminate or cure early signs of lymphedema (Deutsch et al. 2008; Stout et al. 2011; Johansson and Branje 2010), is limited. A new area of promise is surveillance where all women at risk are screened, and, if diagnosed with early-stage BCRL, they receive intervention and treatment. Significant cost savings were found using this surveillance model vs. impairment-based care (Stout et al. 2012).

Table 8.2 Benefits and limitations of breast cancer-related lymphedema diagnostic methods

Diagnostic method	Benefits	Limitations
Water displacement	Accurately estimates arm volume	Causes discomfort for patients Cannot be used if there are open sores/wounds on skin Unable to account for changes in volume caused by muscle tissue versus subcutaneous tissue
Arm circumference measurement	Low cost Easily administered Causes minimal discomfort	Larger inter-rater and intra-rater variability in measurements Measurements assume that the limb is cylindrical
Perometry	Provides precise volume measurements Causes minimal discomfort Minimal risk of infection	Positioning some patients for accurate measurements may be difficult Device is not portable
Dual frequency ultrasound	Allows for the measurement of skin thickness, which is correlated with degree of swelling Causes minimal discomfort	Studies regarding its effectiveness as a diagnostic tool are limited
Bioimpedance Spectroscopy	Directly measures extracellular fluid Has a high specificity and sensitivity Is able to detect small changes in extracellular fluid and therefore detect early stage lymphedema Device is portable Causes minimal discomfort	Cost Lower accuracy for later stage lymphedema

Table 8.3 Benefits and limitations of breast cancer-related lymphedema treatment methods

Treatment method	Benefits	Limitations
Complex decongestive therapy	Considered the "gold standard" of treatment for lymphedema Significantly reduces swelling	Study results have shown that it is no more effective than standard compression therapy Issues with patient adherence
Pneumatic compression	Significantly reduces swelling	Issues with patient adherence
Low-level laser therapy	Significantly reduces swelling Increases mobility	Requires patients to make multiple visits for treatment
Surgery	May reduce swelling but study results have been inconsistent	Not effective for women with mild or severe BCRL
Exercise	May increase arm function	Does not reduce swelling
Stem cell transplantation	Improves pain, sensitivity and mobility	Compression sleeve must be worn constantly to be effective
Extra-corporeal shock wave therapy	Improves angiogenesis and reduces inflammation Reduces swelling Reduces skin thickness	Cost prohibitive

Treatment While there is no cure for lymphedema, there are many treatment strategies, some tested and others utilized but with varying efficacy (Park et al. 2012; Sayko et al. 2013; Norman et al. 2009; Cormier et al. 2010; Sierla et al. 2013). The most common treatment regimens are Complete Decongestive Therapy (CDT) (including bandaging, compression garments, and manual lymphatic drainage), pneumatic compression, low-level laser therapy (LLLT), and surgery. Newer treatments include exercise, stem cell transplant, and shock wave therapy. Recent studies have shown that guided, gradual exercise may increase arm function (Cormie et al. 2013); however, the impact of exercise on the prevention and/or reduction of swelling needs to be further investigated. Evidence from randomized controlled trials (RCTs) shows conflicting evidence on the efficacy of CDT on both arm volume/function and quality of life (King et al. 2012; Badger et al. 2000; Dayes et al. 2013; Huang et al. 2013; Vignes et al. 2013). Pneumatic compression used at home has only been tested in one study and was found to significantly reduce arm volume (Fife et al. 2012). LLLT shows some promise, but no RCTs have been conducted for surgery as a treatment modality. For the newer treatments, only extra-corporeal shock wave therapy has demonstrated promise but it has only been tested in one small study (Bae and Kim 2013). Thus, treatment modalities for lymphedema are woefully understudied. A summary of treatment methods are presented in Table 8.3.

Future Research Opportunities and Challenges

There are many research opportunities to address the many un- and under-studied areas related to prevention (and causation), diagnosis, treatment, surveillance and education. Overall, the current literature in all of these areas is limited by small sample sizes, lack of comparison groups, and short follow-up times. In addition, quality of life and costs, as well as swelling and functioning, need to be included as outcomes within each of these areas.

Prevention and Risk Reduction Strategies While common risk factors for lymphedema, such as ALND, infection and obesity, have emerged, an improved understanding of how these risk factors interact, particularly in underserved populations (e.g., racial/ethnic minorities, urban/rural residents, the elderly, the poor, and persons with disabilities), is desperately needed (Dominick et al. 2013; Meeske et al. 2009; DiSipio et al. 2010). There is a paucity of information about disparities in lymphedema risk and incidence, as well as treatment characteristics, among underserved populations, but it is certainly plausible that lymphedema disparities mirror the trend generally observed in health and health care (i.e., higher incidence and mortality). For example, African Americans have a higher rate of obesity compared to their white counterparts (Ogden et al. 2012), and BMI is a known risk factor for lymphedema. Minority women, particularly African Americans and Hispanics, are also more likely to present with later stage disease and larger tumors (Dehal et al. 2013; American Cancer Society 2013), increasing the likelihood of undergoing ALND (Arrington et al. 2013), which increases the risk for lymphedema.

Another underserved population includes those living in non-urban areas, who have increased odds of undergoing ALND (OR for rural area=2.06), with non-urban areas lagging 2 years behind urban areas with respect to the use of SLND (Arrington et al. 2013). Not only do those living in non-urban areas undergo ALND more often, they also have limited access to trained lymphedema specialists, who are primarily located in urban centers.

There are very few prevention strategies being tested, thus this area is ripe for further investigation (Armer et al. 2011, 2013; Shah et al. 2012a; Soran et al. 2012; Stout et al. 2013; O'Toole et al. 2013; Fu et al. 2012). What makes prevention studies difficult to conduct, however, is the need for long-term follow-up of women which can be difficult and costly. Future interventions should explore the extent to which compression garments should be worn during exercise, the timing of exercise after curative treatment, the varying usefulness of exercise across the clinical progression of BCRL, and the type of safety monitoring needed during exercise among this population (Tam et al. 2012). To incorporate exercise rehabilitation into cancer survivorship care, there is a need to inform both practitioners and patients of the risks and benefits associated with exercise (including strength training), and to provide healthcare providers with streamlined resources to promote the integration of physical rehabilitation into the supportive care paradigm (Meneses et al. 2007). Another unstudied research topic is whether losing weight after breast cancer treatment reduces BCRL risk. If so, post treatment weight loss could be a risk reduction strategy for survivors.

Clinical Practice Strategies for Risk Reduction There are two areas where clinical practice can be impacted regarding BCRL risk reduction—the provider and the patient. Providers frequently counsel patients regarding BCRL risk based on the presence of previously reported risk factors like injury, infection, BMI, age, and surgery. However, recommendations based solely on these factors are unreliable, as evidenced by the multiple studies presenting conflicting data. This suggests that an individualization of risk reduction strategies is needed. Barriers to this approach include lack of time and provider training to discuss individualized risk factors and strategies with patients. Best practice guidelines need to be updated to include baseline measurements prior to treatment, and continued routine measurements should be part of routine survivorship care.

Women need to be educated about lymphedema, risk factors and self-care guidelines. The most frequent action women reported for management of symptoms for BCRL was no action because they did not know what to do (lack of knowledge of helpful methods). Until the last few years, women remained hospitalized for several days following surgical treatment for breast cancer, and in-hospital care focused on regaining arm function. Now, hospital stays are brief (1, maybe 2 days), and the window of opportunity to introduce lymphedema prevention is gone. Studies as to how best to inform women about these risks and practices, and when to inform women about the risk for lymphedema (e.g., at diagnosis or at every follow-up visit) are needed. Integrating lymphedema prevention education into routine follow-up care alongside regular oncology appointments may improve knowledge and awareness of the condition. Training health care providers to provide lymphedema prevention education involves minimal resource investment and may result in reduced incidence and severity of lymphedema over time.

Diagnosis Diagnosis of BCRL represents a significant hurdle to understanding and managing poor outcomes among breast cancer survivors. First, standardization of diagnostic methods is needed, as well as consensus for measurement and diagnostic criteria. Selected method(s) must not be cost prohibitive to providers or patients and should provide improved estimates of the incidence and prevalence of lymphedema, as well as ways to identify women who are at increased risk of developing BCRL. Secondly, developing standardized measurements and surveillance guidelines for BCRL in patients may lead to earlier detection. Standardization of diagnostic criteria will allow for direct comparison of prevention/treatment interventions. Thus, there is a need for comparative effectiveness research to determine the most accurate and cost-efficient diagnostic method or combination of methods.

Treatment The issues with treatment for lymphedema are many—which treatments work best, when, and delivered by whom? Little research has been conducted, except for evaluating CDT, thus the field is wide open. Future studies should include many outcomes, such as reduction of limb swelling, quality of life, cost and function. Once successful treatments are identified, the timing of treatment initiation and continuation needs to be examined. Lastly, various models of care delivery should be explored so that all women, regardless of socioeconomic status and insurance coverage, can receive treatment. This implies dissemination of best practices, as well as training for lymphedema providers to provide the best comprehensive care.

Future Directions

Future directions for research in lymphedema should focus in several areas.

Prevention and Risk Reduction Strategies While few areas have demonstrated reduction in the risk of lymphedema (e.g., sentinel node biopsy), there are many opportunities to: (1) test the dissemination of risk reduction strategies into clinical practice (e.g., infection prevention, awareness/education); and (2) find new promising risk reduction strategies (e.g., weight reduction, physical activity, prophylactic compression garments). Ways to financially cover effective strategies for lymphedema prevention also need to be implemented.

Quality of Life and Physical Function Many studies have identified the negative effects of lymphedema on quality of life, physical function and body image. No studies have solely addressed these endpoints in studies, i.e., among women with lymphedema. This area is important to investigate and test interventions which, once effective, should be disseminated in clinical practice.

Surveillance Model The prospective surveillance of BCRL had been increasingly advocated for breast cancer patients. In 2012, the National Lymphedema Network encouraged regular BCRL screening as a method to detect and subsequently treat BCRL at an early, or even subclinical stage, to reverse the progression of BCRL to a chronic, irreversible condition. However, this model of early identification has yet to be fully evaluated for its application, cost, and efficacy. Although initial studies are promising, more research is needed to fully investigate the feasibility, applicability, and outcomes of a BCRL early surveillance program (Stout et al. 2012; Armer et al. 2013).

Patient Education The importance of educating breast cancer patients about their risk of BCRL is paramount. There is also a need for future studies to rigorously evaluate the timing, method, and content of disseminating BCRL educational information. An area that should be considered is the post-operative model of care where patients can be informed about lymphedema, the risk factors of lymphedema, and self-care from healthcare professionals. Limited research has been done on interventions to increase patient knowledge of lymphedema. One promising study, conducted by the Cancer and Leukemia Group B (CALGB), is currently testing the efficacy of a comprehensive program of tailored exercise, patient education, and counseling versus patient education only in reducing the incidence of BCRL in women with stage I–III breast cancer who are undergoing ALND. Additional rigorous studies are needed to help increase patient knowledge about their risk factors, particularly modifiable risk factors, promote behaviors that reduce BCRL risk, and improve the quality of life for breast cancer survivors.

Diagnosis Given that there is no consistent, accepted definition for lymphedema, one needs to be developed and accepted by the medical community, and disseminated and implemented across all relevant specialty clinics. A comparison of the effectiveness and costs associated with different diagnostic methods also needs to be developed. This aim follows the surveillance and education piece as these prompt the need for early detection. In addition, ways of assuring coverage of the costs of diagnostic tests for lymphedema can only come from validated diagnostic modalities.

Treatment New treatments need to be developed, perhaps looking to animal models for direction. Treatment effectiveness in the presence of comorbidities, particularly among elderly, minority, and underserved survivors, needs to be explored. Along with examining treatment efficacy in different population groups, personalized care based on patient and disease characteristics needs to become standard of care. An examination of these areas would also allow for the assessment of the cost-effectiveness of treatments. Lastly, there would need to be expansion of workforce capacity to provide the needed lymphedema treatment.

These areas represent a spectrum along the cancer control continuum from prevention and early detection to diagnosis and treatment. This comprehensive approach is needed as prevention and early detection (through surveillance) are the only ways to assure quality treatment and outcomes (e.g., lymphedema, quality of life, function, cost) for all breast cancer survivors.

References

Adriaenssens N, Belsack D, Buyl R et al (2012) Ultrasound elastography as an objective diagnostic measurement tool for lymphoedema of the treated breast in breast cancer patients following breast conserving surgery and radiotherapy. Radiol Oncol 46:284–295

Ahmed RL, Thomas W, Yee D, Schmitz KH (2006) Randomized controlled trial of weight training and lymphedema in breast cancer survivors. J Clin Oncol 24:2765–2772

American Cancer Society (2013) Breast cancer facts & figures 2013–2014. American Cancer Society, Atlanta, GA

Armer J, Fu MR (2005) Age differences in post-breast cancer lymphedema signs and symptoms. Cancer Nurs 28:200–207

Armer JM, Brooks CW, Stewart BR (2011) Limitations of self-care in reducing the risk of lymphedema: supportive-educative systems. Nurs Sci Q 24:57–63

Armer J, Hulett J, Bernas M, Ostby P, Stewart BR, Cormier JN (2013) Best-practice guidelines in assessment, risk reduction, management, and surveillance for post-breast cancer lymphedema. Curr Breast Cancer Rep 5:134–144

Arrington AK, Kruper L, Vito C, Yim J, Kim J, Chen SL (2013) Rural and urban disparities in the evolution of sentinel lymph node utilization in breast cancer. Am J Surg 206:674–681

Badger CM, Peacock JL, Mortimer PS (2000) A randomized, controlled, parallel-group clinical trial comparing multilayer bandaging followed by hosiery versus hosiery alone in the treatment of patients with lymphedema of the limb. Cancer 88:2832–2837

Bae H, Kim HJ (2013) Clinical outcomes of extracorporeal shock wave therapy in patients with secondary lymphedema: a pilot study. Ann Rehabil Med 37:229–234

Bernas M (2013) Assessment and risk reduction in lymphedema. Semin Oncol Nurs 29:12–19

Bernas M, Askew RL, Armer J, Cormier JN (2010) Lymphedema: how do we diagnose and reduce the risk of this dreaded complication of breast cancer treatment? Curr Breast Cancer Rep 2:53–58

Cassileth BR, Van Zee KJ, Yeung KS et al (2013) Acupuncture in the treatment of upper-limb lymphedema: results of a pilot study. Cancer 119:2455–2461

Chen YW, Tsai HJ, Hung HC, Tsauo JY (2008) Reliability study of measurements for lymphedema in breast cancer patients. Am J Phys Med Rehabil 87:33–38

Clark B, Sitzia J, Harlow W (2005) Incidence and risk of arm oedema following treatment for breast cancer: a three-year follow-up study. QJM 98:343–348

Cormie P, Galvao DA, Spry N, Newton RU (2013) Neither heavy nor light load resistance exercise acutely exacerbates lymphedema in breast cancer survivor. Integr Cancer Ther 12:423–432

Cormier JN, Xing Y, Zaniletti I, Askew RL, Stewart BR, Armer JM (2009) Minimal limb volume change has a significant impact on breast cancer survivors. Lymphology 42:161–175

Cormier JN, Askew RL, Mungovan KS, Xing Y, Ross MI, Armer JM (2010) Lymphedema beyond breast cancer: a systematic review and meta-analysis of cancer-related secondary lymphedema. Cancer 116:5138–5149

Cornish BH, Chapman M, Hirst C et al (2001) Early diagnosis of lymphedema using multiple frequency bioimpedance. Lymphology 34:2–11

Courneya KS, Segal RJ, Mackey JR et al (2007) Effects of aerobic and resistance exercise in breast cancer patients receiving adjuvant chemotherapy: a multicenter randomized controlled trial. J Clin Oncol 25:4396–4404

Czerniec SA, Ward LC, Refshauge KM et al (2010) Assessment of breast cancer-related arm lymphedema–comparison of physical measurement methods and self-report. Cancer Invest 28:54–62

Dayes IS, Whelan TJ, Julian JA et al (2013) Randomized trial of decongestive lymphatic therapy for the treatment of lymphedema in women with breast cancer. J Clin Oncol 31:3758–3763

Dehal A, Abbas A, Johna S (2013) Racial disparities in clinical presentation, surgical treatment and in-hospital outcomes of women with breast cancer: analysis of nationwide inpatient sample database. Breast Cancer Res Treat 139:561–569

Deutsch M, Land S, Begovic M, Sharif S (2008) The incidence of arm edema in women with breast cancer randomized on the national surgical adjuvant breast and bowel project study B-04 to radical mastectomy versus total mastectomy and radiotherapy versus total mastectomy alone. Int J Radiat Oncol Biol Phys 70:1020–1024

DiSipio T, Hayes SC, Newman B, Aitken J, Janda M (2010) Does quality of life among breast cancer survivors one year after diagnosis differ depending on urban and non-urban residence? A comparative study. Health Qual Life Outcomes 8:3

Dominick SA, Madlensky L, Natarajan L, Pierce JP (2013) Risk factors associated with breast cancer-related lymphedema in the WHEL Study. J Cancer Surviv 7:115–123

Erickson VS, Pearson ML, Ganz PA, Adams J, Kahn KL (2001) Arm edema in breast cancer patients. J Natl Cancer Inst 93:96–111

Fife CE, Davey S, Maus EA, Guilliod R, Mayrovitz HN (2012) A randomized controlled trial comparing two types of pneumatic compression for breast cancer-related lymphedema treatment in the home. Support Care Cancer 20:3279–3286

Fu MR, Ryan JC, Cleeland CM (2012) Lymphedema knowledge and practice patterns among oncology nurse navigators. J Oncol Navig Surviv 3(4):9–15

Fu MR, Ridner SH, Hu SH, Stewart BR, Cormier JN, Armer JM (2013) Psychosocial impact of lymphedema: a systematic review of literature from 2004 to 2011. Psychooncology 22:1466–1484

Golshan M, Smith B (2006) Prevention and management of arm lymphedema in the patient with breast cancer. J Support Oncol 4:381–386

Graham PH (2002) Compression prophylaxis may increase the potential for flight-associated lymphedema after breast cancer treatment. Breast 11(1):66–71

Hayes SC, Janda M, Cornish B, Battistuatta D, Newman B (2008) Lymphedema after breast cancer: incidence, risk factors, and effect on upper body function. J Clin Oncol 26(21):3536–3542

Huang TW, Tseng SH, Lin CC et al (2013) Effects of manual lymphatic drainage on breast cancer-related lymphedema: a systematic review and meta-analysis of randomized controlled trials. World J Surg Oncol 11:15

Jammallo LS, Miller CL, Singer M (2013) Impact of body mass index and weight fluctuation on lymphedema risk in patients treated for breast cancer. Breast Cancer Res Treat 142:59–67

Johansson K, Branje E (2010) Arm lymphoedema in a cohort of breast cancer survivors 10 years after diagnosis. Acta Oncol 49:166–173

Jonsson C, Johansson K (2009) Pole walking for patients with breast cancer-related arm lymphedema. Physiother Theory Pract 25:165–173

Katz E, Dugan NL, Cohn JC, Chu C, Smith RG, Schmitz KH (2010) Weight lifting in patients with lower-extremity lymphedema secondary to cancer: a pilot and feasibility study. Arch Phys Med Rehabil 91:1070–1076

Kilbreath SL, Ward LC, Lane K, McNeely M, Dylke ES et al (2010) Effect of air travel on lymphedema risk in women with history of breast cancer. Breast Cancer Res Treat 120:649–654

King M, Deveaux A, White H, Rayson D (2012) Compression garments versus compression bandaging in decongestive lymphatic therapy for breast cancer-related lymphedema: a randomized controlled trial. Support Care Cancer 20:1031–1036

Mak SS, Yeo W, Lee YM et al (2008) Predictors of lymphedema in patients with breast cancer undergoing axillary lymph node dissection in Hong Kong. Nurs Res 57:416–425

McLaughlin SA, Wright MJ, Morris KT et al (2008) Prevalence of lymphedema in women with breast cancer 5 years after sentinel lymph node biopsy or axillary dissection: objective measurements. J Clin Oncol 26:5213–5219

McLaughlin SA, Bagaria S, Gibson T et al (2013) Trends in risk reduction practices for the prevention of lymphedema in the first 12 months after breast cancer surgery. J Am Coll Surg 216:380–389

McNeely ML, Campbell K, Ospina M (2010) Exercise interventions for upper-limb dysfunction due to breast cancer treatment. Cochrane Database Syst Rev 6, CD005211

McWayne J, Heiney SP (2005) Psychologic and social sequelae of secondary lymphedema: a review. Cancer 104:457–466

Meeske KA, Sullivan-Halley J, Smith AW (2009) Risk factors for arm lymphedema following breast cancer diagnosis in black women and white women. Breast Cancer Res Treat 113:383–391

Meneses KD, McNees P, Loerzel VW, Su X, Zhang Y, Hassey LA (2007) Transition from treatment to survivorship: effects of a psychoeducational intervention on quality of life in breast cancer survivors. Oncol Nurs Forum 34:1007–1016

Mortimer PS (1998) The pathophysiology of lymphedema. Cancer 83:2798–2802

Moshiri M, Katz DS, Boris M, Yung E (2002) Using lymphoscintigraphy to evaluate suspected lymphedema of the extremities. AJR Am J Roentgenol 178:405–412

Norman SA, Localio AR, Potashnik SL (2009) Lymphedema in breast cancer survivors: incidence, degree, time course, treatment, and symptoms. J Clin Oncol 27:390–397

Ogden CL, Carroll MD, Kit KB, Flegal KM (2012) Prevalence of obesity in the United States, 2009–2010. NCHS data brief 82:1–8

O'Toole J, Jammallo LS, Skolny MN et al (2013) Lymphedema following treatment for breast cancer: a new approach to an old problem. Crit Rev Oncol Hematol 88:437–446

Ozaslan C, Kuru B (2004) Lymphedema after treatment of breast cancer. Am J Surg 187:69–72

Park JE, Jang HJ, Seo KS (2012) Quality of life, upper extremity function and the effect of lymphedema treatment in breast cancer related lymphedema patients. Ann Rehabil Med 36:240–247

Paskett ED, Dean JA, Oliveri JM, Harrop JP (2012) Cancer-related lymphedema risk factors, diagnosis, treatment, and impact: a review. J Clin Oncol 30:3726–3733

Ridner SH, Dietrich MS, Stewart BR, Armer JM (2011) Body mass index and breast cancer treatment-related lymphedema. Support Care Cancer 19:853–857

Ridner SH, Deng J, Fu MR et al (2012) Symptom burden and infection occurrence among individuals with extremity lymphedema. Lymphology 45:113–123

Rockson SG (2012) Update on the biology and treatment of lymphedema. Curr Treat Options Cardiovasc Med 14:184–192

Rourke LL, Hunt KK, Cormier JN (2010) Breast cancer and lymphedema: a current overview for the healthcare provider. Womens Health 6:399–406

Sagen A, Karesen R, Skaane P, Risberg MA (2009) Validity for the simplified water displacement instrument to measure arm lymphedema as a result of breast cancer surgery. Arch Phys Med Rehabil 90:803–809

Sayko O, Pezzin LE, Yen TW, Nattinger AB (2013) Diagnosis and treatment of lymphedema after breast cancer: a population-based study. PM R 5:915–923

Schmitz KH (2010) Balancing lymphedema risk: exercise versus deconditioning for breast cancer survivors. Exerc Sport Sci Rev 38:17–24

Schmitz KH, Ahmed RL, Troxel A (2009) Weight lifting in women with breast-cancer-related lymphedema. N Engl J Med 361:664–673

Schmitz KH, Ahmed RL, Troxel AB et al (2010) Weight lifting for women at risk for breast cancer-related lymphedema: a randomized trial. JAMA 304:2699–2705

Schwartz AL (2012) Safety, injury prevention, and emergency procedures. In: Irwin ML (ed) ACSM's guide to exercise and cancer survivorship. Human Kinetics, Champaign, IL, p 153–160

Shah C, Vicini FA (2011) Breast cancer-related arm lymphedema: incidence rates, diagnostic techniques, optimal management and risk reduction strategies. Int J Radiat Oncol Biol Phys 81:907–914

Shah C, Arthur D, Riutta J, Whitworth P, Vicini FA (2012a) Breast-cancer related lymphedema: a review of procedure-specific incidence rates, clinical assessment AIDS, treatment paradigms, and risk reduction. Breast J 18:357–361

Shah C, Wilkinson JB, Baschnagel A et al (2012b) Factors associated with the development of breast cancer-related lymphedema after whole-breast irradiation. Int J Radiat Oncol Biol Phys 83:1095–1100

Sherman KA, Koelmeyer L (2011) The role of information sources and objective risk status on lymphedema risk-minimization behaviors in women recently diagnosed with breast cancer. Oncol Nurs Forum 38:E27–E36

Shigaki CL, Madsen R, Wanchai A, Stewart BR, Armer JM (2013) Upper extremity lymphedema: presence and effect on functioning five years after breast cancer treatment. Rehabil Psychol 58:342–349

Shih YC, Xu Y, Cormier JN et al (2009) Incidence, treatment costs, and complications of lymphedema after breast cancer among women of working age: a 2-year follow-up study. J Clin Oncol 27:2007–2014

Sierla R, Lee TS, Black D, Kilbreath SL (2013) Lymphedema following breast cancer: regions affected, severity of symptoms, and benefits of treatment from the patients' perspective. Clin J Oncol Nurs 17:325–331

Soran A, D'Angelo G, Begovic M et al (2006) Breast cancer-related lymphedema – what are the significant predictors and how they affect the severity of lymphedema? Breast J 12:536–543

Soran A, Finegold DN, Brufsky A (2012) Lymphedema prevention and early intervention: a worthy goal. Oncol 26:249, 254, 256

Stout Gergich NL, Pfalzer LA, McGarvey C, Springer B, Gerber LH, Soballe P (2008) Preoperative assessment enables the early diagnosis and successful treatment of lymphedema. Cancer 112:2809–2819

Stout NL, Pfalzer LA, Levy E et al (2011) Segmental limb volume change as a predictor of the onset of lymphedema in women with early breast cancer. PM R 3:1098–1105

Stout NL, Pfalzer LA, Springer B et al (2012) Breast cancer-related lymphedema: comparing direct costs of a prospective surveillance model and a traditional model of care. Phys Ther 92:152–163

Stout NL, Weiss R, Feldman JL et al (2013) A systematic review of care delivery models and economic analyses in lymphedema: health policy impact (2004–2011). Lymphology 46:27–41

Szuba A, Strauss W, Sirsikar SP, Rockson SG (2002) Quantitative radionuclide lymphoscintigraphy predicts outcome of manual lymphatic therapy in breast cancer-related lymphedema of the upper extremity. Nucl Med Commun 23:1171–1175

Tam EK, Shen L, Munneke JR (2012) Clinician awareness and knowledge of breast cancer-related lymphedema in a large, integrated health care delivery setting. Breast Cancer Res Treat 131:1029–1038

Vignes S, Blanchard M, Arrault M, Porcher R (2013) Intensive complete decongestive physiotherapy for cancer-related upper-limb lymphedema: 11 days achieved greater volume reduction than 4. Gynecol Oncol 131:127–130

Ward LC, Bunce IH, Cornish BH, Mirolo BR, Thomas BJ, Jones LC (1992) Multi-frequency bioelectrical impedance augments the diagnosis and management of lymphoedema in postmastectomy patients. Eur J Clin Invest 22:751–754

Chapter 9
Symptoms: Menopause, Infertility, and Sexual Health

Debra L. Barton and Patricia A. Ganz

Abstract By 2022, the number of survivors is expected to grow to nearly 18 million. Therefore, addressing acute and chronic negative sequelae of a cancer diagnosis and its treatments becomes a health imperative. For women with a history of breast cancer, one of the common goals of treatment and prevention of recurrence is to reduce circulating concentrations of estradiol, especially in women with hormone receptor positive breast cancer. Hormone deprivation after a diagnosis of breast cancer impacts physiological targets other than in the breast tissue and can result in unwanted side effects, all of which can negatively impact quality of life and function and cause distress. Symptoms that are most strongly linked by evidence to hormone changes after cancer diagnosis and treatment include hot flashes, night sweats, sleep changes, fatigue, mood changes, and diminishing sexual function, including vaginal atrophy (decreased arousal, dryness and dyspareunia), infertility, decreased desire and negative self-image. Weight gain and resulting body image changes are often concomitants of the abrupt onset of treatment-induced menopause.

The purpose of this chapter is to briefly review what is known about the advent of premature menopause in women treated for breast cancer, menopausal symptoms that are exacerbated by endocrine treatments for breast cancer, and the associated concerns of hot flashes and related menopausal symptoms, sexual health and fertility issues. We will discuss limitations in the current research and propose strategies that address current limitations in order to move the science forward.

Keywords Menopause • Hot flashes • Infertility • Sexual health • Breast neoplasms

D.L. Barton, R.N., Ph.D., A.O.C.N., F.A.A.N. (✉)
Mary Lou Willard French Professor of Nursing, University of Michigan School of Nursing,
Ann Arbor, MI, USA
e-mail: debbartn@med.umich.edu

P.A. Ganz, M.D.
UCLA Schools of Medicine and Public Health, Jonsson Comprehensive
Cancer Center, Los Angeles, CA, USA
e-mail: pganz@mednet.ucla.edu

© Breast Cancer Research Foundation 2015   115
P.A. Ganz (ed.), *Improving Outcomes for Breast Cancer Survivors*,
Advances in Experimental Medicine and Biology 862,
DOI 10.1007/978-3-319-16366-6_9

The Challenge of Symptom Complexity

There are estimated to be over 13 million cancer survivors alive as of January, 2012, more than half of whom are women; 22 % are breast cancer survivors (de Moor et al. 2013). By 2022, the number of survivors is expected to grow to nearly 18 million (Siegel et al. 2012). Therefore, addressing acute and chronic negative sequelae of a cancer diagnosis and its treatments becomes a health imperative.

For women with a history of breast cancer, one of the common goals of treatment and prevention of recurrence is to reduce circulating concentrations of estradiol, especially in women with hormone receptor positive breast cancer. Accomplishment of this goal can result in unwanted side effects, since there are estrogen receptors throughout a woman's body. Hence, hormone deprivation after a diagnosis of breast cancer impacts physiological targets other than in the breast tissue and can result in unwanted side effects.

Symptoms in women with a history of breast cancer that are most strongly linked by evidence to hormone changes after cancer diagnosis and treatment include hot flashes, night sweats, sleep changes, fatigue, mood changes, and diminishing sexual function, including vaginal atrophy (decreased arousal, dryness and dyspareunia), decreased desire and negative self-image (Rogers and Kristjanson 2002; Ganz et al. 1998, 2003; Young-McCaughan 1996; No Authors 2005). Weight gain and resulting body image changes are often concomitants of the abrupt onset of treatment-induced menopause (Goodwin et al. 1999). Many of these symptoms can persist for long periods of time (such as hot flashes and weight gain), and some can become more severe over time (such as vaginal atrophy). Symptoms can co-occur (e.g., sleep disturbance and hot flashes, or depression, pain and fatigue); they can be related to each other and yet have distinct etiologies. Although clearly related to estrogen deprivation, symptoms such as hot flashes, sleep disturbance and decreases in sexual health, more often than not, have multiple causes which are conceptually a combination of physiologic and psychosocial domains. In many cases, the precise cause and risk factors, as well as the natural course over time are not definitively known. These features make symptom management difficult from a clinical perspective and challenging from a research perspective.

The purpose of this chapter is to briefly review what is known about the advent of premature menopause in women treated for breast cancer, menopausal symptoms that are exacerbated by endocrine treatments for breast cancer, and the associated concerns of hot flashes and related menopausal symptoms, sexual health and fertility issues. We will discuss limitations in the current research and propose strategies that address current limitations in order to move the science forward.

Addressing Life Stage

One common consequence of treatment for breast cancer is hormone depletion resulting in premature menopause for women under the mean menopause age of 51 (Gracia and Freeman 2004; Ganz et al. 2003). For women in their third or fourth decade of life, menopause is an early intruder that can be a negative reminder of their cancer experience. The risk of premature menopause related to chemotherapy is greatest in women 40 and older (Murthy and Chamberlain 2012). In one study that evaluated menstrual changes longitudinally during a treatment trial (B-30) for premenopausal women with node positive breast cancer, investigators report the rate of amenorrhea at 24 months in those receiving doxorubicin and cyclophospha- mide followed by docetaxel as 54.7 % in those under 40 years of age, 89.1 % in those 40–50 years and 96.8 % in those over 50 years (Swain et al. 2009; Ganz et al. 2011). The use of cyclophosphamide and tamoxifen, however, significantly increased rates of amenorrhea compared to those receiving only doxorubicin and docetaxel and no tamoxifen (Ganz et al. 2011). Interestingly, in this set of reports from the NSABP B-30 trial, amenorrhea and tamoxifen did not significantly predict symptom severity. Rather, the type of chemotherapy did, with those receiving doxo- rubicin and cyclophosphamide followed by docetaxel having more prolonged symptom severity (Ganz et al. 2011). The reason for this is not clear.

Although menopause is a well-known bridge women cross in life, going through this event a decade or so earlier, than others in one's age group, can cause distress and negatively impact body image. Associated with menopause and hormone with- drawal, due to the fact that there are hormone receptors throughout the body, are skin changes (decreased elasticity and increased dryness), vaginal atrophy, changes in hair consistency, and mood changes, to name a few. In short, women who con- front breast cancer treatment in their premenopausal years can experience a more rapid aging phenomenon due to physiologic changes from cancer treatment.

Depending on the life stage and social circumstances of the premenopausal woman, she may accept these changes gracefully or experience tremendous disrup- tions. Those women who are married, closer to the age of natural menopause, and who have completed their families may be trying to do everything possible to have extended survival. The development of early onset menopause might seem like a small price to pay in this setting. In contrast, the younger women who may have recently married, who now have uncertainty about their fertility when they become transiently amenorrheic after chemotherapy, may have considerable anger about this additional burden of the cancer diagnosis. Paradoxically, post-treatment amen- orrhea has an important survival benefit for women with hormone receptor positive breast cancers (Swain et al. 2010); however, younger women may or may not appre- ciate the value of this therapeutic advantage and, instead, have anger related to their daily symptoms and loss of potential fertility (see discussion later).

Another group of women who are important to consider are those who are post- menopausal at breast cancer diagnosis and who have been on long-term hormone therapy (HT), often started at the perimenopause or natural menopause stage to manage vasomotor symptoms, mood, insomnia, and general well-being, or for what was assumed to be cardiovascular or cognitive benefit. Since we have now learned that the potential harms outweigh the benefits of postmenopausal HT, those women who persisted in this therapy have done so in spite of the medical evidence, and may suffer substantially when HT is withdrawn at the time of the breast cancer diagno- sis. These women may experience vasomotor symptoms from the sudden withdrawal of HT and then this can be exacerbated by the use of aromatase inhibitors, which decrease endogenous levels of estrogen even further. Other psychological and physical effects from the withdrawal of HT include concerns about skin, body image, vaginal dryness (see below), joint aches and pains, which add to the distress associated with the cancer diagnosis. These women may have difficulties adhering to endocrine directed breast cancer treatment, and sometimes resume their HT.

Challenges of Managing Menopausal Symptoms

There are several challenges in managing symptoms related to hormone deprivation such as hot flashes, decreased sexual desire, and difficulties with sexual arousal. One challenge is that there is a dearth of research that describes the physiologic etiology and biologic mechanisms of these types of symptoms. For example, animal models for hot flashes use ovariectomized rats. This is not a sufficient model for either natural menopause or chemotherapy induced menopause. Non-human primates offer more relevant insights, but studies with these animals are lacking and translation to women is still largely untested (Appt and Ethun 2010). While what is known about hot flash physiology is currently based on limited laboratory studies in women (Freedman 2001) and points to estrogen withdrawal resulting in a loss of regulation of the thermoregulatory zone and a rising core body temperature (Freedman 2001), there is a newer hypothesis that proposes an imbalance in parasympathetic/sympathetic activity and this is not fully explored, nor are the nuances of the hypothesis proven (Thurston et al. 2012; Freedman et al. 2011).

Another challenge of managing symptoms related to menopause, including fertility, is that though there is undoubtedly a physiologic etiology (despite it being not clearly described), there are also important psychosocial contributors that add to the symptom burden. Insight from studies done in the general population can help inform hypotheses to test in women with breast cancer. In a cross sectional study of 494 women, investigators evaluated attitudes and menopausal symptoms. Lower levels of education, lack of insurance and more negative relationships with children were associated with more severe menopausal symptoms. Negative attitudes toward menopause were also a factor in greater symptom burden (Yanikkerem et al. 2012). A second study in 182 women with dyspareunia revealed that rather than estrogen concentrations, pain was associated with cognitive, affective and dyadic variables (Kao et al. 2012). In research to date, studies generally address one or the other of these types of etiologies, but rarely examine how biologic and psychosocial factors may be additive or synergistic. Interventions are rarely multi-faceted to address more than one focal cause of a symptom, and when they use multiple intervention strategies, there can be a "kitchen sink" approach rather than a rational development of a complex intervention that addresses specific unique and overlapping etiologic variables. In short, research has been reductionist which has limited the ability to fully understand the phenomenon of interest and approach it with strategies that can move the science forward by leaps instead of the current baby steps.

The information contained in this chapter will include examples and thoughts about how research in symptom management requires an informed, multi-component strategy, and we hope to provide food for thought that will help our fellow researchers develop innovative studies that will advance the science in the area of infertility, menopause and sexual health.

Menopause: More than Estrogen

Defining the menopausal state in research has not been consistent and has focused primarily on physiology since there are wide variations in symptoms related to menopause. Although this inconsistency may not have led to erroneous or misleading information (Phipps et al. 2010), readers of the literature could benefit from standardization of definitions. Clearly defining menopause may be particularly important in studies with populations of women with breast cancer due to the some-times late resumption of menses after treatment. Some interventions may only work at certain stages of the transition, therefore, a clear and accurate definition would facilitate this research. Table 9.1 defines menopause according to the Stages of Reproductive Aging Workshop (STRAW) (Soules et al. 2001) enhanced with additional data regarding broader hormonal changes, behavioral correlates and known predictors to date (Ganz et al. 2011; Soules et al. 2001; Hale and Burger 2009; Freeman et al. 2008; Gracia et al. 2007; Nappi et al. 2010; Buijs et al. 2008; Cohen et al. 2002; Gibbs et al. 2013; Sigmon et al. 2004; Stone et al. 2013). Most of the data are drawn from the general population with a sprinkling of data from the population with breast cancer. Despite that, researchers can derive testable hypotheses from related populations. It is interesting to note that early postmenopause is defined as the period through 4 years after the last menses and late postmenopause begins after 4 years of amenorrhea. Exploring differences in factors between those two postmenopausal periods and how those factors may influence response to various interventions or the severity and frequency of menopause related symptoms, particularly in women post treatment for breast cancer, would be an interesting endeavor.

Physiologic changes in menopause, including chemotherapy-induced, surgical, and natural, primarily focus on the withdrawal and gradual depletion of estradiol (Hale and Burger 2009; Yoo et al. 2013). As the follicles become depleted, anti-mullerian hormone decreases and follicle stimulating hormone concentrations rise resultant from decreases in estradiol (Hunter and Rendall 2007; Harlow et al. 2013). Although estrogens post-menopause are still produced from conversion of dehydroepiandosterone from the adrenal gland, androstenedione in fat cells, and from ovarian androgens (if ovaries are present), the amount of estrogen is vastly and sharply decreased (Hunter and Rendall 2007). Estrogen depletion is directly associated with hot flashes, vaginal atrophy and the loss of fertility; however, specific estrogen concentrations have not been highly correlated with symptom severity (Gracia and Freeman 2004). Less is known about the other sex steroid hormones and their relationship to the symptoms experienced during the post-menopausal state; related hormones in chemotherapy induced menopause have been largely unexplored.

Table 9.1 Definitions, correlates and predictors of reproductive stages

Reproductive stage (STRAW)	Known physiology	Behavioral correlates	Known predictors of menopause transition or behavioral correlates
Reproductive early to late	Normal to elevated FSH Menstrual cycles obtain regularity; later AMH drops	Mood swings, headaches, water retention varies with cycle	History of depression, smoking, lower education, not employed outside the home, copying style
Early menopause transition	Increased FSH, estradiol levels are maintained, AMH and inhibin B decrease, irregular menstrual cycles occur	Hot flashes, night sweats, depression or negative mood increases, irritability, sleep dysregulation	Smoking, tamoxifen
Late menopause transition	Increased FSH, estradiol begins to decline, more irregular menstrual cycles	Hot flashes, night sweats, depression or negative mood increases, irritability, sleep dysregulation	Smoking, physical symptoms during pregnancy, history of premenstrual dysphoric disorder, tamoxifen
Early post menopause (first 4 years after menses cease)	Increased FSH, decreased estradiol, amenorrhea	Hot flashes, night sweats, depression or negative mood increases, irritability, sleep dysregulation, fatigue, vaginal dryness	Age, BMI, chemotherapy, mood/attitude, smoking, BMI, age, tamoxifen, DHEA-S, FSH, anxiety, history of PMS
Late post menopause (after 4 years of amenorrhea)	Increased FSH, increased LH, undetectable inhibin B, decreased estradiol, amenorrhea	Hot flashes, night sweats, depression or negative mood increases, irritability, sleep dysregulation, vaginal atrophy, dyspareunia	Aromatase inhibitors, age, chemotherapy, mood/attitude, anxiety, DHEA-S, FSH, perceived stress, BMI, history of premenstrual dysphoric disorder, tamoxifen

Abbreviations: AMH antimullerian hormone, *FSH* follicle stimulating hormone, *LH* luteinizing hormone

Recent research indicates that, in addition to follicular senescence due to chemotherapy, there may also be stromal degradation as well, leading to decreases in androgens (Barton et al. 2007a, 2012). Evidence for this hypothesis is demonstrated by translational data collected for a study done, by the North Central Cancer Treatment Group, evaluating transdermal testosterone for libido in women with a history of breast or gynecologic cancer. At baseline and after 4 weeks of testosterone use, blood was collected to analyze changes in sex steroid hormone concentrations. At baseline, the mean bioavailable testosterone concentration was 3.18 % (normal range 8–10 %), mean free testosterone was .56 ng/dl (norms 0.3–1.9 ng/dl) with 53 % of the women having free testosterone at 0.3 ng/dl and below (Barton et al. 2007a). A longitudinal study, following 20 premenopausal women through chemotherapy and 6 months beyond. demonstrated that women 40 and over years of age who remained amenorrheic at 6 months after chemotherapy had significantly lower androgen levels (in addition to estrogen) compared to the other women who had resumed menses (Barton et al. 2012). Concentrations of DHEA-S were not different between those who ceased versus continued their menses suggesting that the adrenal function was not impacted. Therefore, chemotherapy induced amenorrhea/menopause may be more like surgical menopause than natural menopause, with broad decreases in sex steroid hormones possibly accounting for the more severe experience of symptoms. This hypothesis needs to be explored further and put into context with the life stage and psychosocial factors surrounding menopause.

Interrelatedness and Co-occurrence of Symptoms

Symptom clusters have become a popular concept in oncology, however, this concept can be misunderstood. One definition of a symptom cluster is a group of two , three or more concurrent symptoms that are related to each other (Miaskowski et al. 2007). This relationship can constitute several different things; there can be some shared mechanisms, correlations in severity, synergistic or additive burden or emotional distress. However, it does not generally mean that all of the symptoms have the same origin and/or can be ameliorated with the same treatment. One example of the potential heterogeneity of symptom clusters is demonstrated by a study from Freedman and Roehrs (2007), who sought to uncover the source of sleep problems in healthy peri and post menopausal women. These investigators found a significant sleep disturbance in 102 women, whose mean age was 50. Overall the women slept only 6½ hours per night. They were awake over an hour sometime during the night and took longer than half an hour to fall asleep. Some elements of their sleep disturbance were due to periodic limb movements and sleep apnea while others were related to mood and hot flash issues. Different etiologies call for different approaches to management, and often, both physiologic and psychosocial variables are contributing to the symptom experience.

Symptom clusters can change throughout the trajectory of the cancer experience and the symptoms within a cluster can vary in severity and prevalence over time

(Kim et al. 2009; Dodd et al. 2005). Therefore, the phenomenon of symptom clusters contributes to the complexity inherent in symptom management research. The complexity of symptom relationships is further exemplified by a study in 69 women with early stage breast cancer. Data were collected at seven points from pre chemotherapy through cycle 4 of chemotherapy. Sleep, menopausal symptoms and depression were evaluated in the context of menopausal status based on self-reported menses, or absence thereof. Overall, women experienced a combination of depressive symptoms, poor sleep and vasomotor symptoms. Though those who became perimenopausal had increased vasomotor symptoms, this symptom was not related to sleep and moreover, in all groups, depressive symptoms did not appear to be related to sleep (Rissling et al. 2011).

Current Research Strategies and Their Limitations

Hot Flashes

There has been limited longitudinal research in hot flashes and related menopausal symptoms in cancer that defines when the most problematic symptoms begin, which women experience hot flashes the longest and what the predictors of response to various treatments are. In one cross sectional internet based survey of women who were diagnosed with breast cancer at 40 years of age or younger, cognitive symptoms were more prevalent than hot flashes. Of 371 women with a mean age of 33, 81 % of the sample reported forgetfulness as a bothersome symptom, 72 % concentration difficulties, 71 % distractability and 46 % reported bothersome hot flashes, using the Breast Cancer Prevention Treatment Checklist to measure symptoms (Leining et al. 2006). In contrast, in an earlier longitudinal European treatment trial where women were randomized to high dose versus conventional chemotherapy (Malinovszky et al. 2006), both groups of women reported increases in night sweats and hot flashes throughout the first year, maintaining high levels of those symptoms throughout the 5 years of follow up. A second longitudinal study followed women on the NSABP B-30 trial for 24 months. Vasomotor symptoms (hot flashes, night sweats and cold sweats) were common in both women who had stopped menses and those who continued menstruating. As early as day 1 of cycle 4 of chemotherapy, 74 % of women reported hot flashes. At 6 months, 85 % of women who were amenorrheic and 89 % of those who were still menstruating, reported vasomotor symptoms. At 12 months, of the women who ceased menses, 90 % reported symptoms and of those who were menstruating, 55 % reported vasomotor symptoms (Swain et al. 2009). Research indicates that hot flashes begin during chemotherapy and increase and continue throughout 2 years of follow up (Barton et al. 2009).

Pharmacologic treatment with estrogen has been a common treatment for healthy women, but that may not be a safe option in women who have a history of breast cancer. During the 1990s, in the period before the results of the Women's Health Initiative hormone trials, bothersome hot flashes were perceived as another trauma of the cancer diagnosis, since women with breast cancer were being denied a therapy that was routinely recommended in healthy mid-life women. Thus, there was a strong sense of urgency to find alternative strategies to manage hot flashes in breast cancer patients and survivors (Loprinzi et al. 2008). Serendipitous findings, and rigorous placebo controlled clinical trials, demonstrated the treatment benefits of serotonin reuptake inhibitor antidepressants and gabapentin for hot flash relief (Loprinzi et al. 2008, 2009; Barton and Loprinzi 2004). Subsequent mechanistic studies related to these agents have been pursued. These agents now have the strongest evidence to date for non-hormonal treatment of hot flashes.

None of these non-hormonal agents, though, have reduced hot flashes beyond about 60 %. Further, pharmacologic treatments are wrought with unwanted side effects or unwanted stigma. Many times women do not want to take an antidepressant and women who have gone through treatment for breast cancer often do not want to take "yet another pill," as taking medication is reminiscent of "being ill". Research has also not provided insight into who does or does not respond to various antidepressant therapies. It is hypothesized that serotonin is the active ingredient in antidepressants for the amelioration of hot flashes but this has not been proven and there is less known about why gabapentin helps hot flashes. One thing that has been clearly proven with the hot flash research is that neither the population (naturally menopausal, chemotherapy induced or surgically induced) nor the hot flash etiology (tamoxifen, aromatase inhibitors, or just menopausal status) has differentially impacted response to the evidence-based treatments to date (Loprinzi et al. 2008; Bardia et al. 2009).

Mind-body, psycho-educational and cognitive-behavioral interventions have also been studied. These intervention modalities are interesting as they represent ways for women to self-manage and also have little in the way of unwanted side effects. Unfortunately, the evidence is mixed with regard to these behaviorally based therapies and are plagued by small sample sizes, poor effect sizes and lack of appropriate control groups. Recent randomized trials have evaluated cognitive behavioral therapy (CBT) for hot flashes, and at least three have been done in women with breast cancer. Most of these interventions have utilized a combination of cognitive and behavioral approaches, most commonly, paced breathing and relaxation, education about menopause, cognitive strategies to address negative thinking or attitudes and catastrophizing, and behaviors to improve sleep and manage stress and anxiety (Ayers et al. 2012; Duijts et al. 2012; Mann et al. 2012; Tremblay et al. 2008; Balabanovic et al. 2012). Many of the studies have used usual care or "no treatment" control groups. In addition, some of the studies used a support group approach to deliver the intervention, while others used one on one time with clinical psychologists and/or social workers. The intervention time was often 90 min for 6 weeks. Most of these studies have demonstrated improvements in the distress and bother related to hot flashes , but not the number or severity of hot flashes themselves (Ayers et al. 2012; Duijts et al. 2012; Mann et al. 2012; Tremblay et al. 2008; Balabanovic et al. 2012). One study, using a cognitive behavioral intervention for hot flashes in women with breast cancer, included a qualitative interview to learn about women's perception of the effect of the intervention on their symptoms

(Balabanovic et al. 2012). Women talked about having a different attitude toward their symptoms, coping better, feeling distracted from their symptoms, and gaining control over their lives. They also talked about the importance of the group support. This study provides some insight into the elements of a cognitive behavioral intervention that may be more important in achieving wanted results. Interestingly, to date, there has been little research done to capitalize upon the potential synergy or additive effect of non-pharmacologic and pharmacologic therapies in such a way as to essentially eliminate side effects while improving effects.

Pharmacologic research for hot flash control has demonstrated a placebo effect of about 25–30 %, but this varies across studies (Loprinzi et al. 2008; Bardia et al. 2009). The mechanism by which the placebo improves hot flashes has not been investigated and would provide insight. It is important, though, to include an appropriate control group when evaluating interventions for hot flashes and related menopausal symptoms. It could be said that there is a placebo effect in much of symptom research, which makes appropriate control groups necessary, even in behavioral research, in order to understand the benefit of the intervention evaluated.

In summary, much of the research in hot flashes has been narrowly focused and has neither addressed menopausal symptoms broadly nor incorporated complementary mechanistic approaches (pharmacologic with behavioral). Research is needed to address relationships between symptoms and respective responses to tailored treatment.

Sexual Health

There is a surprising amount of research in sexual health that encompasses descriptive studies, psychological interventions for overall sexual health and pharmacologic interventions for vaginal symptoms. Much of the research in this area, however, suffers from small sample sizes, small effect sizes and a lack of control groups to account for non-specific effects of group and provider interactions. Most studies focus on three groups of survivors, breast, gynecologic and prostate cancer (Brotto et al. 2010; Taylor et al. 2011). In cancer survivors, sexual health research is largely represented by cross-sectional studies or very small longitudinal research. What is known about sexual health in women with breast cancer is that, in age matched studies, women with breast cancer report worse functioning (Howard-Anderson et al. 2012; Basson 2010; Speer et al. 2005) and that women who have undergone treatment for breast cancer (including surgery, tamoxifen or chemotherapy) report more sexual concerns than those women with breast cancer who have not had these treatments (Gilbert et al. 2010). Women who are younger and those with more advanced disease may experience the most disruption of their sexual health (Andersen et al. 2007). Though sexual health may decline during treatment, there is some improvement gradually when treatment ends, but data do not support that function returns to baseline levels (Krychman and Millheiser 2013). However, it is not known in which individuals function returns to baseline and for whom concerns persist or even increase. The prevalence of sexual health concerns in published data ranges from 30 to 100 % (Speer et al. 2005; Gilbert et al. 2010; Andersen et al. 2007; Burwell et al. 2006; Krychman and Millheiser 2013; Biglia et al. 2010) and generally consists of problems with lubrication, dyspareunia, desire, body image and relationship concerns (Burwell et al. 2006). Like other symptoms, such as fatigue where research is growing to provide new insights, sexual health concerns may be more pervasive, start earlier, and last longer than we currently know.

One source of evidence is a longitudinal study in 35 premenopausal women diagnosed with breast cancer (Biglia et al. 2010). These women reported below normal sexual activity on the McCoy Female Sexual Questionnaire, as early as their first post-surgical visit. Sexual scores decreased further during chemotherapy and even further one year later. Specific areas which were negatively impacted included activity, desire, arousability, quality of partner relationship and body image (Biglia et al. 2010). On the other end of the spectrum of study sizes, a survey study of breast cancer survivors (N = 1,134) had participants complete self-report questionnaires to identify variables that predicted sexual health (Ganz et al. 1999). Predictors of sexual interest included body image and mental health, as well as having a new partner since being diagnosed, and predictors of decreased sexual function included vaginal dryness, past chemotherapy, and having a new partner since being diagnosed (Ganz et al. 1999).

A comprehensive review of the literature between 1998 and 2010 summarizes the breadth and complexity of the issues surrounding sexual health in women after a diagnosis of breast cancer. The list includes sexual function disturbances (arousal, lubrication, orgasm, desire and pleasure), but also lists psychological issues of negative body image, feeling sexually unattractive, loss of femininity, anxiety, depression and changes in one's sense of sexual self (Gilbert et al. 2010). Likewise, a meta-synthesis of 30 qualitative studies, representing 795 women, supports the concepts of "redefining self" in terms of body image and womanhood/femaleness as a pervasive, critical issue in sexual health and functioning in women with breast cancer (Bertero and Chamberlain Wilmoth 2007). Estimates of the prevalence of body image concerns range from 31 to 67 %, and the prevalence of those reporting arousal or interest issues is 46 to 56 %, respectively (Fobair and Spiegel 2009).

Thought provoking results emanate from one European longitudinal study (Malinovszky et al. 2006). Three hundred ninety women randomized to conventional or high dose chemotherapy for high risk, node positive breast cancer completed the sexual activity questionnaire at baseline, after surgery but before treatment, at 6 and 12 months and yearly out to 5 years. Despite the findings that vaginal dryness and dyspareunia occurred during the first year and persisted throughout the 5 years and significantly increased compared to baseline, the numbers of women who engaged in sexual activity and the frequency of sexual activity did not significantly change from 12 months and beyond. Pleasure was also significantly lower at every time point, when compared to baseline. This was not significantly different based on high dose or conventional dose chemotherapy (Malinovszky et al. 2006). Therefore, women in this study were engaging in behavior that was increasingly difficult and unpleasant, suggesting a critical need for research to address this unmet need.

It is important to note that intervention research in sexual health in the general population cannot likely be extrapolated to the cancer population, which is admittedly different than the research on hot flashes. This lesson is demonstrated by the fact that there are 11 positive randomized controlled trials of transdermal testosterone in various non-cancer populations of women for improving libido (Davis et al. 2006, 2008a, b; Goldstat et al. 2003; Shifren et al. 2000, 2006; Simon et al. 2005; Braunstein et al. 2005; Buster et al. 2005; Nathorst-Boos et al. 2006; Chudakov et al. 2007) while the one large study that evaluated transdermal testosterone in female cancer survivors was decidedly negative (Barton et al. 2007b). Interestingly, the lack of benefit was seen despite similar testosterone doses and improvement in testosterone concentrations for the intervention group (Barton et al. 2007b). This may be because women who have chemotherapy induced menopause are hormonally depleted more severely and more broadly than the women on these positive trials. In fact, in one subanalysis, women who had had bilateral oophorectomies did not experience the same benefit in the primary outcome of sexually satisfying events as women who had were naturally postmenopausal (Davis et al. 2008b), thus supporting the idea that the degree to which hormones are depleted makes a difference in outcomes.

Though there are studies that provide evidence of the areas of sexual health that are negatively impacted as a result of the cancer experience, there is little research that teases out specific predictors in subgroups of women longitudinally. There is even less research evaluating comprehensive interventions to address the complexities of sexual health. One early and important study in this area, that was clearly ahead of its time, was (Ganz et al. 2000; Zibecchi et al. 2003) a comprehensive menopausal assessment intervention. The intervention was developed to address three symptoms (hot flashes, vaginal dryness and urinary incontinence). An advanced practice nurse assessed each woman's needs and developed a tailored intervention, including pharmacologic and behavioral interventions for these three main issues. At the time of the study, there were not extremely effective interventions for any of these problems. Despite this, the investigators reported significant improvements in sexual health as measured by the sexual summary scale from the Cancer Rehabilitation Evaluation System (CARES) over the usual care control group. This significant improvement was still present at the 2 month follow up.

There is a fair amount of research on psychological interventions for sexual health (Brotto et al. 2010; Taylor et al. 2011). These studies are designed to deliver the interventions mostly in person, but at least one tested a telephone intervention (Salonen et al. 2009). The content of the psychological interventions included education about managing symptoms and distress related to symptoms and body image changes, behaviors to improve sexual response, communication skills and, where couples were involved, how to cope as a couple (Brotto et al. 2010; Taylor et al. 2011). Physical exercise was also often included (Taylor et al. 2011). Yet, research has not been done to identify and build on the most effective strategies for sexual health, nor has much of this research been appropriately controlled for non-specific, provider or group effects.

For vaginal symptoms, some research has focused on evaluating the lowest dose of estrogen that has the potential to improve symptoms of dryness and dyspareunia without impacting systemic estradiol concentrations (Krychman and Millheiser 2013; Tan et al. 2012; Goldfarb et al. 2013). There has been little research that has taken a systematic approach to addressing the multiple etiologies that contribute to decreases in sexual health. In addition, the research in this area appears disparate, without evidence of an attempt to build on and expand on previous findings. Hence, more research is needed to clarify the etiologies of various aspects of sexual health changes after cancer and intervention research should be individualized to target more than one aspect of this problem.

Fertility Preservation: Practice and Research

Among a substantial number of younger women with breast cancer, the likelihood of infertility after chemotherapy treatment, and/or the delay in potential attempts at pregnancy due to 5 years of tamoxifen therapy is a significant concern (Senkus et al. 2014; Partridge et al. 2004). Young women's attitudes are most influenced by whether or not they have already had children, as well as their desire to have future children. There appears to be considerable variability in the frequency with which physicians discuss fertility issues with premenopausal women before initiating cancer treatments (Duffy et al. 2005; Quinn et al. 2007, 2009). To some extent, this may relate to lack of knowledge by the oncologist, but also the lack of access to reproductive endocrinology specialists to assist in the care of these patients. In addition, there are substantial financial barriers to receiving these medical services, as they may not be covered through health insurance. Embryo storage may also be costly. In addition, women who do not have a partner may not perceive that it is feasible, and methods of storing oocytes or ovarian tissue may not be as successful (Waimey et al. 2013). The American Society of Clinical Oncology has published fertility preservation guidelines emphasizing the importance of these pre-treatment discussions and the offering of fertility preservation services (Loren et al. 2013). Organizations such as LIVESTRONG and the Oncofertility Consortium (http://www.fertilehope.org/tool-bar/referral-guide.cfm; http://oncofertility.northwestern.edu/) can provide some financial and professional assistance for patients who wish to pursue these options, as well as providing extensive educational and resource information.

The technical and logistical aspects of fertility preservation in the setting of breast cancer has become somewhat easier in large institutions where dedicated teams exist to make this happen (Reinecke et al. 2012). This often includes having a nurse or other professional on call to facilitate the pre-treatment counseling with the patient and the prompt referral to the reproductive endocrinology service (Lambertini et al. 2013). Currently, it may take a few weeks to do preoperative evaluation and consultation for breast surgery (especially with reconstructive surgeons and radiation oncologists), and in this time the reproductive endocrinologist can be consulted and ovarian stimulation started so that in some cases oocyte retrieval can coincide with definitive breast cancer surgery or before the initiation of chemotherapy (Westphal and Wapnir 2012; Baynosa et al. 2009).

While historically there has been some concern about the safety of pregnancy after a breast cancer diagnosis, recent studies have not supported adverse outcomes (Azim et al. 2011, 2013; Kroman et al. 2008), and thus younger women should be given the opportunity to pursue this as a future option, by having pre-treatment counseling.

Moving the Science Forward

Using a Theoretical Framework

The use of a theoretical framework to guide research is a helpful tool that provides a lens through which the investigative team can focus their research strategy. Two theories that have been instructive in symptom research include the Theory of Unpleasant Symptoms by Elizabeth Lenz (Lenz et al. 1997) and the Revised Symptom Management Conceptual Model developed by nurse scientists at the University of California San Francisco (Dodd et al. 2001).

Both of these frameworks provide for psychosocial as well as physiologic influences on the symptom experience. Importantly, they also clearly articulate that people experience symptoms in a situation specific context (age, life stage, developmental stage) and bring to the perception of their symptoms their own history of experiences, self-management, and coping strategies. These variables are not trivial and need to be considered when developing studies to improve or prevent unwanted symptoms related to cancer. These theoretical frameworks can assist the investigator in thinking through potential mediators and moderators of a comprehensive intervention and, in this way, can facilitate a more realistic approach to symptom management research.

Comprehensive Interventions

In intervention research, it is common for investigators to define the problem narrowly, target a narrow population, apply a single intervention and measure one main outcome. Further, studies have often been relatively small and been in single institutions. This approach results in effect sizes that are small and the inability to define characteristics of populations that benefit most from the intervention. Important intervention components are generally not identified and long term outcomes are unknown. While comprehensiveness is critical, it is also important that investigators not develop intervention studies that include "everything but the kitchen sink" because they don't know what will and won't impact their desired outcomes.

Intervention research requires clearly-articulated rationale and etiologically-based components that can address more than one factor that contributes to the symptom experience at hand. Examples of implementing this strategy are provided for hot flash related symptoms and sexual health below.

Specific Strategies

Hot Flash Related Symptoms

Research in menopause needs to focus on developing interventions that can address both the physiologic and psychosocial correlates of menopausal symptoms. Hot flashes have been shown to contribute to many other issues such as mood, sleep and fatigue. As such, interventions targeting hot flashes need to measure effects on this symptom cluster to determine what components are helpful in addressing the breadth of the menopausal symptom experience.

One promising mind body therapy is hypnosis. Collaboration with a clinical psychologist and hypnotherapist from Baylor University, Dr. Gary Elkins, has provided the opportunity to build and evaluate multi-component interventions centered on hypnosis for menopausal symptoms of hot flashes, mood, sleep and fatigue. Dr. Elkins has demonstrated the ability for a hypnotic relaxation intervention alone to decrease hot flashes by about 70 %, in post menopausal women (not breast cancer survivors). The study was a randomized controlled trial using an attention control group that received equal interactions in terms of number and time with study personnel. This 70 % reduction is greater than that seen with other non-hormonal approaches. Importantly, hypnosis, if done by an appropriately trained provider in a person without psychotic risk factors, is safe and without side effects (Elkins et al. 2013). In addition, Dr. Elkins' randomized trial demonstrated significant improvements in sleep quality as measured by the Pittsburgh Sleep Quality Index.

Building on Dr. Elkin's success, a study combining venlafaxine (an effective antidepressant for hot flash relief) with hypnosis in a four arm randomized pilot trial was sponsored by National Center for Complementary and Alternative Medicine (NCCAM) and the National Cancer Institute (NCI) (Barton et al. 2013). This pilot study accomplished some important things. First, it confirmed the development of a viable and believable control for hypnosis (a sham hypnosis condition) and second, led to the knowledge that combining venlafaxine with hypnosis was not better than either intervention alone. Another important lesson from this pilot study was that nurses could efficiently be taught to provide hypnosis and the outcomes from the hypnosis intervention alone were similar to venlafaxine alone. Unlike the other mind-body interventions mentioned earlier, such as paced breathing and psycho-educational programs, hypnosis was able to reduce both the actual severity and frequency of hot flashes as well as the bother/distress associated with this symptom. A follow up study is in development that builds on the findings of this pilot study and expands the outcomes of interest.

Sexual Health

The ability to develop interventions that target related areas in sexual health such as partner communication, vaginal atrophy, self-image and desire, would be an important contribution to the science and, more importantly, to women. To date, intervention research has followed a similar strategy to that of hot flashes, evaluating either behavioral interventions for general sexual improvement or pharmacologic agents for targeted problems such as vaginal dryness or libido. It is time to build on the many positive psychological intervention trials and examine what the strongest effects from this type of approach are, and to evaluate what the critical and necessary components are that need to be brought forward into future research.

For example, one fairly large study randomized women who were distressed about intimacy and/or sexuality to receive a group delivered psychoeducational intervention or to receive printed information on sexual health (control group) (Rowland et al. 2009). Initially, 284 women were randomized to receive the intervention, with 83 agreeing and 72 attending at least one of the 6 two-hour sessions. The psychoeducational sessions addressed body image, sexual anatomy, sexual attitudes and behaviors, menopause, communication and incorporated self-directed future goals. The main outcome, the Mental Health Index, which measures emotional variables, was not significantly impacted by the intervention. However, there were some positive effects on marital and sexual satisfaction for the intervention group compared to the control group (Rowland et al. 2009). It is notable that less than half of the women who were eligible and randomized to the intervention agreed to participate. Reasons for declining were mostly due to convenience of sessions and lack of time. It is not clear what elements of this intervention were most closely aligned with the improvement in sexual satisfaction, but future work to identify critical elements and target elements of the intervention to specific sexual health needs could be pursued. Importantly, simplification in the delivery of the intervention to reduce the time commitment and increase the flexibility of how the intervention is received would be needed. There are many options today for how people access information and care, paving the way for true innovation in the delivery of interventions.

Continuing to evaluate pharmacologic interventions where cognitive behavioral interventions would not be sufficient, such as in vaginal atrophy, is also needed. A large multi-site trial in the cooperative group system has recently been completed evaluating vaginal dehydroepiandosterone for symptoms of dryness and dyspareunia. This study included 364 women who reported moderate or greater severity and bother related to either vaginal dryness or dyspareunia (Clinical Trials.gov identifier NCT01376349). Several measures of sexual health were collected at baseline and at 12 weeks to explore mediators and moderators of sexual function and body image. Variables that are being addressed in this study include relationships as measured with the Revised Dyadic Adjustment Scale (Busby et al. 1995), stress as measured with the Perceived Stress Scale (Cohen et al. 1983), mood as measured with the Profile of Mood States (Curran et al. 1995), energy as measured by the vitality subscale of the SF-36 (Ware 2000), and several outcomes that include function, physical and cognitive aspects as measured with the Female Sexual Function

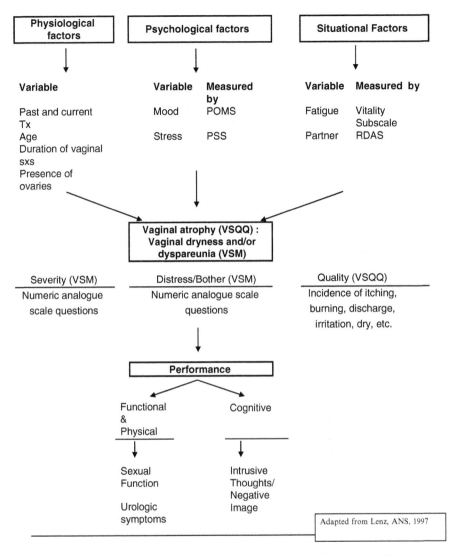

Fig. 9.1 Framework for the development of a complex sexual health intervention. Theory base is the Theory of Unpleasant Symptoms, Lenz, Adv. Nursing Science, 1997

Index (Rosen et al. 2000), Urogenital Atrophy Scale (Lester et al. 2012) and the Impact of Treatment Scale (Frierson et al. 2006). The model guiding this work that is based on Lenz and is depicted above (Fig. 9.1). Current analyses are ongoing to explore relationships between the variables in the model and to identify critical variables that predict body image stress, relationship issues, and sexual function. This information will add to the already published data on predictors and will guide future research.

Fertility Work

To have greater impact on fertility preservation we must focus our efforts on the delivery of high quality cancer care for breast cancer patients and survivors, who have a right to be counseled about the likelihood of infertility associated with breast cancer treatments and to take actions should they wish to do so. In a recent report from the ASCO Quality Oncology Practice Initiative (QOPI) conducted between 2006 and 2010, adherence to the quality measure of discussing infertility risk of chemotherapy and discussing fertility preservation, documentation of these conversations in the medical record was very infrequent and did not improve over several rounds of assessment, suggesting the QOPI practices did not act on their poor performance (Neuss et al. 2013). Ensuring that this is a key element of breast cancer survivorship care, as measured through various accrediting bodies, will be very important.

In addition, to be able to deliver this care prospectively will take investment in the organizational structures within health systems to provide services in a timely fashion. For those women who cannot preserve either embryos or oocytes prior to cancer treatment, it may be possible to address this in the post-treatment period. Thus, addressing these issues, in much the same way as breast reconstruction may be handled—either immediately or delayed—may at least give women who missed the pre-treatment setting an opportunity to engage with reproductive specialists at a later time. All of this will be facilitated if some of the costs of these services could be considered as part of cancer rehabilitation. The absolute numbers of individuals (including men who participate in cryopreservation of sperm) is likely to be very small, and would add little to insurance benefit plans. This will be an important policy issue in the future, especially if demand increases as a result of greater pre-treatment counseling.

Looking into the Future

Key strategies for moving the research forward include the need to (a) individualize interventions, (b) develop a better understanding of who responds to what interventions and why, (c) understand better the breadth and consequences of premature aging based on cancer treatment and (d) better understand the role that prevention can play in preserving fertility, maximizing sexual health and preventing bothersome symptoms related to menopause.

Individualizing Interventions

Building and evaluating multi-component interventions can occur from two directions. They can be built, one at a time, with focused interventions being evaluated in rigorously designed trials; then those demonstrating efficacy, based on a predetermined effect sizes, could be added together. Alternatively, several components can be evaluated together and if effective, steps could be taken to deconstruct the intervention to determine whether there are any unneeded elements. Either way, once a multi-component intervention is determined to be helpful, efforts could be made to individualize the intervention, based on specific issues. For example, in a multi-component intervention being built for sexual health, the intervention can have components (already tested and found effective) to address vaginal atrophy, sexual energy, relationships, partner communication, and self-image. The specific intervention for a particular woman, however, would be built from the menu based on relevant concerns, so that the intervention can be tailored accordingly.

Predicting Response

The ability to understand characteristics of people who respond to an intervention or parts of an intervention is critical in order to both individualize the intervention but also to allow others to build on, and apply, the research to other similar populations. In order to do this effectively, studies would likely need to be large, with sample sizes over 100, requiring multi-site networks. If studies in symptom management insist on being powered to only detect large effect sizes and evaluate only one focused intervention on one narrowly defined outcome, it will not be possible to either build effective multi-component interventions or do sub group analyses, as it is unlikely that one single intervention will be strong enough to sufficiently impact a symptom that has multiple etiologies and is highly influenced by personal characteristics. The reductionist strategy is likely the reason for the many negative trials in symptom management.

In the research on hypnosis for hot flashes, investigators are evaluating moderators such as hypnotizability and expectancy to understand their influence on the ability of the intervention to impact the outcomes. In the trial evaluating vaginal DHEA for dyspareunia and/or dryness, the study design controls for the effect of the strength of the relationship with the significant other as measured with the Relationship Dyadic Adjustment Scale to see whether that variable "trumps" the ability of the intervention to impact sexual health (Clinical Trials.gov identifier NCT01376349). These types of explorations are important if we are to advance the science in symptom management in a meaningful way.

Understanding Premature Aging

Although cancer treatments, in particular chemotherapy and radiation, may accelerate the aging process (see especially young adults with cancer), and lead to serious organ damage that my influence comorbid conditions and competing causes of death, relatively little is known about premature ovarian failure in this setting. Studies done by investigators with regard to surgical oophorectomy have shown deleterious health outcomes in such women (Rocca et al. 2006; Shuster et al. 2010). To what extent there may be parallel adverse effects in younger women who become prematurely menopausal with breast cancer treatments is uncertain. Currently, the NSABP B-47 trial that is focused on use of trastuzumab or not in the adjuvant setting of women with HER2 low expressing tumors has an embedded host factor study that is looking at the incidence and prevalence of comorbid conditions, as well as amenorrhea, in the prospective monitoring of outcomes, and this study should provide some insight into the added burden that premature ovarian failure may play in subsequent survivorship outcomes (see ClinicalTrials.gov NCT01275677).

The Role of Prevention

Reducing the untoward effects of cancer treatment on the reproductive health of breast cancer survivors is the ultimate goal. Two possible prime strategies are to (1) prevent the overtreatment of women who are not in need of gonadotoxic therapy with genomic or other prognostic tools, and (2) tailor therapy to meet the preferences of women who may wish to preserve fertility. For example, in the NSABP B-30 trial, investigators found that the patients in the treatment arm that did not have cyclophosphamide had a much lower rate of post-treatment amenorrhea, compared to the two treatment arms that contained this therapy. The differences in disease-free survival outcomes between the treatment arms were very small, and thus this alternative treatment should be discussed with patients who wish to reduce their risk for premature ovarian failure (Swain et al. 2010). Similarly, there are encouraging data that GnRH analogs may offer protection against premature ovarian failure, with a new large trial from SWOG whose results are pending. Should this be proven effective, then patient's should be offered such therapy if they are concerned about future fertility. The primary prevention assumption we must make at diagnosis is that the patient will be a survivor, and anticipating this as part of treatment planning is essential.

Summary/Conclusion

Menopause related to breast cancer, whether prematurely initiated or exacerbated by the treatment, presents important challenges for women related to daily function, personal relationships and overall feelings of well-being. Menopause can have consequences that can interfere with usual life/developmental stage goals and that is perhaps one of the most difficult issues with which cancer survivors cope with in the long term.

While there is a fair amount of research in the areas of hot flashes, sexual health and fertility, large, rigorous longitudinal descriptive studies and intervention research specifically in the breast cancer population are lacking. If research would definitively identify physiologic and/or psychosocial targets for treatment, the evaluation of interventions likely to be beneficial could increase. Further, studies in the general population can inform testable hypotheses for breast cancer survivors, but extrapolation is not evidence based.

Symptoms and side effects from breast cancer and its treatment are complex in that there are numerous physiologic and psychologic effects that overlap, but are also distinct. Studies to date that have approached the problem from a reductionist perspective have resulted in less than satisfactory solutions with no or small effects on outcomes.

From a scientific perspective, it is time to change, (not merely tweak), the research paradigm. We must be willing to embrace the complexity of the human condition with our research designs and consider social, psychologic, physiologic, and environmental influences on the concept of interest (ie: hot flashes, sexual health, fertility). We must be willing to target more than one etiology and evaluate complex interventions. It is time to move into study designs that allow for individualization of treatment. More research is needed to provide information on understanding response. Perhaps pooled and/or meta-analyses can begin to look at the question of who responds and why, instead of simply being a means to improve power to add statistical significance to small or unclear effect sizes. There needs to be increased research from a systems perspective to define what effect hormone deprivation has on a woman's overall physiology, neurology and psychology long term and understand premature aging effects. Finally, we must think about preventing unwanted long term sequelae of treatment. Sometimes, that may mean a better understanding of individual risk/benefit perceptions and decisions at the outset to avoid treatment that will unnecessarily decrease a woman's quality of survivorship. It is in this way that we will be able to make clinically meaningful strides in breast cancer treatment as we keep an eye on the quality of a woman's life as a long term survivor.

References

Andersen BL, Carpenter KM, Yang HC, Shapiro CL (2007) Sexual well-being among partnered women with breast cancer recurrence. J Clin Oncol 25(21):3151–3157

Appt SE, Ethun KF (2010) Reproductive aging and risk for chronic disease: Insights from studies of nonhuman primates. Maturitas 67(1):7–14

Ayers B, Smith M, Hellier J, Mann E, Hunter MS (2012) Effectiveness of group and self-help cognitive behavior therapy in reducing problematic menopausal hot flushes and night sweats (MENOS 2): a randomized trial. Menopause 19(7):749–759

Azim HA Jr, Santoro L, Pavlidis N, Gelber S, Kroman N, Azim H, Peccatori FA (2011) Safety of pregnancy following breast cancer diagnosis: a meta-analysis of 14 studies. Eur J Cancer 47(1):74–83

Azim HA Jr, Kroman N, Paesmans M, Gelber S, Rotmensz N, Ameye L, De Mattos-Arruda L, Pistilli B, Pinto A, Jensen MB, Cordoba O, de Azambuja E, Goldhirsch A, Piccart MJ, Peccatori FA (2013) Prognostic impact of pregnancy after breast cancer according to estrogen receptor status: a multicenter retrospective study. J Clin Oncol 31(1):73–79

Balabanovic J, Ayers B, Hunter MS (2012) Women's experiences of group cognitive behaviour therapy for hot flushes and night sweats following breast cancer treatment: an interpretative phenomenological analysis. Maturitas 72(3):236–242

Bardia A, Novotny P, Sloan J, Barton D, Loprinzi C (2009) Efficacy of nonestrogenic hot flash therapies among women stratified by breast cancer history and tamoxifen use: a pooled analysis. Menopause 16(3):477–483

Barton D, Loprinzi CL (2004) Making sense of the evidence regarding nonhormonal treatments for hot flashes. Clin J Oncol Nurs 8(1):39–42

Barton DLC, Atherton P, Sloan J, Dalton R, Balcueva E, Carpenter P (2007a) The significance of serum testosterone concentrations from female cancer survivors. Oncol Nurs Forum 34(1):170

Barton DL, Wender DB, Sloan JA, Dalton RJ, Balcueva EP, Atherton PJ, Bernath AM Jr, DeKrey WL, Larson T, Bearden JD 3rd, Carpenter PC, Loprinzi CL (2007b) Randomized controlled trial to evaluate transdermal testosterone in female cancer survivors with decreased libido; North Central Cancer Treatment Group protocol N02C3. J Natl Cancer Inst 99(9):672–679

Barton DTA, Atherton P, Collins M, Sloan J (2009) The menopausal experience of premenopausal women receiving adjuvant chemotherapy for breast cancer. Oncol Nurs Forum 36(3):21–22

Barton DL, Thompson SL, Senn-Reeves JN, Satele DV, Frost M (2012) Effects of chemotherapy on the ovary: what you didn't know. Cancer Res 72(24 Suppl 3):2-11-01

Barton D, Fee-Schroeder K, Linquist B, Keith T, Wolf S, Abboud L, Elkins G (2013) Pilot study of a biobehavioral treatment for hot flashes. Ann Behav Med 45(S33):Abstract A-130

Basson R (2010) Sexual function of women with chronic illness and cancer. Womens Health (Lond Engl) 6(3):407–429

Baynosa J, Westphal LM, Madrigrano A, Wapnir I (2009) Timing of breast cancer treatments with oocyte retrieval and embryo cryopreservation. J Am Coll Surg 209(5):603–607

Bertero C, Chamberlain Wilmoth M (2007) Breast cancer diagnosis and its treatment affecting the self: a meta-synthesis. Cancer Nurs 30(3):194–202, quiz 203–204

Biglia N, Moggio G, Peasno E, Sgandurra P, Ponzone R, Nappi RE, Sismondi P (2010) Effects of surgical and adjuvant therapies for breast cancer on sexuality, cognitive functions, and body weight. J Sex Med 7(5):1891–1900

Braunstein GD, Sundwall DA, Katz J, Shifren JL, Buster JE, Simon JA, Bachman G, Aguirre OA, Lucas JD, Rodenberg C, Buch A, Watts NB (2005) Safety and efficacy of a testosterone patch for the treatment of hypoactive sexual desire disorder in surgically menopausal women: a randomized, placebo-controlled trial. Arch Intern Med 165(14):1582–1589

Brotto LA, Yule M, Breckon E (2010) Psychological interventions for the sexual sequelae of cancer: a review of the literature. J Cancer Surviv 4(4):346–360

Buijs C, de Vries EG, Mourits MJ, Willemse PH (2008) The influence of endocrine treatments for breast cancer on health-related quality of life. Cancer Treat Rev 34(7):640–655

Burwell SR, Case LD Kaelin C, Avis NE (2006) Sexual problems in younger women after breast cancer surgery. J Clin Oncol 24(18):2815–2821

Busby D, Christensen C, Crane R, Larson J (1995) A revision of the dyadic adjustment scale for use with distressed and nondistressed couples: construct hierarchy and multidimensional scales. J Marital Fam Ther 21(3):289–303

Buster JE, Kingsberg SA, Aguirre O, Brown C, Breaux JG, Buch A, Rodenberg CA, Wekselman K, Casson P. (2005) Testosterone patch for low sexual desire in surgically menopausal women: a randomized trial. Obstet Gynecol 105(5 Pt 1):944–952

Chudakov B, Ben Zion IZ, Belmaker RH (2007) Transdermal testosterone gel prn application for hypoactive sexual desire disorder in premenopausal women: a controlled pilot study of the effects on the Arizona sexual experiences scale for females and sexual function questionnaire. J Sex Med 4(1):204–208

Cohen S, Kamarck T, Mermelstein R (1983) A global measure of perceived stress. J Health Soc Behav 24(4):385–396

Cohen LS, Soares CN, Otto MW, Sweeney BH, Liberman RF, Harlow BL (2002) Prevalence and predictors of premenstrual dysphoric disorder (PMDD) in older premenopausal women. The Harvard study of moods and cycles. J Affect Disord 70(2):125–132

Curran S, Andrykowsky M, Studts J (1995) Short form of the profile of mood states (POMS-SF): psychometric information. Psychol Assess 7(1):80–83

Davis SR, van der Mooren MJ, van Lunsen RH, Lopes P, Ribot C, Rees M, Moufarege A, Rodenberg C, Buch A, Purdie DW (2006) Efficacy and safety of a testosterone patch for the treatment of hypoactive sexual desire disorder in surgically menopausal women: a randomized, placebo-controlled trial. Menopause 13(3):387–396

Davis S, Papalia MA, Norman RJ, O'Neill S, Redelman M, Williamson M, Stuckey BG, Wlodarczyk J, Gard'ner K, Humberstone A (2008a) Safety and efficacy of a testosterone metered-dose transdermal spray for treating decreased sexual satisfaction in premenopausal women: a randomized trial. Ann Intern Med 148(8):569–577

Davis SR, Moreau M, Kroll R, Bouchard C, Panay N, Gass M, Braunstein GD, Hirschberg AL, Rodenberg C, Pack S, Koch H, Moufarege A, Studd J, Aphrodite Study Team (2008b) Testosterone for low libido in postmenopausal women not taking estrogen. N Engl J Med 359(19):2005–2017

deMoor JS, Mariotto AB, Parry C, Alfano CM, Padgett L, Kent EE, Forsythe L, Scoppa S, Hachey M, Rowland JH (2013) Cancer survivors in the United States: prevalence across the survivorship trajectory and implications for care. Cancer Epidemiol Biomarkers Prev 22(4):561–570

Dodd M, Janson S, Facione N, Faucett J, Froelicher ES, Humphreys J, Lee K, Miaskowski C, Puntillo K, Rankin S, Taylor D (2001) Advancing the science of symptom management. J Adv Nurs 33(5):668–676

Dodd MJ, Cho MH, Cooper B, Miaskowski C, Lee KA, Bank K (2005) Advancing our knowledge of symptom clusters. J Support Oncol 3(6 Suppl 4):30–31

Duffy CM, Allen SM, Clark MA (2005) Discussions regarding reproductive health for young women with breast cancer undergoing chemotherapy. J Clin Oncol 23(4):766–773

Duijts SF, van Beurden M, Oldenburg HS, Hunter MS, Kieffer JM, Stuiver MM, Gerritsma MA, Menke-Pluymers MB, Plaisier PW, Rijna H, Lopes Cardozo AM, Timmers G, van der Meij S, van der Veen H, Bijker N, de Widt-Levert LM , Geenen MM, Heuff G, van Dulken EJ, Boven E, Aaronson NK (2012) Efficacy of cognitive behavioral therapy and physical exercise in alleviating treatment-induced menopausal symptoms in patients with breast cancer: results of a randomized, controlled, multicenter trial. J Clin Oncol 30(33):4124–4133

Elkins GR, Fisher WL, Johnson AK, Carpenter JS, Keith TZ (2013) Clinical hypnosis in the treatment of postmenopausal hot flashes: a randomized controlled trial. Menopause 20(3):291–298

Fobair P, Spiegel D (2009) Concerns about sexuality after breast cancer. Cancer J 15(1):19–26

Freedman RR (2001) Physiology of hot flashes. Am J Hum Biol 13(4):453–464

Freedman RR, Roehrs TA (2007) Sleep disturbance in menopause. Menopause 14(5):826–829

Freedman RR, Kruger ML, Wasson SL (2011) Heart rate variability in menopausal hot flashes during sleep. Menopause 18(8):897–900

Freeman EW, Sammel MD, Lin H, Gracia CR, Kapoor S (2008) Symptoms in the menopausal transition: hormone and behavioral correlates. Obstet Gynecol 111(1):127–136

Frierson G, Thiel D, Andersen B (2006) Body change stress for women with breast cancer: the breast-impact of treatment scale. Ann Behav Med 32(1):77–81

Ganz PA, Rowland JH, Desmond K, Meyerowitz BE, Wyatt GE (1998) Life after breast cancer: understanding women's health-related quality of life and sexual functioning. J Clin Oncol 16(2):501–514

Ganz PA, Desmond KA, Belin TR, Meyerowitz BE, Rowland JH (1999) Predictors of sexual health in women after a breast cancer diagnosis. J Clin Oncol 17(8):2371–2380

Ganz PA, Greendale GA, Petersen L, Zibecchi L, Kahn B, Belin TR (2000) Managing menopausal symptoms in breast cancer survivors: results of a randomized controlled trial. J Natl Cancer Inst 92(13):1054–1064

Ganz PA, Greendale GA, Petersen L, Kahn B, Bower JE (2003) Breast cancer in younger women: reproductive and late health effects of treatment. J Clin Oncol 21(22):4184–4193

Ganz PA, Land SR, Geyer CE Jr, Cecchini RS, Costantino JP, Pajon ER, Fehrenbacher L, Atkins JN, Polikoff JA, Vogel VG, Erban JK, Livingston RB, Perez EA, Mamounas EP, Wolmark N,

Swain SM (2011) Menstrual history and quality-of-life outcomes in women with node-positive breast cancer treated with adjuvant therapy on the NSABP B-30 trial. J Clin Oncol 29(9):1110–1116

Gibbs Z, Lee S, Kulkarni J (2013) Factors associated with depression during the perimenopausal transition. Womens Health Issues 23(5):e301–e307

Gilbert E, Ussher JM, Perz J (2010) Sexuality after breast cancer: a review. Maturitas 66(4):397–407

Goldfarb S, Muhall J, Nelson C, Kelvin J, Dickler M, Carter J (2013) Sexual and reproductive health in cancer survivors. Semin Oncol 40(6):726–744

Goldstat R, Briganti E, Tran J, Wolfe R, Davis SR (2003) Transdermal testosterone therapy improves well-being, mood, and sexual function in premenopausal women. Menopause 10(5):390–398

Goodwin PJ, Ennis M, Pritchard KI, Trudeau M, Hood N (1999) Adjuvant treatment and onset of menopause predict weight gain after breast cancer diagnosis. J Clin Oncol 17(1):120–129

Gracia CR, Freeman EW (2004) Acute consequences of the menopausal transition: the rise of common menopausal symptoms. Endocrinol Metab Clin North Am 33(4):675–689

Gracia CR, Freeman EW, Sammel MD, Lin H, Mogul M (2007) Hormones and sexuality during transition to menopause. Obstet Gynecol 109(4):831–840

Hale GE, Burger HG (2009) Hormonal changes and biomarkers in late reproductive age, menopausal transition and menopause. Best Pract Res Clin Obstet Gynaecol 23(1):7–23

Harlow SD, Karvonen C, Bromberger J, Cauley J, Gold E, Matthews K (2013) Menopause: its epidemiology in women and health. Elsevier, Amsterdam

Howard-Anderson J, Ganz PA, Bower JE, Stanton AL (2012) Quality of life, fertility concerns, and behavioral health outcomes in younger breast cancer survivors: a systematic review. J Natl Cancer Inst 104(5):386–405

Hunter M, Rendall M (2007) Bio-psycho-socio-cultural perspectives on menopause. Best Pract Res Clin Obstet Gynaecol 21(2):261–274

Kao A, Binik YM, Amsel R, Funaro D, Leroux N, Khalife S (2012) Biopsychosocial predictors of postmenopausal dyspareunia: the role of steroid hormones, vulvovaginal atrophy, cognitive-emotional factors, and dyadic adjustment. J Sex Med 9(8):2066–2076

Kim E, Jahan T, Aouizerat BE, Dodd MJ, Cooper BA, Paul SM, West C, Lee K, Swift PS, Wara W, Miaskowski C (2009) Changes in symptom clusters in patients undergoing radiation therapy. Support Care Cancer 17(11):1383–1391

Kroman N, Jensen MB, Wohlfahrt J, Ejlertsen B, Danish Breast Cancer Cooperative Group (2008) Pregnancy after treatment of breast cancer–a population-based study on behalf of Danish Breast Cancer Cooperative Group. Acta Oncol 47(4):545–549

Krychman M, Millheiser LS (2013) Sexual health issues in women with cancer. J Sex Med 10(Suppl 1):5–15

Lambertini M, Anserini P, Levaggi A, Poggio F, Del Mastro L (2013) Fertility counseling of young breast cancer patients. J Thorac Dis 5(Suppl 1):S68–S80

Leining MG, Gelber S, Rosenberg R, Przypyszny M, Winer EP, Partridge AH (2006) Menopausal-type symptoms in young breast cancer survivors. Ann Oncol 17(12):1777–1782

Lenz ER, Pugh LC, Milligan RA, Gift A, Suppe F (1997) The middle-range theory of unpleasant symptoms: an update. ANS Adv Nurs Sci 19(3):14–27

Lester J, Bernhard L, Ryan-Wenger N (2012) A self-report instrument that describes urogenital atrophy symptoms in breast cancer survivors. West J Nurs Res 34(1):72–96

Loprinzi CL, Barton DL, Sloan JA, Novotny PJ, Dakhil SR, Verdirame JD, Knutson WH, Kelaghan J, Christensen B (2008) Mayo Clinic and North Central Cancer Treatment Group hot flash studies: a 20-year experience. Menopause 15(4 Pt 1):655–660

Loprinzi CL, Sloan J, Stearns V, Slack R, Iyengar M, Diekmann B, Kimmick G, Lovato J, Gordon P, Pandya K, Guttuso T Jr, Barton D, Novotny P (2009) Newer antidepressants and gabapentin for hot flashes: an individual patient pooled analysis. J Clin Oncol 27(17):2831–2837

Loren AW, Mangu PB, Beck LN, Brennan L, Magdalinski AJ, Patriddge AH, Quinn G, Wallace WH, Oktay K, American Society of Clinical Oncology (2013) Fertility preservation for patients with cancer: American Society of Clinical Oncology clinical practice guideline update. J Clin Oncol 31(19):2500–2510

Malinovszky KM, Gould A, Foster E, Cameron D, Humphreys A, Crown J, Leonard RC, Anglo Celtic Co-operative Oncology Group (2006) Quality of life and sexual function after high-dose or conventional chemotherapy for high-risk breast cancer. Br J Cancer 95(12):1626–1631

Mann E, Smith MJ, Hellier J, Balabanovic JA, Hamed H, Grunfeld EA, Hunter MS (2012) Cognitive behavioral treatment for women who have menopausal symptoms after breast cancer treatment (MENOS 1): a randomized controlled trial. Lancet Oncol 13(3):309–318

Miaskowski C, Aouizerat BE, Dodd M, Cooper B (2007) Conceptual issues in symptom clusters research and their implications for quality-of-life assessment in patients with cancer. J Natl Cancer Inst Monogr 37:39–46

Murthy V, Chamberlain R (2012) Menopausal symptoms in young survivors of breast cancer: a growing problem without an ideal solution. Cancer Control 19(4):317–329

Nappi RE, Albani F, Santamaria V, Tonani S, Magri F, Martini E, Chiovato L., Polatti F (2010) Hormonal and psycho-relational aspects of sexual function during menopausal transition and at early menopause. Maturitas 67(1):78–83

Nathorst-Böös J, Flöter A, Jarkander-Rolff M, Carlström K, Schoultz Bv (2006) Treatment with percutaneous testosterone gel in postmenopausal women with decreased libido–effects on sexuality and psychological general well-being. Maturitas 53(1):11–18

Neuss MN, Malin JL, Chan S, Kadlubek PJ, Adams JL, Jacobson JO, Blayney DW, Simone JV (2013) Measuring the improving quality of outpatient care in medical oncology practices in the United States. J Clin Oncol 31(11):1471–1477

No Authors (2005) National Institutes of Health State-of-the-Science Conference statement: management of menopause-related symptoms. Ann Intern Med 142(12):1003–1013

Partridge AH, Gelber S, Peppercorn J, Sampson E, Knudsen K, Laufer M, Rosenberg R, Przypyszny M, Rein A, Winer EP (2004) Web-based survey of fertility issues in young women with breast cancer. J Clin Oncol 22(20):4174–4183

Phipps AI, Ichikawa L, Bowles EJ, Carney PA, Kerlikowske K, Miglioretti DL, Buist DS (2010) Defining menopausal status in epidemiologic studies: a comparison of multiple approaches and their effects on breast cancer rates. Maturitas 67(1):60–66

Quinn GP, Vadaparampil ST, Gwede CK, Miree C, King LM, Clayton HB, Wilson C, Munster P (2007) Discussion of fertility preservation with newly diagnosed patients: oncologists' views. J Cancer Surviv 1(2):146–155

Quinn GP, Vadaparampil ST, Lee JH, Jacobsen PB, Bepler G, Lancaster J, Keefe DL, Albrecht TL (2009) Physician referral for fertility preservation in oncology patients: a national study of practice behaviors. J Clin Oncol 27(35):5952–5957

Reinecke JD, Kelvin JF, Arvey SR, Quinn GP, Levine J, Beck LN, Miller A (2012) Implementing a systematic approach to meeting patients' cancer and fertility needs: a review of the Fertile Hope Centers of Excellence program. J Oncol Pract 8(5):303–308

Rissling MB, Liu L, Natarajan L, He F, Ancoli-Israel S (2011) Relationship of menopausal status and climacteric symptoms to sleep in women undergoing chemotherapy. Support Care Cancer 19(8):1107–1115

Rocca WA, Grossardt BR, de Andrade M, Malkasian GD, Melton LJ 3rd (2006) Survival patterns after oophorectomy in premenopausal women: a population-based cohort study. Lancet Oncol 7(10):821–828

Rogers M, Kristjanson LJ (2002) The impact on sexual functioning of chemotherapy-induced menopause in women with breast cancer. Cancer Nurs 25(1):57–65

Rosen R, Brown C, Heiman J, Leiblum S, Meston C, Shabsigh R, Ferguson D, D'Agostino R Jr (2000) The Female Sexual Function Index (FSFI): a multidimensional self-report instrument for the assessment of female sexual function. J Sex Marital Ther 26(2):191–208

Rowland JH, Meyerowitz BE, Crespi CM, Leedham B, Desmond K, Belin TR, Ganz PA (2009) Addressing intimacy and partner communication after breast cancer: a randomized controlled group intervention. Breast Cancer Res Treat 118(1):99–111

Salonen P, Tarkka MT, Kellokumpu-Lehtinen PL, Astedt-Kurki P, Luukkaala T, Kaunonen M (2009) Telephone intervention and quality of life in patients with breast cancer. Cancer Nurs 32(3):177–190, quiz 191–192

Senkus E, Gomez H, Dirix L, Jerusalem G, Murray E, Van Tienhoven G, Westernberg AH, Bottomonley A, Rapion J, Bogaerts J, Di Leo A, Nešković-Konstantinović Z (2014) Attitudes of young patients with breast cancer toward fertility loss related to adjuvant systemic therapies. EORTC study 10002 BIG 3-98. Psychooncology 23(2):173–182

Shifren JL, Braunstein GD, Simon JA, Casson PR, Buster JE, Redmond GP, Burki RE, Ginsburg ES, Rosen RC, Leiblum SR, Caramelli KE, Mazer NA (2000) Transdermal testosterone treatment in women with impaired sexual function after oophorectomy. N Engl J Med 343(10):682–688

Shifren JL, Davis SR, Moreau M, Waldbaum A, Bouchard C, DeRogatis L, Derzko C, Bearnson P, Kakos N, O'Neill S, Levine S, Wekselman K, Buch A, Rodenberg C, Kroll R (2006) Testosterone patch for the treatment of hypoactive sexual desire disorder in naturally menopausal women: results from the INTIMATE NM1 Study. Menopause 13(5):770–779

Shuster LT, Rhodes DJ, Gostout BS, Grossardt BR, Rocca WA (2010) Premature menopause or early menopause: long-term health consequences. Maturitas 65(2):161–166

Siegel R, DeSantis C, Virgo K, Stein K, Mariotto A, Smith T, Cooper D, Gansler T, Lerro C, Fedewa S, Lin C, Leach C, Cannady RS, Cho H, Scoppa S, Hachey M, Kirch R, Jemal A, Ward E (2012) Cancer treatment and survivorship statistics, 2012. CA Cancer J Clin 62(4):220–241

Sigmon ST, Whitcomb-Smith SR, Rohan KJ, Kendrew JJ (2004) The role of anxiety level, coping styles, and cycle phase in menstrual distress. J Anxiety Disord 18(2):177–191

Simon J, Braunstein G, Nachtigall L, Utian W, Katz M, Miller S, Waldbaum A, Bouchard C, Derzko C, Buch A, Rosenberg C, Lucas J, Davis S (2005) Testosterone patch increases sexual activity and desire in surgically menopausal women with hypoactive sexual desire disorder. J Clin Endocrinol Metab 90(9):5226–5233

Soules MR, Sherman S, Parrott E, Rebar R, Santoro N, Utian W, Woods N (2001) Executive summary: Stages of Reproductive Aging Workshop (STRAW). Climacteric 4(4):267–272

Speer JJ, Hillenberg B, Sugrue DP, Blacker C, Kresge CL, Decker VB, Zakalik D, Decker DA (2005) Study of sexual functioning determinants in breast cancer survivors. Breast J 11(6):440–447

Stone SE, Mazmanian D, Oinonen KA, Sharma V (2013) Past reproductive events as predictors of physical symptom severity during the menopausal transition. Menopause 20(8):831–839

Swain SM, Land SR, Ritter MW, Costantino JP, Cecchini RS, Manounas EP, Wolmark N, Ganz PA (2009) Amenorrhea in premenopausal women on the doxorubicin-and-cyclophosphamide-followed-by-docetaxel arm of NSABP B-30 trial. Breast Cancer Res Treat 113(2):315–320

Swain SM, Jeong JH, Geyer CE Jr, Costantino JP, Pajon ER, Fehrenbacher L, Atkins JN, Polikoff J, Vogel VG, Erban JK, Rastogi P, Livingston RB, Perez EA, Mamounas EP, Land SR, Ganz PA, Wolmark N (2010) Longer therapy, iatrogenic amenorrhea, and survival in early breast cancer. N Engl J Med 362(22):2053–2065

Tan O, Bradshaw K, Carr BR (2012) Management of vulvovaginal atrophy-related sexual dysfunction in postmenopausal women: an up-to-date review. Menopause 19(1):109–117

Taylor S, Harley C, Ziegler L, Brown J, Velikova G (2011) Interventions for sexual problems following treatment for breast cancer: a systematic review. Breast Cancer Res Treat 130(3):711–724

Thurston RC, Christie IC, Matthews KA (2012) Hot flashes and cardiac vagal control during women's daily lives. Menopause 19(4):406–412

Tremblay A, Sheeran L, Aranda S (2008) Psychoeducational interventions to alleviate hot flashes: a systematic review. Menopause 15(1):193–202

Waimey KE, Duncan FE, Su HI, Smith K, Wallach H, Jona K, Coutifaris C, Gracia CR, Shea LD, Brannigan RE, Chang RJ, Zelinski MB, Stouffer RL, Taylor RL, Woodruff TK (2013) Future directions in oncofertility and fertility preservation: a report from the 2011 Oncofertility Consortium Conference. J Adolesc Young Adult Oncol 2(1):25–30

Ware JE Jr (2000) SF-36 health survey update. Spine 25(24):3130–3139

Westphal LM, Wapnir IL (2012) Integration and safety of fertility preservation in a breast cancer program. Gynecol Oncol 124(3):474–476

Yanikkerem E, Koltan SO, Tamay AG, Dikayak Ş (2012) Relationship between women's attitude towards menopause and quality of life. Climacteric 15(6):552–562

Yoo C, Yun MR, Ahn JH, Jung KH, Kim HJ, Kim JE, Park JY, Park KO, Yoon DH, Kim SB (2013) Chemotherapy-induced amenorrhea, menopause-specific quality of life, and endocrine profiles in premenopausal women with breast cancer who received adjuvant anthracycline-based chemotherapy: a prospective cohort study. Cancer Chemother Pharmacol 72(3):565–575

Young-McCaughan S (1996) Sexual functioning in women with breast cancer after treatment with adjuvant therapy. Cancer Nurs 19(4):308–319

Zibecchi L, Greendale GA, Ganz PA (2003) Continuing education: comprehensive menopausal assessment: an approach to managing vasomotor and urogenital symptoms in breast cancer survivors. Oncol Nurs Forum 30(3):393–407

Chapter 10
Host Factors and Risk of Breast Cancer Recurrence: Genetic, Epigenetic and Biologic Factors and Breast Cancer Outcomes

Christine B. Ambrosone, Chi-Chen Hong, and Pamela J. Goodwin

Abstract Among women with breast cancer, there is wide variability in outcomes, both in treatment-related toxicities and disease-free survival (DFS). Primary predictors of DFS are those related to the extent of the disease and tumor characteristics, associated not only with tumor aggressiveness, but also responsiveness to targeted therapies. Inherited germline variation may also play a role in cancer treatment outcomes, and there have been studies targeting drug metabolism and other candidate pathways as well as genome-wide association studies (GWAS), which take a more agnostic approach and interrogate hundreds of thousands single nucleotide polymorphisms (SNPs) to determine those that modify response to breast cancer treatment. While this field of pharmacogenetics and pharmacogenomics has held exciting promise for personalized medicine, the results have not been as consistent, or the effects as profound, as first hoped. An emerging field in studies of cancer prognosis is epigenetics, which regulates DNA expression and can be influenced by numerous biologic processes as well as environmental exposures. Although young, this field of research likely holds promise for understanding of epigenetic mechanisms driving cancer and cancer outcomes, with a potential to modify these factors through drugs or other approaches. Finally, circulating markers in blood that reflect some lifestyle factors have also been studies in relation to cancer outcomes, particularly Vitamin D. In this chapter, we highlight advances in the areas noted above, and comment on factors that can impact interpretation of results from observational studies. We also discuss future directions, and avenues necessary to move the field forward.

Keywords Breast cancer • Prognosis • Tumor heterogeneity • Pharmacogenetics • Epigenetics • Vitamin D

C.B. Ambrosone, Ph.D. (✉) • C.-C. Hong, Ph.D.
Department of Cancer Prevention and Control, Roswell Park Cancer Institute,
Elm & Carlton Streets, Buffalo, NY 14263, USA
e-mail: Christine.ambrosone@roswellpark.org; chi-chen.hong@roswellpark.org

P.J. Goodwin, M.D., M.Sc., F.R.C.P.C.
Lunenfeld-Tanenbaum Research Institute, Mount Sinai Hospital,
1284-600 University Avenue, Toronto, ON, Canada, M5G 1X5
e-mail: pgoodwin@mtsinai.on.ca

© Breast Cancer Research Foundation 2015   143
P.A. Ganz (ed.), *Improving Outcomes for Breast Cancer Survivors*,
Advances in Experimental Medicine and Biology 862,
DOI 10.1007/978-3-319-16366-6_10

Tumor characteristics impact cancer prognosis, and also indicate treatments to be given. However, efficacy, as well as side effects of treatment, may be affected by genetic, epigenetic, and non-genetic factors, as shown in Fig. 10.1.

Breast Cancer Is Not One Disease

Over the last two decades, breast cancer research at the cellular and molecular level has allowed for better understanding of the extensive heterogeneity of breast cancer, with wide differences identified between tumors among populations, and also molecular heterogeneity within tumors. Molecular characterization of tumors has informed likely prognostic outcomes, and also led to targeted therapies. Tumor characteristics indicate treatments to be given, but efficacy, as well as side effects of treatment, may be affected by genetic, epigenetic, and non-genetic factors, as shown in Fig. 10.1.

Investigations of the estrogen receptor (ER) began in the early 1970s (McGuire 1975; Jensen 1975), and within less than a decade, the anti-estrogen, tamoxifen, was being used to treat ER positive breast cancer (Fisher et al. 1981). Discovery of the HER2/neu proto-oncogene in the 1980s and identification of its important role in

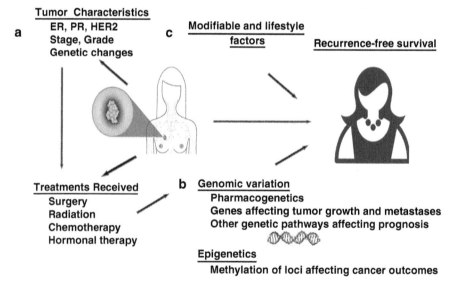

Fig. 10.1 Factors affecting breast cancer prognosis. (**a**) Characteristics of the tumor will affect likelihood of recurrence and metastasis, and will also determine treatments to be given. (**b**) The effects of treatments on outcomes may be modified by genomic variation in drug metabolism and other pathways, as well as epigenetic silencing our activation of important pathways. (**c**) Treatment outcomes may also be modified by numerous lifestyle factors, including physical activity, body size, and dietary factors

breast cancer prognosis then led to development of trastuzumab, a monoclonal antibody directed against HER2 (Slamon and Pegram 2001), which has greatly improved survival for women with HER2 positive breast cancer (Baselga et al. 2006). For many years, testing for ER, progesterone receptor (PR) and HER2 has guided breast cancer treatments, in addition to standard chemotherapy regimens. Even with ER+ breast cancer, however, there are notable differences in treatment outcomes, and additional molecular tests, such as Oncotype Dx recurrence score, have been used to further stratify patients for adjuvant chemotherapy treatments (Paik et al. 2004).

Finer classifications of breast cancer subtypes were identified with the advent of multi-gene arrays and expression analyses (van de Vijver et al. 2002; Perou et al. 2000), and the intrinsic subtypes have been shown to be associated with breast cancer prognosis (Carey et al. 2006). Importantly, classifications obtained using these arrays can be approximated using immunohistochemical (IHC) markers to classify ER+ breast cancer into Luminal A and Luminal B, with the latter having more proliferative indices and associated with poorer prognosis than Luminal A. Further refinement of 'triple negative' breast cancer (ER−, PR−, HER2−) into basal-like cancers (ER−, PR−, HER−, ck5/6+, EGFR+) with poorer prognosis is also possible using IHC markers. More recently, the PAM50 assay, which can now be performed using formalin-fixed paraffin-embedded tissue, builds upon classifications based on IHC markers, with reassignment of a fair proportion of tumors to other intrinsic subtype groups based upon the more detailed analyses, further refining prognostic estimates (Nielsen et al. 2010; Cheang et al. 2012; Caan et al. 2014).

Recent research from the Molecular Taxonomy of Breast Cancer International Consortium (METABRIC) in the United Kingdom and Canada, and the NCI-led Tumor Cancer Genome Atlas (TCGA) Network has provided more comprehensive portraits of breast cancer, with classifications into subgroups. With fresh frozen tumor samples from more than 2,000 women with breast cancer, METABRIC examined copy number and gene expression in discovery and validation sets (Curtis et al. 2012). Analyzing paired DNA and RNA samples, they identified novel subgroups with different clinical outcomes, including a high-risk ER+ subgroup, and a group with better prognosis whose tumors had no copy number variants. Their work highlighted a limited number of gene regions that likely harbor 'driver' genes. The next step recommended by the authors is to follow up with sequencing efforts for mutational profiles, particularly in cancers with no copy number aberrations.

In the TCGA, breast tumor and germline samples were available from 825 patients, and were analyzed on a number of platforms for assessment of copy number variants, DNA methylation, exome sequencing, messenger RNA arrays, and analysis of microRNAs and proteins (Cancer Genome Atlas Network 2012). Combining data from several platforms, tumors were classified into four main classes, although there was extensive heterogeneity within these groups. In fact, mutations were more diverse and recurrent in luminal A and luminal B tumors than within basal-like and HER2 enriched. The most frequently mutated genes in luminal A tumors were PIK3CA (45 %) and others including MAP2K4, which was also identified as a key cancer gene in the METABRIC analysis (Curtis et al. 2012). In basal-like tumors, 80 % of the cases had p53 mutations. These projects have provided a wealth of data and information which helps to elucidate breast cancer subtypes and may also provide clues for therapeutic targets to be followed. The TCGA study also showed a number of similarities between basal-like tumors and serous ovarian cancer, suggesting common therapeutic approaches.

This advanced molecular work using a number of platforms supports the initial classification of the intrinsic breast cancer subgroups, but also points to the significant heterogeneity within classes. Further research along these lines will hopefully not only inform our understanding of etiologic pathways, but perhaps lend guidance for development of targeted therapeutics. For cancer prevention and control, however, it is unclear how fine-grained classification of tumors needs to be to categorize for studies of lifestyle or other interventions. There are a growing number of studies showing, for example, that PAM50 classifications better predict treatment outcomes in breast cancer patients than IHC subgroups alone. Would this more refined classification also better inform studies evaluating the effects of, for example, physical activity and recurrence? These are studies that will likely need to be done to be able to best target those most likely to benefit from interventions.

Does Genetic Make-up Influence Recurrence and Survival?

For many years, scientists focused on characteristics of breast tumors as predictors of cancer outcomes. Although there had been awareness of the concept of pharmacogenetics, genetic variability in drug metabolism, from before the 1950s, it was primarily in relation to adverse outcomes for subsets of the population when being treated with drugs, such as isoniazid (Weber and Cohen 1968). It is only within the last two decades that there has been growing interest in the role of genetic variability in relation to breast cancer treatment outcomes. Initial studies investigating the role of genetic variability in relation to treatment outcomes focused on specific drug regimens and their metabolic pathways, taking a candidate gene approach in pathways for cyclophosphamide, anthracyclines and taxanes, with few consistent results [reviewed in Yao et al. (2012); Westbrook and Stearns (2013)].

The anti-estrogen tamoxifen is metabolized by cytochrome p450 enzymes, with CYP2D6 primarily investigated because it produces endoxifen, considered to be the primary activity metabolite responsible for the anti-estrogen activity of tamoxifen (Hoskins et al. 2009). Initially, there was enthusiastic interest and recommendations for genotyping for CYP2D6 variants in the clinic to predict drug efficacy and side effects, with the goal to be able to titrate doses based upon genotypes to enhance efficacy while reducing adverse outcomes, or for selection of alternate agents. This may be particularly important when using tamoxifen in a prevention setting among high risk patients. However, numerous studies have resulted in inconsistent results, leading to some controversy. In commenting on results from two trials showing null results, the accompanying editorial stated that "this matter has likely been laid to rest" (Kelly and Pritchard 2012), but other researchers believe that the lack of replication may be due to a number of methodological issues, including use of tumor DNA and problems with genotyping (Pharoah et al. 2012), as well as potential confounding by use of other medications that may induce or inhibit CYP2D6, or other differences in study populations (Stearns et al. 2003). In particular, a number of serotonin reuptake inhibitors (SSRIs) and norepinephrine reuptake inhibitors (SNRIs) used to treat depression and hot flashes also inhibit CYP2D6 activity (Jin et al. 2005; Borges et al. 2006). In breast cancer patients, CYP2D6 inhibition by co-medication with these drugs results in lower levels of the active metabolite endoxifen and potentially, reduction of efficacy of treatment with tamoxifen (Goetz et al. 2007). Although there is drug label information regarding the potential for drug interactions between tamoxifen and SSRIs and SNRIs, it is likely that these medications are still prescribed together, and may contribute, in part, to the inconsistency in study results regarding CYP2D6 genotypes, tamoxifen, and breast cancer outcomes (Binkhorst et al. 2013).

This example (tamoxifen and CYP2D6) illustrates the challenges faced when hoping to apply pharmacogenetics in a clinical setting to prediction of treatment outcomes. Here was a drug where there was bountiful data showing the functional activity of genotype variants and direct associations between genotypes and levels of the active metabolite. It seemed relatively straightforward to then extrapolate that there would be associations between genotypes and tamoxifen-related side effects as well as outcomes. However, results have been disappointing, perhaps due to the complexity of drug metabolic pathways, interactions between tamoxifen and CYP2D6 inhibitors, issues with study design, and heterogeneity of study populations.

Although investigations of drug metabolism pathways and breast cancer outcomes have not yielded definitive results with direct relevance for the clinic, there has been great anticipation for the use of genome wide association studies (GWAS) to identify key genes and/or gene variants that are associated with treatment side effects and recurrence and survival. Using an agnostic approach, genomic DNA from patients is genotyped for thousands of single nucleotide polymorphisms (SNPs), and genomic profiles compared between patients with and without the outcomes of interest. It is clear that not all patients respond similarly to cancer therapy, and it is likely that genetic variability, in part, plays a role in these differential responses.

GWAS have been used with some success for identification of susceptibility loci for etiology of a number of cancers, many of which are multifactorial and likely caused by numerous exposures and genetic variants. Thus, the thinking has been that genetic factors likely play a large role in differences in experience of grade 3 and 4 toxicities among patients receiving specific chemotherapy agents. Unlike using a candidate gene approach, GWAS may reveal pathways involved in side effects and outcomes that may not have been previously hypothesized. For example, Ingle and colleagues performed a GWAS to identify SNPs that were associated with musculoskeletal adverse events (AEs) among breast cancer patients treated with aromatase inhibitors (AIs) (Ingle et al. 2010). The SNPs identified were near the T-cell leukemia 1A (TCL1A) gene; follow-up with functional studies revealed effects of differential TCL1A expression on cytokine receptor genes and on transcription of NF-kB, indicating that the musculoskeletal AEs are related to an inflammatory response (Liu et al. 2012). Genetic variability in this pathway had not been previously hypothesized to be associated with AI-related side effects, and opens doors for new approaches for prevention of these AEs.

GWAS has also been used to investigate the basis for neurotoxicities often experienced among breast cancer patients treated with taxanes. In a Cancer and Leukemia Group B clinical trial, the loci identified that were associated with paclitaxel-induced neuropathy were in genes involved in axon outgrowth (Baldwin et al. 2012; Chhibber et al. 2014). Although, in retrospect, these findings make sense, they provide a new perspective or paradigm for pharmacogenetics. Previously, pathways that could modify the treatment agent effects were investigated, such as drug activation, detoxification, and DNA repair. These findings regarding neurotoxicity and SNPs in genes in axonal outgrowth, as well as the finding for AIs and musculoskeletal AEs, illustrate the value of GWAS in relation to treatment outcomes. By revealing pathways that were previously not hypothesized, new targets can be identified for prevention efforts.

The Interface Between Genomics and the Environment

Genomic DNA sequences are inherited, are in every cell in the human body, and account for a large portion of variations in phenotypes and conditions. Unlike DNA sequences, however, epigenetics, defined as covalent modifications of DNA base and chromatic alterations, affect DNA function without altering sequence. The most commonly studied epigenetic mechanism is DNA methylation, which is known for its plasticity, and is influenced by genetics as well as external exposures (Bernstein et al. 2007). DNA methylation is tissue specific, undergoing dynamic changes and influenced by factors such as aging, smoking, alcohol, and dietary intake (Rakyan et al. 2011; Langevin and Kelsey 2013; Langevin et al. 2011). There have been a number of studies of DNA methylation in breast tumors in relation to breast cancer characteristics, risk factors and prognosis, the majority of which have been performed targeting genes known to be commonly mutated in breast cancer, such as p16, ER, cyclin D2, RASSF1A, TWIST, RATB and HiN1 (Fackler et al. 2004; Swift-Scanlan et al. 2011; Tao et al. 2009). More recently, platforms have been used to examine thousands of loci for methylation. In the Sister Study, using a 27K platform, 250 differentially methylated loci were identified from blood samples that distinguished women who later developed breast cancer from those who did not (Xu et al. 2013). Using the same platform, Fackler and colleagues found that DNA methylation classified tumors into ER positive and ER negative, with 100 methylated loci significantly associated with disease progression (Fackler et al. 2011). We recently used the Illumina 450K platform and DNA from African-American and European American women, and found that methylation classified tumors according to ER status (Ambrosone et al. 2014), similar to Fackler et al. We also noted that there were more differentially methylated loci by race among women with ER negative breast cancer than those with ER positive disease, suggesting that etiologic pathways of ER negative breast cancer could differ between racial groups (Ambrosone et al. 2014).

With the refinement of approaches to conducting Epi-Genome Wide Associations Studies (EWAS), it is likely that this biomarker, which incorporates genetic and biologic factors with environmental exposures, will be used increasingly to establish risk prediction models and to identify genes that impact the disease process when altered through methylation. Although still in the early stages, there are also groups who are studying changes in methylation over time with cancer therapies and in response to interventions. Because methylation has been shown to differ between current, ex- and never smokers (Harlid et al. 2014), as well as between obese and non-obese individuals (Almén et al. 2014), there are hopes that it may eventually be used to monitor efficacy of interventions to reduce risk of breast cancer recurrence. In fact, in a 6 months exercise intervention, DNA from adipose tissue showed distinct methylation differences before and after the exercise intervention (Rönn et al. 2013). Of interest, the exercise intervention resulted in differential methylation of 39 candidate genes for obesity and type 2 diabetes. Thus, this marker holds promise for prognostic studies among breast cancer survivors, particularly to monitor efficacy of interventions.

Blood Levels of Vitamin D

Host factors that influence prognosis, particularly tumor characteristics and inherited genetic make-up, cannot be modified, but may be used to better understand survival outcomes. As discussed in other chapters, there are a number of behavioral/lifestyle factors that may be relevant for prognosis, and could be undertaken among patients diagnosed with breast cancer to reduce the likelihood of breast cancer recurrence and poorer survival. Blood levels of 25-hydroxyvitamin D (25(OH)D) reflect uptake from diet, supplements, sun exposure, and biologic processes, and may therefore be a better measure for studies of prognosis than assessment of intake. Goodwin et al. were the first to report an association of Vitamin D blood levels with breast cancer outcomes (Goodwin et al. 2009); there have been a number of subsequent studies examining serum 25(OH)D and breast cancer survival, with somewhat inconsistent results. Studies conducted outside of clinical trial settings have fairly consistently identified significant associations of low vitamin D with poor disease-free or overall survival [reviewed in Rose et al. (2013)], while studies conducted in the setting of a clinical trial have failed to identify associations of vitamin D with outcomes (Lohmann et al. 2014; Pritchard et al. 2011). A recent systematic review concluded that circulating 25-OHD levels "may be associated with better prognosis in patients with breast cancer," but the included studies had mixed results (Toriola et al. 2014). One important issue for assessment of serum vitamin D and breast cancer outcomes in observational studies, however, is the time during the clinical course of the disease at which blood samples were drawn. For example, prospective studies may use blood samples that were drawn prior to the occurrence of breast cancer, others have used samples that were drawn after surgery but before adjuvant therapy (Goodwin et al. 2009), and some studies were from well past breast cancer diagnosis and treatment, such as in the Health, Eating, Activity and Lifestyle Study (Villaseñor et al. 2013). The latter design does not allow for examination of associations of Vitamin D with early breast cancer events (as they have already occurred before patients are enrolled); this may be of greatest relevance for triple negative breast cancers that are most likely to recur early. Recently, we examined serum 25-OHD levels in relation to prognosis in a subset of the Pathways Study, a prospective cohort of breast cancer patients enrolled through Kaiser Permanente Northern California (Yao et al. 2014). The vast majority of samples were drawn prior to adjuvant therapy, but after surgery. In these analyses, all women in quartiles above the lowest had improved overall survival, with the greatest risk reduction among women in the highest quartile (adjusted HR=0.57, 95 % CI, 0.37–0.87). Although there were suggestions of reduced risk of disease-free survival, the point estimate was weaker and the confidence interval included unity. Another important consideration in interpretation of the Vitamin D—breast cancer prognosis literature is the differentiation of association from causality. Higher blood levels of Vitamin D may reflect other factors that impact breast cancer outcomes, including normal body size and adoption of healthy behaviors (such as outdoor physical activity, balanced diet and use of supplements) that are the causal basis for the observed association. Although preclinical evidence supports a potential biologic effect of Vitamin D in breast cancer, it cannot be concluded that any association of Vitamin D with outcomes is causal, or that breast cancer patients should take Vitamin D supplements in the hopes of improving their outcomes.

Conclusion

Research is advancing at a rapid pace to better understand host factors that may impact risk of recurrence and mortality from breast cancer. With accelerating knowledge and newer technologies to examine both tumor and host genomes at the molecular level, the promise of personalized medicine becomes further within the reach of the breast cancer research and clinical community. With genomic profiles of tumors, therapies targeting specific mutations may lead to better prognosis, and discoveries of GWAS studies may lead to the right drugs, at the proper doses, for the right patients, to minimize side effects and enhance treatment efficacy. Use of intermediate biomarkers that reflect both genomic and environmental exposures will hopefully lead to further understanding of the role of lifestyle, genetic and non-genetic factors in determination of treatment outcomes among breast cancer patients. With the growing body of research showing associations between non-genetic factors, such as body size and physical activity and breast cancer outcomes, we may be able to incorporate these factors with information on tumor mutations and inherited genetics to provide a more comprehensive picture of prognostic factors, and better recommendations for enhancing breast cancer outcomes.

References

Almén MS, Nilsson EK, Jacobsson JA et al (2014) Genome-wide analysis reveals DNA methylation markers that vary with both age and obesity. Gene 548(1):61–67

Ambrosone CB, Young AC, Sucheston LE et al (2014) Genome-wide methylation patterns provide insight into differences in breast tumor biology between American women of African and European ancestry. Oncotarget 5(1):237–248

Baldwin RM, Owzar K, Zembutsu H et al (2012) A genome-wide association study identifies novel loci for paclitaxel-induced sensory peripheral neuropathy in CALGB 40101. Clin Cancer Res 18(18):5099–5109

Baselga J, Perez EA, Pienkowski T et al (2006) Adjuvant trastuzumab: a milestone in the treatment of HER-2-positive early breast cancer. Oncologist 11(Suppl 1):4–12

Bernstein BE, Meissner A, Lander ES (2007) The mammalian epigenome. Cell 128(4):669–681

Binkhorst L, Mathijssen RHJ, Van Herk-Sukel MPP et al (2013) Unjustified prescribing of CYP2D6 inhibiting SSRIs in women treated with tamoxifen. Breast Cancer Res Treat 139(3):923–929

Borges S, Desta Z, Li L et al (2006) Quantitative effect of CYP2D6 genotype and inhibitors on tamoxifen metabolism: implication for optimization of breast cancer treatment. Clin Pharmacol Ther 80(1):61–74

Caan BJ, Sweeney C, Habel LA et al (2014) Intrinsic subtypes from the PAM50 gene expression assay in a population-based breast cancer survivor cohort: prognostication of short- and long-term outcomes. Cancer Epidemiol Biomarkers Prev 23(5):725–734

Cancer Genome Atlas Network (2012) Comprehensive molecular portraits of human breast tumours. Nature 490(7418):61–70

Carey LA, Perou CM, Livasy CA et al (2006) Race, breast cancer subtypes, and survival in the Carolina Breast Cancer Study. JAMA 295(21):2492–2502

Cheang MCU, Voduc KD, Tu D et al (2012) Responsiveness of intrinsic subtypes to adjuvant anthracycline substitution in the NCIC.CTG MA.5 randomized trial. Clin Cancer Res 18(8):2402–2412

Chhibber A, Mefford J, Stahl EA et al (2014) Polygenic inheritance of paclitaxel-induced sensory peripheral neuropathy driven by axon outgrowth gene sets in CALGB 40101 (Alliance). Pharmacogenomics J 14(4):336–342

Curtis C, Shah SP, Chin S et al (2012) The genomic and transcriptomic architecture of 2,000 breast tumours reveals novel subgroups. Nature 486(7403):346–352

Fackler MJ, McVeigh M, Mehrotra J et al (2004) Quantitative multiplex methylation-specific PCR assay for the detection of promoter hypermethylation in multiple genes in breast cancer. Cancer Res 64(13):4442–4452

Fackler MJ, Umbricht CB, Williams D et al (2011) Genome-wide methylation analysis identifies genes specific to breast cancer hormone receptor status and risk of recurrence. Cancer Res 71(19):6195–6207

Fisher B, Redmond C, Brown A et al (1981) Treatment of primary breast cancer with chemotherapy and tamoxifen. N Engl J Med 305(1):1–6

Goetz MP, Knox SK, Suman VJ et al (2007) The impact of cytochrome P450 2D6 metabolism in women receiving adjuvant tamoxifen. Breast Cancer Res Treat 101(1):113–121

Goodwin PJ, Ennis M, Pritchard KI et al (2009) Prognostic effects of 25-hydroxyvitamin D levels in early breast cancer. J Clin Oncol 27(23):3757–3763

Harlid S, Xu Z, Panduri V et al (2014) CpG sites associated with cigarette smoking: analysis of epigenome-wide data from the sister study. Environ Health Perspect 122(7):673–678

Hoskins JM, Carey LA, McLeod HL (2009) CYP2D6 and tamoxifen: DNA matters in breast cancer. Nat Rev Cancer 9(8):576–586

Ingle JN, Schaid DJ, Goss PE et al (2010) Genome-wide associations and functional genomic studies of musculoskeletal adverse events in women receiving aromatase inhibitors. J Clin Oncol 28(31):4674–4682

Jensen EV (1975) Estrogen receptors in hormone-dependent breast cancers. Cancer Res 35(11 Pt. 2):3362–3364

Jin Y, Desta Z, Stearns V et al (2005) CYP2D6 genotype, antidepressant use, and tamoxifen metabolism during adjuvant breast cancer treatment. J Natl Cancer Inst 97(1):30–39

Kelly CM, Pritchard KI (2012) CYP2D6 genotype as a marker for benefit of adjuvant tamoxifen in postmenopausal women: lessons learned. J Natl Cancer Inst 104(6):427–428

Langevin SM, Kelsey KT (2013) The fate is not always written in the genes: epigenomics in epidemiologic studies. Environ Mol Mutagen 54(7):533–541

Langevin SM, Houseman EA, Christensen BC et al (2011) The influence of aging, environmental exposures and local sequence features on the variation of DNA methylation in blood. Epigenetics 6(7):908–919

Liu M, Wang L, Bongartz T et al (2012) Aromatase inhibitors, estrogens and musculoskeletal pain: estrogen-dependent T-cell leukemia 1A (TCL1A) gene-mediated regulation of cytokine expression. Breast Cancer Res 14(2):R41

Lohmann AE, Chapman J, Burnell MJ et al (2014) Prognostic associations of 25OH vitamin D in NCIC CTG MA.21, a phase III adjuvant RCT of three chemotherapy regimens (EC/T, CEF, AC/T) in high-risk breast cancer (BC). J Clin Oncol 32(15):504

McGuire WL (1975) Current status of estrogen receptors in human breast cancer. Cancer 36(2 Suppl):638–644

Nielsen TO, Parker JS, Leung S et al (2010) A comparison of PAM50 intrinsic subtyping with immunohistochemistry and clinical prognostic factors in tamoxifen-treated estrogen receptor-positive breast cancer. Clin Cancer Res 16(21):5222–5232

Paik S, Shak S, Tang G et al (2004) A multigene assay to predict recurrence of tamoxifen-treated, node-negative breast cancer. N Engl J Med 351(2):2817–2826

Perou CM, Sorlie T, Eisen MB et al (2000) Molecular portraits of human breast tumours. Nature 406(6797):747–752

Pharoah PDP, Abraham J, Caldas C (2012) Re: CYP2D6 genotype and tamoxifen response in postmenopausal women with endocrine-responsive breast cancer: The breast international group 1-98 trial and Re: CYP2D6 and UGT2B7 genotype and risk of recurrence in tamoxifen-treated breast cancer patients. J Natl Cancer Inst 104(16):1263–1264

Pritchard KI, Shepherd LE, Chapman J-W et al (2011) Randomized trial of tamoxifen versus combined tamoxifen and octreotide LAR therapy in the adjuvant treatment of early-stage breast cancer in postmenopausal women: NCIC CTG MA.14. J Clin Oncol 29(29):3869–3876

Rakyan VK, Down TA, Balding DJ et al (2011) Epigenome-wide association studies for common human diseases. Nat Rev Genet 12(8):529–541

Rönn T, Volkov P, Davegårdh C et al (2013) A six months exercise intervention influences the genome-wide DNA methylation pattern in human adipose tissue. PLoS Genet 9(6):e1003572

Rose AAN, Elser C, Ennis M et al (2013) Blood levels of vitamin D and early stage breast cancer prognosis: a systematic review and meta-analysis. Breast Cancer Res Treat 141(3):331–339

Slamon D, Pegram M (2001) Rationale for trastuzumab (Herceptin) in adjuvant breast cancer trials. Semin Oncol 28(1 Suppl 3):13–19

Stearns V, Johnson MD, Rae JM et al (2003) Active tamoxifen metabolite plasma concentrations after coadministration of tamoxifen and the selective serotonin reuptake inhibitor paroxetine. J Natl Cancer Inst 95(2):1758–1764

Swift-Scanlan T, Vang R, Blackford A et al (2011) Methylated genes in breast cancer: associations with clinical and histopathological features in a familial breast cancer cohort. Cancer Biol Ther 11(10):853–865

Tao MH, Shields PG, Nie J et al (2009) DNA hypermethylation and clinicopathological features in breast cancer: the Western New York Exposures and Breast Cancer (WEB) study. Breast Cancer Res Treat 114(3):559–568

Toriola AT, Nguyen N, Scheitler-Ring K et al (2014) Circulating 25-hydroxyvitamin D levels and prognosis among cancer patients: a systematic review. Cancer Epidemiol Biomarkers Prev 23(6):917–933 van de Vijver MJ, He YD, van't Veer LJ et al (2002) A gene-expression signature as a predictor of survival in breast cancer. N Engl J Med 347(2):1999–2009

Villaseñor A, Ballard-Barbash R, Ambs A et al (2013) Associations of serum 25-hydroxyvitamin D with overall and breast cancer-specific mortality in a multiethnic cohort of breast cancer survivors. Cancer Causes Control 24(4):759–767

Weber WW, Cohen SN (1968) The mechanism of isoniazid acetylation by human N-acetyltransferase. Biochim Biophys Acta Enzymol 151(1):276–278

Westbrook K, Stearns V (2013) Pharmacogenomics of breast cancer therapy: an update. Pharmacol Ther 139(1):1–11

Xu Z, Bolick SCE, Deroo LA et al (2013) Epigenome-wide association study of breast cancer using prospectively collected sister study samples. J Natl Cancer Inst 105(10):694–700

Yao S, Maghsoudlou D, Ambrosone CB (2012) Breast cancer pharmacogenetics in the era of personalized medicine. Curr Breast Cancer Rep 4(4):271–281

Yao S, Kwan ML, Ergas IJ et al (2014) The associations of serum 25-hydroxyvitamin D with breast cancer characteristics and prognosis in the Pathways Study. In: 105th Annual meeting of the American Association for Cancer Research, San Diego, CA, 5–9 Apr 2014

Chapter 11
Comorbidities and Their Management: Potential Impact on Breast Cancer Outcomes

Chi-Chen Hong, Christine B. Ambrosone, and Pamela J. Goodwin

Abstract Pre-existing comorbidities negatively impacts overall breast cancer prognosis, increasing both breast cancer specific deaths as well as death from competing causes. Improvements in breast cancer survival in recent decades, however, have primarily been experienced among cancer patients without comorbidities, and less so among those with moderate or severe comorbidities. As guidelines for the treatment of breast cancer are mostly based on studies excluding patients with moderate and severe comorbidities with under-representation of older women with comorbid conditions, information regarding treatment effectiveness in breast cancer patients with comorbidities is currently lacking. This chapter describes the impact of comorbidities on breast cancer treatment and outcomes, previous research approaches taken, and specific populations that may be most susceptible to the effects of comorbidities on breast cancer outcomes. Future research directions are suggested that may help to improve understanding of comorbidity-related factors that underlie disparities in breast cancer outcomes, and to examine the potential role of effective management of comorbidities among breast cancer patients as a strategy to help close gaps in disease prognosis.

Keywords Comorbidities • Medications • Breast cancer survival • Competing cause mortality

C.-C. Hong, Ph.D. (✉) • C.B. Ambrosone, Ph.D.
Department of Cancer Prevention and Control, Roswell Park Cancer Institute,
Elm & Carlton Streets, Buffalo, NY 14263, USA
e-mail: Chi-Chen.Hong@RoswellPark.org; Christine.Ambrosone@RoswellPark.org

P.J. Goodwin, M.D., M.Sc., F.R.C.P.C.
Lunenfeld-Tanenbaum Research Institute, Mount Sinai Hospital,
1284-600 University Avenue, Toronto, ON, Canada, M5G 1X5
e-mail: pgoodwin@mtsinai.on.ca

© Breast Cancer Research Foundation 2015
P.A. Ganz (ed.), *Improving Outcomes for Breast Cancer Survivors*,
Advances in Experimental Medicine and Biology 862,
DOI 10.1007/978-3-319-16366-6_11

Introduction

Pre-existing comorbidities are increasingly recognized to negatively impact overall survival in breast cancer patients (Ording et al. 2013; Sogaard et al. 2013; Patnaik et al. 2011a; Ring et al. 2011) and was highlighted as a pressing issue in the most recent Annual Report to the Nation on the Status of Cancer (Edwards et al. 2013). The negative impact of comorbidities on breast cancer outcomes is substantial and can be as important as stage in predicting survival (Patnaik et al. 2011b). Breast cancer patients with comorbidities are less likely to receive definitive treatment (Louwman et al. 2005; Griffiths et al. 2014), and have higher overall mortality compared to those without comorbidities. Similar to the rest of the US population, breast cancer patients bear substantial comorbidity burdens, particularly as they age, with rates of severe comorbidities rising to over 30 % among women age 65 and older (Edwards et al. 2013; Cho et al. 2013). Rising rates of breast cancer risk factors, such as obesity, metabolic syndrome, and reduced levels of physical activity may further contribute to high rates of comorbidity in breast cancer patients (Guh et al. 2009; Berrino et al. 2014; Hair et al. 2014). Improvements in breast cancer survival in recent decades, however, have primarily been experienced among cancer patients without comorbidities, and less so among those with moderate or severe comorbidities (Cronin-Fenton et al. 2007; Land et al. 2012a). As guidelines for the treatment of breast cancer are mostly based on studies excluding patients with moderate and severe comorbidities with under-representation of older women, who are more likely to have comorbid conditions (Hutchins et al. 1999), information regarding treatment effectiveness in breast cancer patients with comorbidities is currently lacking and the potential role that effective management and control of comorbidities play on breast cancer treatment and outcomes are largely unknown. This has fueled increasing research attention in the past decade on the impact of comorbidities on cancer outcomes, and going forward, how these relationships might be modified to improve disease prognosis among women with comorbid conditions. The goals of this chapter will be to highlight the impact of comorbidities on breast cancer treatment and outcomes, discuss how comorbidities are being researched and how this might be expanded, point out specific populations that may be most susceptible to the effects of comorbidities on breast cancer outcomes, and suggest future research directions that may improve our understanding of factors that underlie the disparities in breast cancer outcomes experienced by women with comorbidities and provide insights into strategies needed to close these gaps in disease prognosis. The conceptual outline and key points raised in this chapter are presented in Fig. 11.1.

Current Research

Comorbidities and Survival Outcomes

There is ample evidence indicating that breast cancer patients with comorbidities have poorer overall disease prognosis, which includes increased breast cancer specific deaths as well as death from other causes (Sogaard et al. 2013; Edwards et al. 2013;

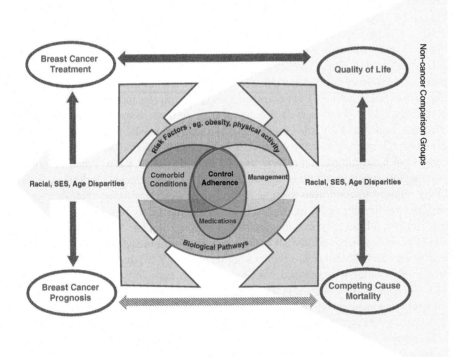

Fig. 11.1 Relationships between comorbidities, breast cancer treatment and breast cancer outcomes. Comorbid conditions among breast cancer survivors can negatively influence breast cancer treatment and patient quality of life, increasing breast cancer mortality by 20–50 %, and competing cause mortality by up to sixfold. The large influence of comorbidities on competing cause mortality suggests that early stage breast cancer patients are more likely to die from competing causes than from breast cancer, and that addressing comorbid conditions effectively will be important to further gains in improving breast cancer prognosis. Research is needed to understand how effective control of comorbid conditions, as an interplay of management approach, choice of medications used, and patient adherence to treatment of comorbid conditions, affects breast cancer treatment, quality of life, breast cancer prognosis, and competing cause mortality, and reciprocally, how a diagnosis of breast cancer affects comorbid conditions, their management, and control. The influence of specific comorbidities and various management approaches used to treat these conditions, including choice of medications used, also needs to be evaluated. These questions are particularly important for African Americans, older women, and women of lower socioeconomic status (SES) who bear higher comorbidity burdens, experience worse breast cancer prognosis, and potentially utilize health care differently compared to the general population. Studies aimed at understanding the pattern of comorbid conditions among breast cancer patients, the larger set of lifestyle and biological risk factors contributing to these conditions, and their impact on quality-of-life and competing cause mortality in these women will be strengthened by including comparison samples of women without a history of breast cancer with similar burdens of comorbidity. This knowledge, particularly the interplay of factors that contribute to the various breast cancer outcomes, and how relationships between breast cancer treatment, quality-of-life, breast cancer prognosis, and competing risk mortality are potentially modified by comorbidity and their management will be instrumental in reducing disparities in disease prognosis experienced by breast cancer patients with comorbidities

Patnaik et al. 2011b; Land et al. 2012a, b; Berglund et al. 2012; Bush et al. 2011). In a US population of older breast cancer patients, women with stage 1 tumor and a comorbid condition had similar or poorer overall survival compared with patients with stage 2 cancer and no comorbid conditions (Patnaik et al. 2011a). In a cohort of ~125,000 breast cancer patients aged 65 years of age or older, diagnosed between 1992 and 2005 residing in 11 Surveillance, Epidemiology, and End Results (SEER) areas, the prevalence of 16 comorbidities that contribute to the Charlson Comorbidity Index was considerable with 32.2 % of women having 1 or more conditions, similar to the prevalence (31.8 %) observed among women without breast cancer receiving Medicare benefits (Edwards et al. 2013). Most women with 1 or more comorbid condition fell into the severe comorbidity group, which referred to illnesses, such as congestive heart failure and chronic renal failure that often led to organ failure or systemic dysfunction requiring adjustments in cancer treatment. Moderate comorbidity referred to conditions such as diabetes and vascular disease that sometimes required modifying cancer treatment, while low comorbidity referred to conditions that usually did not require adjustments to cancer treatment. Among women aged 66–74 years in this cohort, the probability of dying from breast cancer among those with severe comorbidities was twofold higher (6 % vs 3 %) than in women without any comorbidities if diagnosed with local cancer, and 37 % higher (20.2 % vs 14.7 %) if diagnosed with regional cancer. The probability of dying from other causes in this same group of women was substantially raised, with probabilities of dying from other causes observed at 23.3 %, 10.6 %, and 5.1 % among women with severe, low/moderate, and no comorbidities, respectively. As expected, women diagnosed with distant stage disease were most likely to die of their breast cancers (≥69 %) regardless of their comorbidity status, although non-breast cancer related deaths still accounted for 5 to 20 % of deaths in this group. These findings reported in the 2014 Annual Report to the Nation on the Status of Cancer (Edwards et al. 2013) underscore previous findings that breast cancer patients with one or more comorbidities are at substantially increased risk of death from competing causes and at modestly increased risk of breast cancer specific death (Sogaard et al. 2013; Patnaik et al. 2011b; Land et al. 2012a, b; Berglund et al. 2012; Bush et al. 2011), and that breast cancer survivors who are most likely to be impacted by comorbidities are women with early stage breast cancer who have high other cause mortality, who have shown little or modest improvements in breast cancer specific mortality over time (Edwards et al. 2013; Cronin-Fenton et al. 2007; Land et al. 2012a; Izano et al. 2014). Findings from over 15 retrospective cohort studies (Cronin-Fenton et al. 2007; Tammemagi et al. 2005; Yancik et al. 2001a; Schonberg et al. 2010; Carlsen et al. 2008; Dalton et al. 2007; Janssen-Heijnen et al. 2005; Louwman et al. 2005, Houterman et al. 2004; Nagel et al. 2004; Maskarinec et al. 2003; Du et al. 2008; Harris et al. 2008; McPherson et al. 2002; Siegelmann-Danieli et al. 2006) suggest that comorbidity increases risk of competing cause mortality by up to sixfold, while breast cancer specific mortality is increased by 20–50 % (Patnaik et al. 2011a; Berglund et al. 2012; Schonberg et al. 2010; Dalton et al. 2007; Du et al. 2008), although some studies have failed to observe differences in breast cancer recurrence or survival (Tammemagi et al. 2005; Braithwaite et al. 2012; Field et al. 2011).

The larger influence of comorbidities on competing cause mortality compared to breast cancer mortality suggests that most early stage breast cancer patients with comorbidities will die from competing causes before they die of breast cancer, and that the former is a larger contributor to the disparities in overall mortality observed among these women (Ring et al. 2011). This understanding points to the overall importance of addressing comorbid conditions appropriately if further gains are to be made in improving overall survival among breast cancer patients. To date, most studies examining breast cancer outcomes have focused on breast cancer related deaths to the exclusion of competing causes of deaths. Given that most breast cancer patients are diagnosed at an early stage disease due to better screening efforts, and are expected to have good disease prognosis due to advancements in breast cancer treatments, greater understanding of factors contributing to high competing-cause mortality in breast cancer patients needs to become an important research priority (Cho et al. 2013). It should be noted, however, that although comorbidities in early stage breast cancer patients contributes to higher mortality rates among breast cancer survivors, these women are no more likely than the general United States population to die from other conditions (Cho et al. 2013). This comparison, however, may mask the true impact of comorbidities among early stage breast cancer patients (who often find their cancers through screening), since these women may be more likely to engage in healthy behaviors, have higher socioeconomic status, and show greater access to health care, including routine physician monitoring for existing comorbid conditions compared to the general population (Cho et al. 2013; Bush et al. 2011). Even among older women in the SEER-Medicare database, women diagnosed with DCIS or stage 1 breast cancer have slightly lower mortality than non-cancer controls (Schonberg et al. 2011). Early stage breast cancer patients should instead be compared to patients without breast cancer who participate in breast cancer screening programs to determine if early stage breast cancer patients are more likely to die from other conditions compared to a similar group of women without breast cancer. If death rates are found to be higher, this might suggest that further improvements to overall mortality in these patients can be made by reducing deaths due to other causes among women with early stage disease.

The potential long-term impact of comorbidities in combination with a diagnosis of breast cancer on non-breast cancer deaths are also not well understood in relation to the general population. Very few prior studies include comparisons to women without a history of breast cancer (Ording et al. 2013; Cho et al. 2013; Schonberg et al. 2011; Snyder et al. 2013; Hanchate et al. 2010), and virtually none have matched on comorbidity status to help understand potential differences in the long-term impact of comorbidities in combination with a diagnosis of breast cancer in comparison to women in the general population with the same comorbidity (Ording et al. 2013). Studies including a well-characterized comparison group with extended follow-up will help to elucidate key groups at excess risk for poor outcomes among breast cancer survivors.

Effect of Comorbidities During and After Breast Cancer Treatment

Comorbidities may reduce breast cancer specific survival, in part, by reducing the likelihood that these patients receive guideline recommended treatment (Land et al. 2012b, c; Vulto et al. 2006; Jagsi et al. 2009, 2010; Bouchardy et al. 2007; Harlan et al. 2009; Ring 2010; Kimmick et al. 2014; Sabatino et al. 2014; Shayne et al. 2006), which in turn, is linked to higher rates of breast cancer recurrence (Lash et al. 2000). The impact is likely to be strongest among those with early stage breast cancer since the likelihood of a cure is highest in these women and more dependent on treatment decisions. Generally, as comorbidity increases, treatment intensity decreases, including decreased ability to complete prescribed chemotherapy treatments (Lee et al. 2011). Findings from previous studies show that breast cancer patients with comorbidities are less likely to receive surgery, axillary dissections if undergoing breast-conserving surgery, radiotherapy, and adjuvant chemotherapy (Louwman et al. 2005; Griffiths et al. 2014; Vulto et al. 2006; Jagsi et al. 2009, 2010; Harlan et al. 2009; Ring 2010; Kimmick et al. 2014; Sabatino et al. 2014; Land et al. 2012c; Shayne et al. 2006; Bouchardy et al. 2007; Velanovich et al. 2002; Stavrou et al. 2012; Dialla et al. 2012; Garg et al. 2009; Ballard-Barbash et al. 1996). Comorbidities have also been shown to predict nonadherence to tamoxifen and aromatase inhibitors (Hershman et al. 2010), although not in all studies (Hadji et al. 2013). Certain comorbidities, including congestive heart failure, chronic obstructive pulmonary disease, osteoarthritis, autoimmune disease, liver dysfunction, renal disease, and thyroid disorder can elevate risk of developing chemotherapy-induced febrile neutropenia (Chia et al. 2013; Chao et al. 2014; Hosmer et al. 2011), which can lead to chemotherapy dose delays and dose reductions (Shayne et al. 2006; Garg et al. 2009). Pre-existing comorbidities can also increase risk of treatment associated comorbidities. For instance, cardiac dysfunction, diabetes, and hypertension are all associated with greater risk of anthracycline cardiotoxicity (Lotrionte et al. 2013). An important unanswered research question is whether treatment intensity can be safely increased in those with comorbidities and by how much, and whether variations exist according to the type of comorbidity.

Guidelines for the treatment of breast cancer are mostly developed on the basis of findings from clinical trials that exclude patients with moderate and severe comorbidities, to examine the impact of breast cancer treatments without the effect of other health conditions that may interfere with treatment or increase the risk of death. These exclusions mean that participants in randomized controlled trials are generally healthier than the general population. As a result, there are limited data available on the impact of comorbidities on treatment complications among breast cancer patients and the underlying reasons for failure to complete treatment. A recent study, for instance, that evaluated the impact of self-reported comorbidities among older women receiving adjuvant chemotherapy for breast cancer while in the CALGB 49907 and CALGB 361004 clinical trials found comorbidity to be associated with shorter overall survival, but not with toxicity or time to relapse (Klepin et al. 2014), possibly because these women all had good functional status with less severe comorbidity at the time of enrollment since eligible patients could not have a medical condition that would make the protocol hazardous (Klepin et al. 2014). Greater understanding of the degree to which various comorbidities affect breast cancer treatment and ultimately breast cancer survival is a research priority, and can be addressed through both observational studies as well as randomized trials designed to more broadly examine the potential impact of new breast cancer treatments across the entire targeted patient population.

There are very limited data on the effect of breast cancer and its treatment on the development of newly diagnosed comorbidities, and whether these incident comorbidities are associated with poorer outcomes than in a comparable population without a history of breast cancer. Only a few studies have followed breast cancer patients longitudinally and assessed comorbidities at more than one time point. Harlan and colleagues (Harlan et al. 2009) reported that breast cancer patients who received chemotherapy alone, chemotherapy plus radiation or radiation plus tamoxifen were 2–3 times more likely to develop newly diagnosed comorbidities after breast cancer diagnosis than women who did not receive radiation, chemotherapy, or tamoxifen, with arthritis, hypertension and osteoporosis being among those commonly reported (Harlan et al. 2009). A study of 1,361 five year breast cancer survivors aged 65 and older compared to women without breast cancer for a 10 year follow-up period, found that comorbidities included in the Charlson Comorbidity Index were not more likely to develop in breast cancer patients compared to age-matched women free of breast cancer, although breast cancer patients were slightly more likely to die in the 10 year follow-up period beginning 5 years after diagnosis (Jordan et al. 2014), suggesting perhaps for a role for more common comorbidities not represented in the Charlson Comorbidity Index. These findings point to a need to examine the impact of comorbidities on breast cancer treatment and outcomes more broadly, beyond those represented in the commonly used Charlson Comorbidity Index.

Impact of Type of Comorbidities

To date most studies examining the link between comorbidities and breast cancer outcomes have been based on population-based cancer registry data linked with administrative health insurance claims data, with many studies taking advantage of data from the SEER-Medicare database. While these studies have been instrumental for determining the prevalence of comorbidity among older women and their impact on survival outcomes, they have largely focused on the impact of a few select comorbidities available in these databases. The most widely used of these indices is the Charlson Comorbidity Index, along with several adaptations of the Charlson Comorbidity Index, including the National Cancer Institute Comorbidity Index (Klabunde et al. 2007). A few studies have also used the Adult Comorbidities Evaluation Index (ACE-27) (Kimmick et al. 2014; Fleming et al. 2011), which considers a greater number of comorbidities than the Charlson Comorbidity Index and unlike most measures of comorbidity, considers the severity of each condition with three grades of decompensation (Kallogjeri et al. 2014). The ACE-27 method also captures obesity comorbidity, hypertension, and a wider range of cardiovascular diseases not captured by Charlson that may be particularly relevant to breast cancer outcomes. Despite differences in the number, type, and severity of comorbid conditions captured, however, the Charlson and ACE-27 indices perform similarly in predicting 2 year overall survival in cancer patients, and models including both indices produced better predictive models (Kallogjeri et al. 2014). Direct comparisons between the Charlson Comorbidity Index and ACE-27, however, have not been made for breast cancer patients and future research can be directed at testing the predictive ability of these comorbidity measures individually and together on various breast cancer outcomes.

The Charlson score was originally developed in 1987 using medical records to predict 1 year mortality among hospitalized patients, and was later shown to predict risk of death from comorbid disease in a 10 year follow-up study (Charlson et al. 1987). Reflecting the original intent of the index to predict short-term mortality, the 16 comorbidities that contribute to the Charlson Comorbidity Score tend to be more severe, requiring hospitalization, and include myocardial infarction, congestive heart failure, peripheral vascular disease, cerebrovascular disease, dementia, chronic obstructive pulmonary disease, connective tissue disease, peptic ulcer disease, type 2 diabetes, chronic renal disease, paralysis, malignant lymphoma, solid tumor, liver disease and acquired immunodeficiency syndrome (AIDS). Comorbidities are assigned a weight between 1 and 6, reflecting likelihood of dying from the disease. This was later expanded to incorporate physician claims in addition to inpatient data from Medicare files since most individuals will have comorbidities that do not require hospitalization. This allowed improved prediction of non-cancer mortality and treatment choice for breast cancer patients after development of condition weights specific for breast cancer (Klabunde et al. 2000). While the Charlson Comorbidity Index has been repeatedly shown to be a valid prognostic predictor among breast cancer patients, the index is based on underlying assumptions more relevant to short term mortality risk, with very few patients actually having a high Charlson Index score in most early stage breast cancer populations. Consequently, an important limitation of the Charlson Index is that the score tends to classify a large proportion of breast cancer patients as having no comorbid conditions. Nevertheless, the hypertension-augmented comorbidity index, an extension of the Charlson index, has been shown to be a significant predictor of overall survival, breast cancer specific, and competing cause survival in breast cancer patients (Braithwaite et al. 2009). Also, given dramatic improvements in the prognosis of individuals with AIDS in the past 20 years, the need for reappraising how AIDS is weighted in the Charlson Comorbidity Index has been raised (Zavascki and Fuchs 2007). This reassessment may be particularly important in breast cancer studies focused on women with higher relative incidence of positive HIV status and AIDS, such as young African Americans (Center for Disease Control, *HIV surveillance report* 2010).

Conceivably, certain comorbidities may have different effects on breast cancer treatment, quality-of-life, and survival outcomes (Louwman et al. 2005; Braithwaite et al. 2009). Very little research to date has assessed associations between individual comorbid conditions and their impact on breast cancer prognosis (Patnaik et al. 2011a, b; Yancik et al. 2001b), and whether these relationships might be modified by other prognostic factors such as estrogen receptor status or tumor subtypes. Studies that have examined specific comorbidities have largely focused on comorbidities contributing to the Charlson Comorbidity Index (Patnaik et al. 2011a, b; Yancik et al. 2001b). Patnaik et al. (2011a) showed in a large cohort of >63,000 breast cancer cases, using SEER-Medicare linked data, that breast cancer patients with any of the comorbidities comprising the Charlson Comorbidity Index had lower survival rates compared to patients with no comorbidities, and that liver disease, chronic renal failure, dementia, and congestive heart failure were associated with the highest all-cause mortality, while cardiovascular disease, COPD, and diabetes, specifically raised breast cancer deaths by 10–25 % (Patnaik et al. 2011a, b), presumably due to less intensive treatment and/or to direct biologic effects, e.g. diabetes is associated with reduced likelihood of receiving chemotherapy and increased glucose and insulin which have been associated with poorer outcomes (Goodwin et al. 2012; Gold et al. 2014; Peairs et al. 2011).

Generally, cancer patients who report more comorbid conditions report lower quality of life, including poorer physical and mental health (Smith et al. 2008). Specific comorbidities have been shown to increase adverse effects of breast cancer therapy although most of this research has focused on the effects of obesity and related cardiovascular risk factors (Schmitz et al. 2013). Diabetes for instance is a risk factor for paclitaxel neuropathy and increased risk of neuropathic pain following breast surgery (Lee and Swain 2006; Wilson et al. 2013). Hypertension and obesity are risk factors for development of heart failure with trastuzumab, and development of postoperative lymphedema, fatigue and worse functional health (Schmitz et al. 2013; Helyer et al. 2010; Perez et al. 2008).

The effects of specific comorbid conditions on various breast cancer endpoints, including quality of life, needs to be further examined, although, going forward, comorbidities considered should be expanded beyond those in the Charlson Comorbidity Index to include major chronic health conditions that are highly prevalent in the United States' population (US Burden of Disease Collaborators 2013) and among breast cancer patients (Piccirillo et al. 2008; Sarfati et al. 2013), including obesity, high blood pressure, diabetes, metabolic syndrome, cardiovascular disease, respiratory disease, and psychiatric diseases. Such research may be aided by recent development of the Chronic Condition Warehouse (Centers for Medicare and Medicaid Services, *Chronic Condition Warehouse, accessed 10/11/14*), which combines Medicare, Medicaid, and Part D Prescription Drug Events data and makes these datasets available for research. The Chronic Conditions Warehouse was designed to support studies on improving care for chronically ill beneficiaries and contains 27 annual chronic condition flags indicating the presence of specific diagnostic codes on Medicare claims. These include chronic conditions such as asthma, anemia, depression, Alzheimer's, hyperlipidemia, osteoporosis, arthritis, and diabetes. Understanding which comorbid conditions have the greatest impact on breast cancer specific outcomes may provide insights into common etiological risk factors shared between the comorbidity and breast cancer, and suggest improved management strategies that offer the best gains in disease outcomes.

Use of Cancer Registry and Administrative Claims Data to Study Comorbidities

While use of cancer registry and administrative claims data has helped to define the link between comorbidities and breast cancer outcomes at the population level, the scope of questions that can be posed in studying the effects of comorbidity on breast cancer is constrained by a number of limitations inherent in these databases (Riley 2009). Presently cancer registries do not routinely collect data on comorbidities, although for some populations, these data can be obtained by linking with Medicare or Medicaid data, hence the popularity of using linked SEER-Medicare data. Secondly, as discussed above, a very limited number of comorbid conditions are usually considered and many of the more common, minor, chronic conditions are not assessed. Development of the Chronic Condition Warehouse linking Medicare and Medicaid data, however, can help facilitate the study of how common chronic conditions impact cancer outcomes. Other challenges include examining the impact of disease duration and severity, which is difficult to gauge because changes in claims for a specific comorbidity may be a function of payment rules rather than variability of the comorbidity over time. Incident disease in claims databases are hard to identify, and limited availability of clinical information in these databases means that the underlying reason for service and outcomes are unavailable. Some conditions, particularly less severe ones, tend to be under-diagnosed and under-reported in insurance claim data, and comorbidities might be missed if only inpatient care is considered. These include conditions such as osteoporosis, dementia, arthritis, and low back pain, which are usually treated in outpatient settings, are not associated with short-term mortality, and often do not require hospitalization. Patient movement in and out of insurance claims databases may also limit the utility of these data for prospective comorbidity studies, making populations who do not have continuous health coverage difficult to study.

If using Medicare data, one problem with studying women close to age 65 will be that these women have less "at risk" time to appear in Medicare claims. One study found that 12 % of people enrolled in Medicare at age 65 waited more than 2 years before making their first use of Part B services, which includes medically necessary services and preventive services (Sloan et al. 2012). Use of SEER-Medicare data also excludes examination of comorbidities among women who are diagnosed with breast cancer at younger ages, who are more likely to have aggressive estrogen receptor negative breast cancers. SEER areas are also known to have lower proportions of Caucasians, to be more urbanized, and to have fewer people living in poverty, which may make findings less generalizable (Warren et al. 2002).

Future studies on the impact of comorbidities on breast cancer treatment and outcomes will need to use study approaches that complement findings obtained by studying large administrative databases, which have not been able to provide data on the impact of comorbidities on treatment delivery, complications, toxicities, and patient tolerance of treatments, nor on quality-of-life in these women. Some of these questions can only be answered with prospective studies of breast cancer patients.

Findings from these studies will be able to provide information on the duration and severity of comorbidities that affect cancer treatment and outcomes, and how these relationships are potentially modified by management and control of coexisting conditions. Such studies will also be able to address potential confounders, including functional status and lifestyle factors such as smoking, diet, and physical activity that are not available in most administrative databases. Thus to improve research on the impact of comorbidity on breast cancer outcomes, an expansion of study approach is needed along with collection of information from a greater number of data sources. This includes the use of survey data, administrative data, detailed clinical data, prescription records, and patient medical records from all health care providers.

Research Priorities

Management and Control of Comorbidities and Impact on Breast Cancer Outcomes

The majority of breast cancer patients have at least one chronic disease condition at the time of diagnosis, but management of these conditions may be overlooked during survivorship care, leading to poorer outcomes (Weaver et al. 2013). Consequently, an important research priority will be to determine whether adequate management and control of comorbid conditions among breast cancer patients is associated with greater likelihood of receiving guideline-recommended breast cancer treatment, better quality-of-life, and better survival outcomes, including better breast cancer survival as well as competing cause survival. Studies, including those using a randomized clinical trial design, are needed to assess the importance of primary care physician involvement in the care of breast cancer patients with co-morbidities to ensure that co-morbidities are optimally diagnosed and managed, and to facilitate collaborative care between the oncologist and primary care provider (Oeffinger and McCabe 2006) as an essential component of survivorship planning identified in the 2005 Institute of Medicine report From Cancer Patient to Cancer Survivor: Lost in Transition (Hewitt et al. 2005). Studies using administrative data suggest that breast cancer survivors who see both their oncologist and primary care providers are more likely to receive preventive health services such as cholesterol screening, mammograms, and flu vaccination (Snyder et al. 2009), and breast cancer patients who have 5–10 primary care physician visits in the 2 year period prior to their breast cancer diagnosis have lower breast cancer mortality and all-cause mortality compared to those who had 0 or 1 primary care physician visit, which was only partly explained by greater use of screening mammography (Fisher et al. 2013).

The management and control of traditional risk factors for cardiovascular disease and their impact on breast cancer outcomes will be particularly important to understand since individuals diagnosed with early stage breast cancer will more often die of cardiovascular disease than from breast cancer recurrence (Patnaik et al. 2011b; Weaver et al. 2013), and cardiovascular risk factors, including obesity, hypertension, and diabetes are more common among breast cancer survivors than the general population (Weaver et al. 2013). These comorbidities may be particularly important among African American women, who have high rates of obesity, hypertension and diabetes, and may account for some of the survival disparity observed between African American and Caucasian women (Tammemagi et al. 2005; Braithwaite et al. 2009; Polednak 2004).

A related research priority will be to understand how breast cancer impacts the care and control of comorbid conditions, which may include increasing non-adherence to chronic disease medications. In a study of 1,393 women with breast cancers who were also statin users (Calip et al. 2013), the percent of women who were adherent with statin use was 67 % prior to breast cancer diagnosis, fell to 52 % during the breast cancer treatment period, and remained low in the years that followed breast cancer treatment. Similarly, the percent of women adherent with use of oral type 2 diabetes medications declined from 75 % prior to breast cancer diagnosis to 25 % during breast cancer treatment, and rose up to 32 % three years post treatment, but never returned to baseline levels. This coincided with declines in glycemic control, with the proportion of women with percent glycosylated hemoglobin levels (HbA1C) ≤ 7 dropping from 65 % in the year prior to diagnosis to 52 % during treatment and 45 % three years post-treatment (Calip et al. 2014). Compared to adherent users during the breast cancer treatment period, non-adherent users of oral diabetes medications tended to have higher stage breast cancers, were more likely to have been treated with chemotherapy, and were more likely to have ≤ 1 visit to their primary care provider within the year following breast cancer diagnosis.

A few studies have examined whether breast cancer modifies management of comorbid conditions among older adults. A recent study found no differences between breast cancer survivors and age-matched controls, with breast cancer survivors appearing to have similar or better quality of care (Hanchate et al. 2010). Snyder and colleagues using the national SEER-Medicare database found that breast cancer survivors received care comparable to non-cancer controls for both chronic and acute conditions using indicators of care quality (Snyder et al. 2013). The study, however, using administrative data was only able to look at the frequency of visits to health care providers and could not simultaneously assess the degree to which the condition was medically controlled. Less is understood of the impact of breast cancer on management of comorbid condition in more disadvantaged groups, who tend to have higher burdens of comorbidities and simultaneously less access to health care. Also, whether breast cancer survivors receive comparable chronic disease care compared to women with similar disease burdens is not clear because comorbidity has not been consistently used as a matching variable in most studies (Earle et al. 2003). A large study of >23,000 breast cancer survivors compared to comorbidity controls (i.e. Chronic obstructive pulmonary disease, congestive heart failure, diabetes) using SEER-Medicare data, did find that survivors were more likely to receive preventive care, which included cholesterol screening and influenza vaccination (Snyder et al. 2009). Generally breast cancer survivors as a group receive high-quality health care, at least among older adults with Medicare, with breast cancer patients displaying enhanced participation in the health care system. Nevertheless, inequities still exist according to race and socioeconomic status and it is not clear if breast cancer impacts health care utilization differently in these groups, and in younger breast cancer survivors, who may have more limited access to health care compared to older adults with Medicare.

Potential Independent Effects of Medications

An important research priority will be to delineate the mechanism through which better medication adherence for chronic conditions might improve breast cancer outcomes, i.e. whether through better control of the comorbid condition, direct effects of these medications on pathways implicated in breast cancer progression, and/or better compliance with breast cancer medications/treatment as an extension of good medication adherence for pre-existing chronic conditions. This is particularly important given emerging evidence that a number of commonly prescribed medications for chronic conditions may have direct beneficial effects on breast cancer outcomes, possibly by modulating pathways necessary for breast cancer progression (Holmes and Chen 2012; Vaklavas et al. 2011; Vendramini-Costa and Carvalho 2012; Vinayak and Kurian 2009; Bo et al. 2012). For example, metformin for treatment of type II diabetes may improve insulin and other metabolic parameters that have been associated with poor breast cancer outcomes (Goodwin et al. 2012); the effect of metformin on breast cancer outcomes and on co-morbidities is being examined in a fully accrued Phase III trial of 3,649 women with early stage breast cancer (Goodwin et al. 2011), and has been associated with reduced breast cancer mortality in population-based studies (Zhang et al. 2013; Hou et al. 2013). Other medications that may improve breast cancer outcomes include angiotensin-converting-enzyme (ACE) inhibitors and angiotensin receptor blockers for the treatment of hypertension and diabetic nephropathy (Mc Menamin et al. 2012; Barron et al. 2011), statins for the management of dyslipidemia (Holmes and Chen 2012; Ahern et al. 2011; Kwan et al. 2008; Nickels et al. 2013), and aspirin and NSAIDs for treatment of inflammatory conditions (Holmes and Chen 2012; Kwan et al. 2007; Blair et al. 2007). This raises the possibility that use of these medications for management of comorbidities may have direct beneficial effects on breast cancer outcomes. Thus, comprehensive assessments are needed to simultaneously evaluate the potential beneficial effects of specific medications against the benefits of achieving good control of the comorbid condition to determine their relative importance in improving breast cancer outcomes. To minimize the possibility that specific medications are erroneously identified as potentially benefiting breast cancer outcomes, it may be necessary in future studies to include adjustments for guideline-concordant breast cancer treatment as a potential confounder (Kimmick et al. 2014). For some conditions, such as hypertension, better guideline concordance for breast cancer treatment is observed, possibly because these individuals have better access to health care rather than because they achieved better control of their condition, and this in turn may confound associations suggesting that antihypertensive use improves breast cancer diagnosis (Kimmick et al. 2014).

Comorbidities Among Susceptible Populations

The role of comorbidities on breast cancer outcomes is likely to be most important for older patients, minorities, particularly African Americans, and women of lower socioeconomic status, because these women have greater comorbidity burdens than the general population, are least likely to receive guideline concordant treatment for their breast cancer (Kimmick et al. 2014), and have poorer disease prognosis (Albain et al. 2009; Aizer et al. 2014). Hence, improvements to breast cancer outcomes potentially achieved by better management of comorbid conditions will likely be greatest among these women, making them a research priority.

The potential impact of comorbidities on breast cancer outcomes is important for older women since comorbidities become more common with increasing age, resulting in reduced life expectancy. At the same time, older women are at increased risk of recurrence from breast cancer, which may be due in part to the larger tumor sizes found in older women and greater probability of undertreatment due in part to comorbid conditions (Ring et al. 2011; Bouchardy et al. 2007). While a number of studies have examined the impact of comorbidity on breast cancer outcomes in older women, relatively few have examined the role of comorbidity as a mediator for the survival disparity between younger and older breast cancer survivors. A recent study of 553 women with metastatic breast cancer found that both hypertension and higher Charlson Comorbidity Scores were related to worse overall survival, with hypertension explaining much of the survival disparities observed between young and older women (Jung et al. 2012). If better comorbidity control is indeed linked to better breast cancer outcomes in future studies, older breast cancer patients might be more likely to make positive changes in health behaviors compared to younger women, and may be most likely to benefit from improved care as younger patients may survive many years regardless of health behavior and adherence to comorbidity treatment (Bush et al. 2011).

African American women may be another group that is strongly impacted by comorbidities since these women are more likely to have sub-optimally managed comorbidities because of low medication adherence (Kyanko et al. 2013; Bosworth et al. 2008), which may decline further during breast cancer treatment (Calip et al. 2013, 2014). African American breast cancer patients have more breast cancer recurrence/progression and worse all-cause, breast cancer specific and competing cause survival. A cohort study from the Henry Ford Health System (Tammemagi et al. 2005) that followed women for a median of 10 years found that over 85 % of African American had one or more comorbidities at the time of breast cancer diagnosis, and several studies have found that comorbidity explains 25–50 % of the overall survival disparity observed between African Americans and Caucasian breast cancer patients (Tammemagi et al. 2005; Eley et al. 1994). Among African Americans, comorbidities related to cardiovascular disease, such as hypertension and diabetes, seem to be particularly important in explaining racial disparities in overall breast cancer survival (Tammemagi et al. 2005; Braithwaite et al. 2009). This is important given recent findings that hypertension may be independently related to overall and breast cancer specific mortality (Braithwaite et al. 2012; Jung et al. 2012), an effect that can be attenuated when adjusted for antihypertensive medication (Braithwaite et al. 2012) suggesting that control of comorbidities may modify associations between comorbidities and breast cancer outcomes. Among 416 African-American and 838 White women diagnosed with breast cancer in the Kaiser Permanente Northern California Medical Care Program, Braithwaite and colleagues (2009) found that even after accounting for the effects of age, tumor characteristics and breast cancer treatment, high blood pressure was associated with 60 % increased risk of recurrence and 49 % increased risk of breast cancer specific deaths among African Americans with non-significant effects among Whites, and that this single comorbidity explained 30 % of racial disparities in all-cause mortality and 20 % of racial disparities in breast cancer specific survival. While these findings were adjusted for breast cancer treatment, future studies will need to determine if reductions in treatment intensity, such as chemotherapy dose delays and dose reductions, can explain these survival disparities.

Summary

Over the past decade the use of cancer registry and administrative claims data has helped to establish and define links between comorbidities and poorer breast cancer survival at the population level. Comorbidities have been associated with lower treatment intensities for breast cancer, and increases in overall, breast cancer specific, and competing cause mortality. Based on this knowledge, we are now poised to design comprehensive longitudinal studies to assess the clinical importance of adequate management and control of comorbid conditions on breast cancer treatment, quality-of-life, and breast cancer outcomes. A comprehensive assessment of the role of comorbidities before, during and after breast cancer diagnosis and treatment will be critical for developing strategies to improve breast cancer survival. Findings from such studies will fill current gaps in understanding of how comorbidities and their management affect breast cancer treatments and outcomes, and how relationships between breast cancer treatment, quality-of-life, breast cancer prognosis, and competing risk mortality are potentially modified by comorbidities. This understanding could have a major impact on advancing clinical approaches to breast cancer treatment and survivorship care, with the goal of further improving breast cancer and overall outcomes. Greater understanding of these relationships may be particularly relevant among older women, African Americans, and women of lower socioeconomic status since these women generally have poorer disease prognosis and higher rates of comorbid conditions.

References

Ahern TP, Pedersen L, Tarp M et al (2011) Statin prescriptions and breast cancer recurrence risk: a Danish nationwide prospective cohort study. J Natl Cancer Inst 103(19):1461–1468

Aizer AA, Wilhite TJ, Chen MH et al (2014) Lack of reduction in racial disparities in cancer-specific mortality over a 20-year period. Cancer 120(10):1532–1539

Albain KS, Unger JM, Crowley JJ et al (2009) Racial disparities in cancer survival among randomized clinical trials patients of the Southwest Oncology Group. J Natl Cancer Inst 101(14):984–992

Ballard-Barbash R, Potosky AL, Harlan LC et al (1996) Factors associated with surgical and radiation therapy for early stage breast cancer in older women. J Natl Cancer Inst 88(11):716–726

Barron TI, Connolly RM, Sharp L et al (2011) Beta blockers and breast cancer mortality: a population- based study. J Clin Oncol 29(19):2635–2644

Berglund A, Wigertz A, Adolfsson J et al (2012) Impact of comorbidity on management and mortality in women diagnosed with breast cancer. Breast Cancer Res Treat 135(1):281–289

Berrino F, Villarini A, Traina A et al (2014) Metabolic syndrome and breast cancer prognosis. Breast Cancer Res Treat 147(1):159–165

Blair CK, Sweeney C, Anderson KE et al (2007) NSAID use and survival after breast cancer diagnosis in post-menopausal women. Breast Cancer Res Treat 101(2):191–197

Bo S, Benso A, Durazzo M et al (2012) Does use of metformin protect against cancer in Type 2 diabetes mellitus? J Endocrinol Invest 35(2):231–235

Bosworth HB, Powers B, Grubber JM et al (2008) Racial differences in blood pressure control: potential explanatory factors. J Gen Intern Med 23(5):692–698

Bouchardy C, Rapiti E, Blagojevic S et al (2007) Older female cancer patients: importance, causes, and consequences of undertreatment. J Clin Oncol 25(14):1858–1869

Braithwaite D, Tammemagi CM, Moore DH et al (2009) Hypertension is an independent predictor of survival disparity between African-American and white breast cancer patients. Int J Cancer 124(5):1213–1219

Braithwaite D, Moore DH, Satariano WA et al (2012) Prognostic impact of comorbidity among long-term breast cancer survivors: results from the LACE study. Cancer Epidemiol Biomarkers Prev 21(7):1115–1125

Bush D, Smith B, Younger J et al (2011) The non-breast-cancer death rate among breast cancer patients. Breast Cancer Res Treat 127(1):243–249

Calip GS, Boudreau DM, Loggers ET (2013) Changes in adherence to statins and subsequent lipid profiles during and following breast cancer treatment. Breast Cancer Res Treat 138(1):225–233

Calip GS, Hubbard RA, Stergachis A et al (2014) Adherence to oral diabetes medications and glycemic control during and following breast cancer treatment. Pharmacoepidemiol Drug Saf. doi:10.1002/pds.3660

Carlsen K, Hoybye MT, Dalton SO et al (2008) Social inequality and incidence of and survival from breast cancer in a population-based study in Denmark, 1994-2003. Eur J Cancer 44(14):1996–2002

Center for Disease Control, HIV surveillance report, 2010. http://www.cdc.gov/hiv/topics/surveillance/resources/reports. Accessed 11 Oct 2014

Centers for Medicare and Medicaid Services, Chronic Condition Warehouse. https://www.ccw-data.org/web/guest/home. Accessed 11 Oct 2014

Chao C, Page JH, Yang SJ et al (2014) History of chronic comorbidity and risk of chemotherapy-induced febrile neutropenia in cancer patients not receiving G-CSF prophylaxis. Ann Oncol 25(9):1821–1829

Charlson ME, Pompei P, Ales KL et al (1987) A new method of classifying prognostic comorbidity in longitudinal studies: development and validation. J Chronic Dis 40(5):373–383

Chia VM, Page JH, Rodriguez R et al (2013) Chronic comorbid conditions associated with risk of febrile neutropenia in breast cancer patients treated with chemotherapy. Breast Cancer Res Treat 138(2):621–631

Cho H, Mariotto AB, Mann BS et al (2013) Assessing non-cancer-related health status of US cancer patients: other-cause survival and comorbidity prevalence. Am J Epidemiol 178(3):339–349

Cronin-Fenton DP, Norgaard M, Jacobsen J et al (2007) Comorbidity and survival of Danish breast cancer patients from 1995 to 2005. Br J Cancer 96(9):1462–1468

Dalton SO, Ross L, During M et al (2007) Influence of socioeconomic factors on survival after breast cancer–a nationwide cohort study of women diagnosed with breast cancer in Denmark 1983–1999. Int J Cancer 121(11):2524–2531

Dialla PO, Dabakuyo TS, Marilier S et al (2012) Population-based study of breast cancer in older women: prognostic factors of relative survival and predictors of treatment. BMC Cancer. doi:10.1186/1471-2407-12-472

Du XL, Fang S, Meyer TE (2008) Impact of treatment and socioeconomic status on racial disparities in survival among older women with breast cancer. Am J Clin Oncol 31(2):125–132

Earle CC, Burstein HJ, Winer EP et al (2003) Quality of non-breast cancer health maintenance among elderly breast cancer survivors. J Clin Oncol 21(8):1447–1451

Edwards BK, Noone AM, Mariotto AB et al (2013) Annual Report to the Nation on the status of cancer, 1975-2010, featuring prevalence of comorbidity and impact on survival among persons with lung, colorectal, breast, or prostate cancer. Cancer 120(9):1290–1314

Eley JW, Hill HA, Chen VW et al (1994) Racial differences in survival from breast cancer. Results of the National Cancer Institute Black/White Cancer Survival Study. JAMA 272(12):947–954

Field TS, Bosco JL, Prout MN et al (2011) Age, comorbidity, and breast cancer severity: impact on receipt of definitive local therapy and rate of recurrence among older women with early-stage breast cancer. J Am Coll Surg 213(6):757–765

Fisher KJ, Lee JH, Ferrante JM et al (2013) The effects of primary care on breast cancer mortality and incidence among Medicare beneficiaries. Cancer 119(16):2964–2972

Fleming ST, Sabatino SA, Kimmick G et al (2011) Developing a claim-based version of the ACE-27 comorbidity index: a comparison with medical record review. Med Care 49(8):752–760

Garg P, Rana F, Gupta R et al (2009) Predictors of toxicity and toxicity profile of adjuvant chemotherapy in elderly breast cancer patients. Breast J 15(4):404–408

Gold HT, Makarem N, Nicholson JM et al (2014) Treatment and outcomes in diabetic breast cancer patients. Breast Cancer Res Treat 143(3):551–570

Goodwin PJ, Stambolic V, Lemieux J et al (2011) Evaluation of metformin in early breast cancer: a modification of the traditional paradigm for clinical testing of anti-cancer agents. Breast Cancer Res Treat 126(1):215–220

Goodwin PJ, Ennis M, Pritchard KI et al (2012) Insulin- and obesity-related variables in early-stage breast cancer: correlations and time course of prognostic associations. J Clin Oncol 30(2):164–171

Griffiths RI, Gleeson ML, Valderas JM et al (2014) Impact of undetected comorbidity on treatment and outcomes of breast cancer. Int J Breast Cancer. doi:10.1155/2014/970780

Guh DP, Zhang W, Bansback N et al (2009) The incidence of co-morbidities related to obesity and overweight: a systematic review and meta-analysis. BMC Public Health. doi:10.1186/1471-2458-9-88

Hadji P, Ziller V, Kyvernitakis J et al (2013) Persistence in patients with breast cancer treated with tamoxifen or aromatase inhibitors: a retrospective database analysis. Breast Cancer Res Treat 138(1):185–191

Hair BY, Hayes S, Tse CK et al (2014) Racial differences in physical activity among breast cancer survivors: implications for breast cancer care. Cancer 120(14):2174–2182

Hanchate AD, Clough-Gorr KM, Ash AS et al (2010) Longitudinal patterns in survival, comorbidity, healthcare utilization and quality of care among older women following breast cancer diagnosis. J Gen Intern Med 25(10):1045–1050

Harlan LC, Klabunde CN, Ambs AH et al (2009) Comorbidities, therapy, and newly diagnosed conditions for women with early stage breast cancer. J Cancer Surviv 3(2):89–98

Harris EE, Hwang WT, Urtishak SL et al (2008) The impact of comorbidities on outcomes for elderly women treated with breast-conservation treatment for early-stage breast cancer. Int J Radiat Oncol Biol Phys 70(5):1453–1459

Helyer LK, Varnic M, Le LW et al (2010) Obesity is a risk factor for developing postoperative lymphedema in breast cancer patients. Breast J 16(1):48–54

Hershman DL, Kushi LH, Shao T et al (2010) Early discontinuation and nonadherence to adjuvant hormonal therapy in a cohort of 8,769 early-stage breast cancer patients. J Clin Oncol 28(27):4120–4128

Hewitt M, Greenfield S, Stovall E (2005) From cancer patient to cancer survivor: lost in transition. National Academies Press, Washington, DC

Holmes MD, Chen WY (2012) Hiding in plain view: the potential for commonly used drugs to reduce breast cancer mortality. Breast Cancer Res 14(2):216

Hosmer W, Malin J, Wong M (2011) Development and validation of a prediction model for the risk of developing febrile neutropenia in the first cycle of chemotherapy among elderly patients with breast, lung, colorectal, and prostate cancer. Support Care Cancer 19(3):333–341

Hou G, Zhang S, Zhang X et al (2013) Clinical pathological characteristics and prognostic analysis of 1,013 breast cancer patients with diabetes. Breast Cancer Res Treat 137(3):807–816

Houterman S, Janssen-Heijnen ML, Verheij CD et al (2004) Comorbidity has negligible impact on treatment and complications but influences survival in breast cancer patients. Br J Cancer 90(12):2332–2337

Hutchins LF, Unger JM, Crowley JJ et al (1999) Underrepresentation of patients 65 years of age or older in cancer-treatment trials. N Engl J Med 341(27):2061–2067

Izano M, Satariano WA, Tammemagi MC et al (2014) Long-term outcomes among African-American and white women with breast cancer: what is the impact of comorbidity? J Geriatr Oncol 5(3):266–275

Jagsi R, Abrahamse P, Morrow M et al (2009) Postmastectomy radiotherapy for breast cancer: patterns, correlates, communication, and insights into the decision process. Cancer 115(6):1185–1193

Jagsi R, Abrahamse P, Morrow M et al (2010) Patterns and correlates of adjuvant radiotherapy receipt after lumpectomy and after mastectomy for breast cancer. J Clin Oncol 28(14):2396–2403

Janssen-Heijnen ML, Houterman S, Lemmens VE et al (2005) Prognostic impact of increasing age and co-morbidity in cancer patients: a population-based approach. Crit Rev Oncol Hematol 55(3):231–240

Jordan JH, Thwin SS, Lash TL et al (2014) Incident comorbidities and all-cause mortality among 5-year survivors of Stage I and II breast cancer diagnosed at age 65 or older: a prospective-matched cohort study. Breast Cancer Res Treat 146(2):401–409

Jung SY, Rosenzweig M, Linkov F et al (2012) Comorbidity as a mediator of survival disparity between younger and older women diagnosed with metastatic breast cancer. Hypertension 59(2):205–211

Kallogjeri D, Gaynor SM, Piccirillo ML et al (2014) Comparison of comorbidity collection methods. J Am Coll Surg 219(2):245–255

Kimmick G, Fleming ST, Sabatino SA et al (2014) Comorbidity burden and guideline-concordant care for breast cancer. J Am Geriatr Soc 62(3):482–488

Klabunde CN, Potosky AL, Legler JM et al (2000) Development of a comorbidity index using physician claims data. J Clin Epidemiol 53(12):1258–1267

Klabunde CN, Legler JM, Warren JL et al (2007) A refined comorbidity measurement algorithm for claims-based studies of breast, prostate, colorectal, and lung cancer patients. Ann Epidemiol 17(8):584–590

Klepin HD, Pitcher BN, Ballman KV et al (2014) Comorbidity, chemotherapy toxicity, and outcomes among older women receiving adjuvant chemotherapy for breast cancer on a clinical trial: CALGB 49907 and CALGB 361004 (Alliance). J Oncol Pract 10(5):e285–e292

Kwan ML, Habel LA, Slattery ML et al (2007) NSAIDs and breast cancer recurrence in a prospective cohort study. Cancer Causes Control 18(6):613–620

Kwan ML, Habel LA, Flick ED et al (2008) Post-diagnosis statin use and breast cancer recurrence in a prospective cohort study of early stage breast cancer survivors. Breast Cancer Res Treat 109(3):573–579

Kyanko KA, Franklin RH, Angell SY (2013) Adherence to chronic disease medications among New York City Medicaid participants. J Urban Health 90(2):323–328

Land LH, Dalton SO, Jensen MB et al (2012a) Impact of comorbidity on mortality: a cohort study of 62,591 Danish women diagnosed with early breast cancer, 1990–2008. Breast Cancer ResTreat 131(3):1013–1020

Land LH, Dalton SO, Jorgensen TL et al (2012b) Comorbidity and survival after early breast cancer. A review. Crit Rev Oncol Hematol 81(2):196–205

Land LH, Dalton SO, Jensen MB et al (2012c) Influence of comorbidity on the effect of adjuvant treatment and age in patients with early-stage breast cancer. Br J Cancer 107(11):1901–1907

Lash TL, Silliman RA, Guadagnoli E et al (2000) The effect of less than definitive care on breast carcinoma recurrence and mortality. Cancer 89(8):1739–1747

Lee JJ, Swain SM (2006) Peripheral neuropathy induced by microtubule-stabilizing agents. J Clin Oncol 24(10):1633–1642

Lee L, Cheung WY, Atkinson E et al (2011) Impact of comorbidity on chemotherapy use and outcomes in solid tumors: a systematic review. J Clin Oncol 29(1):106–117

Lotrionte M, Biondi-Zoccai G, Abbate A et al (2013) Review and meta-analysis of incidence and clinical predictors of anthracycline cardiotoxicity. Am J Cardiol 112(12):1980–1984

Louwman WJ, Janssen-Heijnen ML, Houterman S et al (2005) Less extensive treatment and inferior prognosis for breast cancer patient with comorbidity: a population-based study. Eur J Cancer 41(5):779–785

Maskarinec G, Pagano IS, Yamashiro G et al (2003) Influences of ethnicity, treatment, and comorbidity on breast cancer survival in Hawaii. J Clin Epidemiol 56(7):678–685

Mc Menamin UC, Murray LJ, Cantwell MM et al (2012) Angiotensin-converting enzyme inhibitors and angiotensin receptor blockers in cancer progression and survival: a systematic review. Cancer Causes Control 23(2):221–230

McPherson CP, Swenson KK, Lee MW (2002) The effects of mammographic detection and comorbidity on the survival of older women with breast cancer. J Am Geriatr Soc 50(6):1061–1068

Nagel G, Wedding U, Rohrig B et al (2004) The impact of comorbidity on the survival of postmenopausal women with breast cancer. J Cancer Res Clin Oncol 130(11):664–670

Nickels S, Vrieling A, Seibold P et al (2013) Mortality and recurrence risk in relation to the use of lipid-lowering drugs in a prospective breast cancer patient cohort. PLoS One 8(9):e75088

Oeffinger KC, McCabe MS (2006) Models for delivering survivorship care. J Clin Oncol 24(32):5117–5124

Ording AG, Cronin-Fenton DP, Jacobsen JB et al (2013) Comorbidity and survival of Danish breast cancer patients from 2000-2011: a population-based cohort study. Clin Epidemiol 5(Suppl 1):39–46

Patnaik JL, Byers T, Diguiseppi C et al (2011a) The influence of comorbidities on overall survival among older women diagnosed with breast cancer. J Natl Cancer Inst 103(14):1101–1111

Patnaik JL, Byers T, DiGuiseppi C et al (2011b) Cardiovascular disease competes with breast cancer as the leading cause of death for older females diagnosed with breast cancer: a retrospective cohort study. Breast Cancer Res 13(3):R64

Peairs KS, Barone BB, Snyder CF et al (2011) Diabetes mellitus and breast cancer outcomes: a systematic review and meta-analysis. J Clin Oncol 29(1):40–46

Perez EA, Suman VJ, Davidson NE et al (2008) Cardiac safety analysis of doxorubicin and cyclophosphamide followed by paclitaxel with or without trastuzumab in the North Central Cancer Treatment Group N9831 adjuvant breast cancer trial. J Clin Oncol 26(8):1231–1238

Piccirillo JF, Vlahiotis A, Barrett LB et al (2008) The changing prevalence of comorbidity across the age spectrum. Crit Rev Oncol Hematol 67(2):124–132

Polednak AP (2004) Racial differences in mortality from obesity-related chronic diseases in US women diagnosed with breast cancer. Ethn Dis 14(4):463–468

Riley GF (2009) Administrative and claims records as sources of health care cost data. Med Care 47(7 Suppl 1):S51–S55

Ring A (2010) The influences of age and co-morbidities on treatment decisions for patients with HER2-positive early breast cancer. Crit Rev Oncol Hematol 76(2):127–132

Ring A, Sestak I, Baum M et al (2011) Influence of comorbidities and age on risk of death without recurrence: a retrospective analysis of the Arimidex, Tamoxifen alone or in combination trial. J Clin Oncol 29(32):4266–4272

Sabatino SA, Thompson TD, Wu XC et al (2014) The influence of diabetes severity on receipt of guideline-concordant treatment for breast cancer. Breast Cancer Res Treat 146(1):199–209

Sarfati D, Gurney J, Lim BT et al (2013) Identifying important comorbidity among cancer populations using administrative data: prevalence and impact on survival. Asia Pac J Clin Oncol. doi:10.1111/ajco.12130

Schmitz KH, Neuhouser ML, Agurs-Collins T et al (2013) Impact of obesity on cancer survivorship and the potential relevance of race and ethnicity. J Natl Cancer Inst 105(18):1344–1354

Schonberg MA, Marcantonio ER, Li D et al (2010) Breast cancer among the oldest old: tumor characteristics, treatment choices, and survival. J Clin Oncol 28(12):2038–2045

Schonberg MA, Marcantonio ER, Ngo L et al (2011) Causes of death and relative survival of older women after a breast cancer diagnosis. J Clin Oncol 29(12):1570–1577

Shayne M, Crawford J, Dale DC et al (2006) Predictors of reduced dose intensity in patients with early-stage breast cancer receiving adjuvant chemotherapy. Breast Cancer Res Treat 100(3):255–262

Siegelmann-Danieli N, Khandelwal V, Wood GC et al (2006) Breast cancer in elderly women: outcome as affected by age, tumor features, comorbidities, and treatment approach. Clin Breast Cancer 7(1):59–66

Sloan FA, Acquah KF, Lee PP et al (2012) Despite 'welcome to Medicare' benefit, one in eight enrollees delay first use of part B services for at least two years. Health Aff (Millwood) 31(6):1260–1268

Smith AW, Reeve BB, Bellizzi KM et al (2008) Cancer, comorbidities, and health-related quality of life of older adults. Health Care Fin Rev 29(4):41–56

Snyder CF, Frick KD, Kantsiper ME et al (2009) Prevention, screening, and surveillance care for breast cancer survivors compared with controls: changes from 1998 to 2002. J Clin Oncol 27(7):1054–1061

Snyder CF, Frick KD, Herbert RJ et al (2013) Quality of care for comorbid conditions during the transition to survivorship: differences between cancer survivors and noncancer controls. J Clin Oncol 31(9):1140–1148

Sogaard M, Thomsen RW, Bossen KS et al (2013) The impact of comorbidity on cancer survival: a review. Clin Epidemiol 5(Suppl 1):3–29

Stavrou EP, Lu CY, Buckley N et al (2012) The role of comorbidities on the uptake of systemic treatment and 3-year survival in older cancer patients. Ann Oncol 23(9):2422–2428

Tammemagi CM, Nerenz D, Neslund-Dudas C et al (2005) Comorbidity and survival disparities among black and white patients with breast cancer. JAMA 294(14):1765–1772

US Burden of Disease Collaborators (2013) The state of US health, 1990-2010: burden of diseases, injuries, and risk factors. JAMA 310(6):591–608

Vaklavas C, Chatzizisis YS, Tsimberidou AM (2011) Common cardiovascular medications in cancer therapeutics. Pharmacol Ther 130(2):177–190

Velanovich V, Gabel M, Walker EM et al (2002) Causes for the undertreatment of elderly breast cancer patients: tailoring treatments to individual patients. J Am Coll Surg 194(1):8–13

Vendramini-Costa DB, Carvalho JE (2012) Molecular link mechanisms between inflammation and cancer. Curr Pharm Des 18(26):3831–3852

Vinayak S, Kurian AW (2009) Statins may reduce breast cancer risk, particularly hormone receptor-negative disease. Curr Breast Cancer Rep 1(3):148–156

Vulto AJ, Lemmens VE, Louwman MW et al (2006) The influence of age and comorbidity on receiving radiotherapy as part of primary treatment for cancer in South Netherlands, 1995 to 2002. Cancer 106(12):2734–2742

Warren JL, Klabunde CN, Schrag D et al (2002) Overview of the SEER-Medicare data: content, research applications, and generalizability to the United States elderly population. Med Care 40(8 Suppl):IV-3-18

Weaver KE, Foraker RE, Alfano CM et al (2013) Cardiovascular risk factors among long-term survivors of breast, prostate, colorectal, and gynecologic cancers: a gap in survivorship care? J Cancer Surviv 7(2):253–261

Wilson GC, Quillin RC 3rd, Hanseman DJ et al (2013) Incidence and predictors of neuropathic pain following breast surgery. Ann Surg Oncol 20(10):3330–3334

Yancik R, Ganz PA, Varricchio CG et al (2001a) Perspectives on comorbidity and cancer in older patients: approaches to expand the knowledge base. J Clin Oncol 19(4):1147–1151

Yancik R, Wesley MN, Ries LA et al (2001b) Effect of age and comorbidity in postmenopausal breast cancer patients aged 55 years and older. JAMA 285(7):885–892

Zavascki AP, Fuchs SC (2007) The need for reappraisal of AIDS score weight of Charlson comorbidity index. J Clin Epidemiol 60(9):867–868

Zhang P, Li H, Tan X et al (2013) Association of metformin use with cancer incidence and mortality: a meta-analysis. Cancer Epidemiol 37(3):207–218

Chapter 12
Modifiable Lifestyle Factors and Breast Cancer Outcomes: Current Controversies and Research Recommendations

Pamela J. Goodwin, Christine B. Ambrosone, and Chi-Chen Hong

Abstract Lifestyle factors, particularly obesity, have been associated with poor breast cancer outcomes in a large number of observational studies. Despite a growing body of research, controversy exists regarding obesity associations across breast cancer subtypes and the importance of obesity versus physical activity and dietary composition in determining breast cancer outcome. These controversies are reviewed and the complex biologic nature of the association of obesity with breast cancer addressed. Potential mediators, including insulin, estrogens, adipokines and inflammation markers are identified. Relevant prognostic findings of previous research involving dietary, physical activity and weight loss interventions are summarized. A broad-based program of research is outlined, highlighting the need for a randomized trial of weight loss that is adequately powered to examine survival effects, as well as correlative and preclinical research to investigate mediators and mechanisms of obesity effects on breast cancer outcomes. Finally, potential contributions of alcohol intake and tobacco use in breast cancer survivors are discussed.

Keywords Breast cancer • Obesity • Subtype • Prognosis • Diet • Exercise • Research priorities • Biologic mediators

P.J. Goodwin, M.D., M.Sc., F.R.C.P.C. (✉)
Lunenfeld-Tanenbaum Research Institute, Mount Sinai Hospital, University of Toronto, 1284-600 University Avenue, Toronto, ON M5G 1X5, Canada
e-mail: pgoodwin@mtsinai.on.ca

C.B. Ambrosone, Ph.D. • C.-C. Hong, Ph.D.
Department of Cancer Prevention and Control, Division of Cancer Prevention and Population Sciences, Roswell Park Cancer Institute, Elm St, Buffalo, NY 14263, USA
e-mail: christine.ambrosone@roswellpark.org; chi-chen.hong@roswellpark.org

© Breast Cancer Research Foundation 2015
P.A. Ganz (ed.), *Improving Outcomes for Breast Cancer Survivors*,
Advances in Experimental Medicine and Biology 862,
DOI 10.1007/978-3-319-16366-6_12

Introduction

Women diagnosed with breast cancer often ask whether there are any lifestyle changes they can make that will improve their breast cancer outcomes, over and above the benefits of standard medical therapy. There is increasing evidence that patients who have a healthier lifestyle, notably those who maintain a normal weight and are more physically active, may have better outcomes than those who have less healthy lifestyles. Breast cancer diagnosis and treatment has been considered a "teachable moment," (Demark-Wahnefried et al. 2005) a time when women are more receptive to lifestyle change; if outcomes could be improved as a result of these changes, this may represent an untapped opportunity for clinically significant benefit. In this article, our primary focus will be on obesity-associated variables (BMI, physical activity, diet), however, we will also briefly discuss two additional lifestyle attributes (alcohol intake and tobacco exposure) that are of interest to breast cancer survivors; tobacco exposure is of particular concern as it can increase risk of second primary cancers.

A key scientific issue in the area of lifestyle and breast cancer outcome relates to the tension between the modest prognostic associations of lifestyle factors that have been seen in observational studies and the paucity of data from randomized trials supporting beneficial effects of adoption of a healthier lifestyle post-diagnosis. The modestly better outcomes associated with healthier lifestyles (typically a relative improvement of 25–50 %) (Protani et al. 2010) are in a range that could reflect bias and/or confounding; as a result it cannot be concluded that the observed associations are causal. Even if causal, it is not clear whether adoption of a healthier lifestyle post diagnosis will improve outcomes, or whether effects of unhealthy lifestyles are reflected in more aggressive tumor characteristics at diagnosis that have fixed effects on outcome. Data from well-designed and conducted, adequately powered, randomized trials that test whether adoption of a healthier lifestyle improves outcome, would overcome this tension. Such trials present serious challenges in term of feasibility, cost and duration but their conduct would generate sufficiently rigorous evidence that lifestyle change can be recommended to patients. These trials may also identify improvements in non-cancer outcomes, such as cardiovascular disease (the commonest cause of death in breast cancer survivors beyond 10 years post-diagnosis), or in quality of life. The latter may be sufficient for some survivors to adopt a healthier lifestyle in the absence of effects on breast cancer outcomes. Inclusion of a spectrum of outcomes, including overall survival, will be important in any planned trials.

In this article, we briefly review the evidence linking these traditional lifestyle factors to outcome in breast cancer survivors, highlighting areas of controversy. We focus on key research priorities and challenges in this area, outlining potential strategies for moving forward.

Current Controversies Relating to Body Size and Breast Cancer Outcome

Obesity was first reported to be associated with poor breast cancer outcomes in 1976 (Abe et al. 1976). Since then, over 50 studies have examined this association and obesity has become a recognized adverse prognostic factor. Recent meta-analyses (Protani et al. 2010; Chan et al. 2014; Niraula et al. 2012) that included studies published up to 2011 have provided evidence that the risk of breast cancer specific or overall mortality is increased by one-third or more in women who are obese compared to those who are normal weight. BMI measured 1 year after diagnosis may be more strongly associated with outcomes that BMI measured closer to diagnosis (HR 1.29, HR 1.17 respectively per 5 kg/m^2) (Chan et al. 2014). Obesity at diagnosis has been associated with poor outcomes regardless of menopausal status or hormone receptor status in these meta-analyses (Niraula et al. 2012). Results of some studies have provided evidence that the association of body mass index (BMI) with prognosis may be curvilinear (Goodwin et al. 2002; Suissa et al. 1989). The greatest increase in mortality is seen in women with BMI $\geq$ 30 kg/m^2; there is a more modest increase in mortality in those with BMI under 18–20 kg/m^2. The basis for an adverse association of underweight is poorly understood; it is possible that it may reflect subclinical metastatic disease, although there is no evidence to support this contention.

Although the associations of BMI with breast cancer outcomes were similar in the observational studies and randomized trials included in these meta-analyses, recent post hoc analyses conducted in large, cooperative group randomized clinical trials (RCTs), have yielded inconsistent results (see Table 12.1), and some investigators have suggested that obesity associations may be present only in women with hormone receptor positive breast cancer (Pan et al. 2014; Sparano et al. 2012). If correct, this would have implications for potential weight loss intervention trials in breast cancer survivors and for the selection of participants and identification of subgroup hypotheses to be tested in such trials.

Recent RCT based analyses of prognostic associations of BMI in ER+ breast cancer include reports that high BMI was associated with poor outcome in the ATAC and BIG 1-98 trials (Sestak et al. 2010; Ewertz et al. 2012) which involved only women with ER+ breast cancer receiving tamoxifen or aromatase inhibitors. Analysis of completed ECOG (E1199, E5188) (Sparano et al. 2012) and NSABP studies (B30, B38) (Cecchini et al. 2013) as well as a recent meta-analysis conducted by the Early Breast Cancer Clinical Trialists Collaborative Group (Pan et al. 2014) also identified an increased risk of recurrence or death in obese (vs. non-obese) women with hormone receptor positive breast cancer (premenopausal only in the latter). A meta-analysis involving 8,874 women enrolled onto seven German adjuvant trials identified adverse prognostic associations of BMI in hormone receptor positive cases (Pajares et al. 2013). These results are consistent with results of earlier meta-analyses (Niraula et al. 2012).

Results of similar post hoc RCT analyses in women with hormone receptor negative, triple negative or HER2 positive breast cancer have been less consistent. North American investigators, using data from both ECOG (Sparano et al. 2012)

Table 12.1 Recent inconsistent results of BMI—prognostic associations

Citations		Setting	n	Results
HR-				
Pajares et al. (2013)	2013	GEICAM RCTS (all anthracycline)	1,502	Worse OS, BCS if BMI > 35
Cecchini et al. (2013)	2013	NSABP RCTs	Not stated	No difference in recurrence, OS by BMI
Pan et al. (2014)	2014	EBCTCG	19,618	No difference in BCS
TN				
Turkoz et al. (2013)	2013	Non RCT (Turkey)	193	Worse DFS, OS in obese
Sparano et al. (2012)	2012	ECOG RCTs (all anthracycline)	878	No difference in DFS, OS by BMI
Fontanella et al. (2013)	2013	Neoadjuvant RCTs (Germany)	1,570	Lower pCR, worse DFS, OS in obese (BSA capped at 2.0 m² in 3 of 7 trials)
HER2+				
Turkoz et al. (2013)	2013	Non RCT (Turkey)	238	No difference in DFS, OS by BMI
Pajares et al. (2013)	2013	GEICAM RCTs	830	Worse OS if BMI > 35 n/s Worse BCS if BMI > 35
Crozier et al. (2013)	2013	RCT (N9031)	3,017	DFS worse in OW, OB
Mazzarella et al. (2013)	2013	Non RCT (Italy)	1,250	ER neg: OS, DFS worse in OB ER pos: No difference in OS, DFS
Sparano et al. (2012)	2012	ECOG RCTS	940	No difference in DFS, OS

Abbreviations: RCT = randomized clinical trial; OS = overall survival; BCS = breast cancer survival; pCR = pathologic complete response; DFS = disease free survival; BSA = body surface area; n/s = non significant; ER = estrogen receptor; neg = negative; pos = positive; BMI = body mass index; ECOG = Eastern Oncology Co-operative Group; GEICAM = Spanish Breast Cancer Research Group; EBCTCG = Early Breast Cancer Trialists Co-operative Group; NSABP = National Surgical Adjuvant Breast and Bowel Project

and NSABP (Cecchini et al. 2013) RCTs (E3189, B30, B31, B34, B38) failed to identify significant prognostic associations of BMI in those with hormone receptor negative breast cancer. In contrast, Fontanella et al. (2013) identified adverse prognostic associations of obesity in women with triple negative breast cancers participating in a group of German neoadjuvant RCTs (chemotherapy dose was capped at 2.0 m² in three of these trials; this may have contributed to adverse obesity associations) while Pajares et al. (2013) identified worse overall and breast cancer specific survival in triple negative breast cancer patients with BMI > 35 kg/m² enrolled in a series of GEICAM RCTs. In HER2 positive patients, a significantly worse outcome in heavier women with HER2+ breast cancer was identified in two RCTs; (Pajares et al. 2013; Crozier et al. 2013) in an observational study, Mazzarella et al. (2013) identified a similar association that was present only when cancers were also estrogen receptor negative. In contrast, Sparano et al. (2012) and Turkoz et al. (2013)

identified no associations of BMI with disease-free or overall survival in women with HER2+ breast cancer enrolled onto RCTs or an observational study.

In summary, adverse associations of BMI with breast cancer outcomes have been repeatedly reported in all breast cancer subtypes. It is not clear whether the inconsistency of recent data may relate to differences in study design (discussed below) or to true biologic differences in BMI associations across breast cancer subtypes. The latter should be explored in preclinical studies and in adequately powered clinical datasets that include a full, and representative, spectrum of breast cancer patients.

The more consistent results reported in ER+ breast cancer may reflect, at least in part, higher estrogen levels in obese postmenopausal women, leading to enhanced signaling through estrogen pathways in obese women. Because BMI is associated with prognosis in women receiving tamoxifen and aromatase inhibitors (Sestak et al. 2010; Ewertz et al. 2012), these treatments do not appear to fully overcome effects of higher BMI, suggesting that other obesity associated factors, such as insulin or inflammatory mediators, contribute to the BMI-prognosis association in these patients.

The less consistent results in triple negative breast cancer in particular may reflect capping of BMI at arbitrary levels (e.g. $2.0\ m^2$, $2.2\ m^2$) when calculating chemotherapy doses [a practice that has been less common in recent years and avoided in modern RCTs and advised against in a recent American Society of Clinical Oncology guideline (Lyman and Sparreboom 2013)], leading to BMI associations that reflect under-treatment rather than biologic effects in earlier studies. This practice may have had the greatest impact in triple negative breast cancer in which chemotherapy is the primary adjuvant approach, and targeted treatments, which may overcome effects of under-dosing to some extent, are not available. The observation that BMI is associated with prognosis in recent cohorts and RCTs that avoided dose capping suggest these factors do not fully account for BMI associations. One alternative explanation is that the underlying aggressiveness of advanced triple negative breast cancers in some studies, leading to poor outcomes, may be associated with reduced prognostic impact of obesity.

Different temporal patterns of relapse of ER+, triple negative and HER2+ breast cancers and differing durations of follow-up in reported studies are unlikely to be the primary cause of inconsistent results—for example, our group has demonstrated that obesity effects are constant in periods up to 5 years, and 5–10 years and beyond in a long-term prospective study (Goodwin et al. 2012).

Inclusion of locoregional events (which contribute a greater proportion of events in the modern era of breast conserving therapy and effective systemic adjuvant therapies) in outcome measures in recent trials may have introduced noise and led to reduced power in some studies as these events have not been associated with BMI (Ewertz et al. 2012). The analysis of BMI as a categorical (vs. continuous) variable in statistical analyses, or the modelling of associations as linear (vs. quadratic which allows a curvilinear association which has been demonstrated in several studies) may also have reduced power. Importantly, power to detect associations may have been lower in subsets of receptor negative, triple negative and HER2+ breast cancer, due to smaller numbers of these cancers in some RCTs.

It is also possible that unappreciated differences in the study populations contributed to inconsistencies. Many of the earlier observational studies were population or institution based and included all women diagnosed with breast cancer, regardless of the presence or absence of associated medical conditions. Many recent RCTs involved cardiotoxic medications (e.g. anthracyclines, HER-2 targeted agents) and women with cardiac morbidity (or cardiac risk factors such as hypertension, dyslipidemia, diabetes) were commonly excluded, either explicitly through entry criteria or as a safety precaution by physicians (and patients) wanting to avoid cardiotoxicity of unproven treatments. In trials involving taxanes, women with diabetes were often excluded because of the need for steroid pre-medications; they may also have been less likely to be enrolled because of concerns about neurotoxicity. Cardiovascular disease, dysglycemia, hyperlipidemia and hypertension are components of the insulin resistance (or metabolic) syndrome; (Alberti et al. 2009) physiologic components of this syndrome (e.g. insulin, glucose, inflammation) may mediate the association of obesity with breast cancer outcomes (see below) and it is possible these recent trials preferentially enrolled metabolically healthy women who do not have the physiologic attributes that mediate obesity-breast cancer associations. This selection process has not been investigated in a breast cancer population, however, Kramer et al. (2013) have shown that obese individuals in the general population with any one of hypertension, abnormal lipids, central obesity, abnormal glucose/ diabetes or high C-reactive protein (CRP—a marker of inflammation) have significantly higher greater levels of insulin resistance [reflected by homeostasis model assessment (HOMA) scores] than those who do not have any of these attributes. This issue is of relevance not only to understanding the inconsistency of recent reports; it could also impact the design of weight loss intervention trials in breast cancer survivors. If adverse associations of BMI are present only in metabolically unhealthy women, such trials should be designed to enrich for this population.

Thus, although the associations of obesity with outcome may truly differ across breast cancer subtypes, adverse associations have been repeatedly identified in all subtypes. Design differences across studies may have contributed to the identified inconsistencies.

Obesity Versus Physical Activity

Body size reflects the net balance of energy intake vs. energy expenditure. Energy expenditure occurs as a result of resting metabolism, dietary thermogenesis and physical activity—changes in the latter (occupational and/or recreational) can help to regulate body size. Understanding the relative contribution of obesity vs. physical activity has potential implications for intervention research and patient care—for example, is physical activity in the presence of overweight or obesity sufficient to improve breast cancer outcomes? Overweight women who are physically active have cardiovascular outcomes similar to normal weight women—is the same true for breast cancer prognosis?

The association of physical activity, undertaken either before or after breast cancer diagnosis, with breast cancer specific or overall mortality has been examined in over 15 studies. Ballard-Barbash et al. (2012) recently reviewed this evidence. Modest, largely non-significant associations of pre-diagnosis physical activity with reduced breast cancer specific or overall mortality were identified (the point estimate of the HR of death was between 0.5 and 1 in virtually all studies). A somewhat larger proportion of studies reported greater physical activity post-diagnosis to be associated with reduced overall mortality; again, HRs were in the range of 0.5–1 and were not always significantly different from 1. There was little evidence that physical activity associations differed by menopausal status, tumor stage, hormone receptor status, comorbidity, race or ethnicity, or BMI (although variable BMI subgroup effects have been reported, with stronger and weaker effects seen in obese women in different studies). The available data are not sufficient to conclude a causal association exists. They may reflect (1) greater physical activity in otherwise healthy women (reverse causation bias), (2) a recall bias when physical activity is reported years after breast cancer diagnosis, or (3) adverse effects of more toxic therapy given to women with higher risk of recurrence leading to lower levels of physical activity, rather than a causal effect of physical activity on breast cancer outcomes.

Small randomized trials of physical activity in breast cancer survivors have demonstrated beneficial effects of physical activity on quality of life, treatment toxicity and fitness. Some have examined effects of physical activity on a number of biomarkers. Consistent improvements (significant or marginally significant) have been seen in biomarkers of the insulin pathway (including insulin-like growth factor-1) after physical activity interventions; these improvements may be greatest in obese and/or sedentary women. Weaker effects have been seen on markers of inflammation (CRP or interleukin-6) and circulating levels of markers of cell mediated immunity. In one trial that compared effects of physical activity alone versus dietary restriction with or without physical activity in healthy women, changes in key biomarkers postulated to mediate the obesity-breast cancer prognosis association (insulin, hsCRP, estrogens) were significantly greater in either dietary intervention arm were greater than in the physical activity only arms (e.g. insulin and estrogen decreased >20 vs. <5 %), suggesting dietary restriction leading to weight loss may be key to the link with breast cancer outcomes (Mason et al. 2011; Imayama et al. 2012; Campbell et al. 2012; Abbenhardt et al. 2013).

These observations suggest that physical activity may be most relevant as a contributor to weight management (where it may be most important in maintenance of weight loss) rather than as an independent predictor of outcome, however, they do not preclude an independent effect, particularly in women who are metabolically healthy but overweight, in whom changes in the metabolic factors discussed above may not be key mediators of a physical activity-prognosis association. Future observational and intervention research into physical activity associations with breast cancer outcomes should be prospective, use validated comprehensive assessments of physical activity, and should examine potential contributions of different types (e.g. aerobic, resistance), intensity and duration of physical activity. This research should include embedded correlative studies that prospectively examine effects of physical activity on key biomarkers (discussed below), notably insulin related factors (Ballard-Barbash et al. 2012; Lof et al. 2012), that may mediate physical activity associations with obesity and breast cancer outcomes. Finally, although sedentary behavior, independent of physical activity, may be associated with risk of some cancers (e.g. colorectal) sedentary behavior has not been examined in relation to breast cancer prognosis; this issue could also be addressed in prospective studies of physical activity.

Does Dietary Composition Contribute to Breast Cancer Outcomes?

Caloric intake exceeding energy expenditure contributes to obesity; reduction in caloric intake is a key component of weight loss interventions. It has also been suggested that dietary composition, particularly dietary fat content, may be linked to breast cancer outcomes, independent of total caloric intake. Two randomized trials (Chlebowski et al. 1992; Pierce et al. 2007) conducted in the mid to late 1990s examined the effects of (1) dietary fat reduction in isolation or (2) a complex dietary intervention that included reduction in fat intake, increases in fruits, vegetable and grains (See Table 12.2).

The Women's Intervention Nutrition Study (WINS) (Chlebowski et al. 1992) randomized 2,437 postmenopausal women within 1 year of breast cancer diagnosis to a 15 % fat diet or a control arm. At 12 months, intervention subjects lowered fat intake significantly and lost a mean of 2.1 kg (2.8 %) while control subjects gained

Table 12.2 Differing designs and results of the WINS vs. WHEL RCTs

	WINS (Chlebowski et al. 1992)		WHEL (Pierce et al. 2007)
Population			
Number	2,437		3,088
Enrollment period	Up to 1 year post diagnosis		Up to 4 years post diagnosis
Menopausal status	Post		Pre and post
Age	48–79		18–70
Intervention group			
Fat intake	Reduction maintained		Transient reduction
Weight change	2.3 kg (3.2 %) relative loss		Modest weight gain
DFS	All	HR 0.76 (0.60–0.98)	HR 0.96 (0.80–1.14)
	ER-	HR 0.58 (0.37–0.91)	
	ER+	HR 0.85 (0.63–1.14)	
	BMI < 25 kg/m^2	HR 0.83 (0.54–1.27)	
	BMI 25–30 kg/m^2	HR 0.77 (0.51–1.18)	
	BMI > 30 kg/m^2	HR 0.66 (0.41–1.0)	

Abbreviations: WINS = Women's Intervention Nutrition Study; WHEL = Women's Healthy Eating and Living Study; DFS = disease free survival; ER = estrogen receptor; BMI = body mass index; HR = hazard ratio a mean of 0.2 kg (0.3 %). At 60 months, a significant improvement in relapse-free survival was identified (HR 0.76, 95 % CI 0.6–0.98, 2-tailed p = 0.034) in women randomized to the reduced fat diet. In unplanned subset analyses, this effect appeared to be greatest in patients with ER- cancer (HR 0.58, 95 % CI 0.37–0.91, p = 0.018 vs. HR 0.85, 95 % CI 0.63–1.14, p = 0.277 in ER+ women) and in those with the highest BMI (HR 0.83, 95 % CI 0.54–1.27; HR 0.77, 95 % CI 0.51–1.18; HR 0.66, 95 % CI 0.41–1.0 for BMI < 25, 25–30 and $\geq$30 kg/m^2, respectively). In contrast, the Women's Healthy Eating and Living Study (WHEL) (Pierce et al. 2007) randomized 3,088 pre- and postmenopausal women up to 4 years post-diagnosis to a complex dietary intervention that included reduced intake of fat and increased intake of fruit, vegetables and grains. Effects of the intervention on diet were greater at 12 months than at 72 months. There was no evidence of weight loss in the intervention group and there was no effect of the intervention on disease-free (HR 0.96, 95 % CI 0.81–1.14) or overall survival (HR 0.91, 95 % CI 0.72–1.15) at 5 years.

Although there were multiple differences between these two studies, including the nature of the intervention and interval post diagnosis allowed for enrolment, both involved reduction in dietary fat and only the WINS study identified a significant benefit. It has been postulated that this may reflect the weight loss observed in women in the WINS study; it is also possible that early recurrences in ER negative women were missed in the WHEL study. The WINS intervention has not been incorporated into clinical practice; total caloric intake rather than fat intake has been the focus of more recent intervention research.

Observational research has failed to identify consistent associations of specific dietary composition (e.g. saturated vs. unsaturated fats, protein sources, types of carbohydrates and fiber) with breast cancer outcomes (Kampman et al. 2012). A recent analysis of diet quality in women participating in the Women's Health Initiative who developed breast cancer provided evidence that better diet quality was associated with reduced overall mortality and non-breast cancer related mortality; it was not associated with reduced breast cancer mortality (George et al. 2014). These results underscore the importance of differentiation of associations with breast cancer vs. non-breast cancer deaths is essential in lifestyle studies. Although improvement in overall survival in breast cancer survivors is clearly of interest, it is unlikely that the impact of diet composition on non-breast cancer related outcomes differs in these survivors compared to the general population. Confirmation of this would allow data generated in the general population to be applied to breast cancer survivors, at least in relation to non-breast cancer outcomes.

Biologic Mediators of the Obesity-Prognosis Association

The biologic basis for the obesity-cancer relationship is likely multifactorial, with inter-related contributions of multiple factors whose individual contributions may vary across breast cancer subtypes (Goodwin and Stambolic 2015). Enhanced insight into the biology of this association would advance understanding of the differential contributions of obesity, physical activity and excess caloric intake to breast cancer outcomes and it would contribute to resolution of controversies regarding differential effects in breast cancer subtypes. This insight will come from preclinical as well as clinical research, including RCTs of weight loss interventions.

Obesity is a complex physiologic state that is commonly associated with the metabolic syndrome (particularly when the obesity is centrally located). The metabolic syndrome (Alberti et al. 2009), also known as the insulin resistance syndrome, is characterized by high levels of insulin due to insulin resistance (insulin levels may fall after diagnosis of diabetes as the pancreas fails), dysglycemia (with frank hyperglycemia when diabetes is present), dyslipidemia (high total and LDL cholesterol, low HDL cholesterol), hypertension and a chronic inflammatory state (which is commonly evaluated using hsCRP, a systemic marker of chronic inflammation), however, these patterns are not present to the same extent in all overweight or obese individuals. Obesity is also associated with inflammation within adipose tissue (including in the breast) which may lead to high local levels of cytokines, adipokines (such as leptin) and other inflammatory factors (e.g., TNF-alpha), resulting in a pro-carcinogenic state; these factors may also be elevated systemically. Together, these factors activate many biologic processes associated with cancer progression (Goodwin and Stambolic 2015; Gilbert and Slingerland 2013), including growth pathways (e.g. PI3K, ras-raf-MAPK, JAK-STAT) and cell metabolism (e.g. shunt from oxidative phosphorylation to aerobic glycolysis, the Warburg effect). Many of these biologic correlates of obesity (e.g. insulin, glucose, insulin resistance reflected by HOMA, leptin, hsCRP) have been associated with poor breast cancer outcomes (Hazard Ratios for risk or recurrence or death of 1.5–3 after adjustment for traditional prognostic factors) and it is possible they interact to mediate the association of obesity with poor outcomes. Higher circulating estrogen levels present in obese postmenopausal women may also contribute to poor outcomes although their effects may be reduced by the administration of hormonal interventions such as tamoxifen and aromatase inhibitors.

Putting It All Together: Weight Loss Through Lifestyle Change

Recent focus has shifted from isolated dietary or physical activity interventions to more comprehensive interventions designed to promote weight loss through reduction in caloric intake, increases in physical activity and behavioral counselling to promote adherence to lifestyle change. Small intervention trials have demonstrated the feasibility of weight loss in breast cancer patients; face to face and remotely delivered (telephone, mail) interventions have been tested (Reeves et al. 2014; Goodwin et al. 2014; Rock et al. 2013). Both approaches lead to weight loss that is comparable to similar interventions in other populations (Pi-Sunyer et al. 2007)— the degree of weight loss is approximately 5 % using older approaches and up to 7–10 % using more intensive approaches developed in the last 5 years. A key concern in all of these interventions is maintenance of weight loss; in most studies there is modest regain beginning after the first year, although differences between intervention and control groups persist to 2 years and longer.

There is major interest in the conduct of well-designed and adequately powered trials that will formally test the impact of lifestyle based weight loss after breast cancer diagnosis on breast cancer outcomes. Two such trials are underway in Europe, one testing a lifestyle based approach to weight loss (Rack et al. 2010) and the other a Mediterranean diet (Villarini et al. 2012), however it is unclear whether they are adequately powered for breast cancer outcomes. Key issues in the design of such trials include the expected magnitude of weight loss given currently validated intervention approaches (and whether it is sufficient to impact breast cancer outcomes), the target population (e.g. inclusion of overweight vs. obese women only, incorporation of an attribute of poor metabolic health into inclusion criteria), the potential for differential effects in breast cancer subtypes as well as the optimal method of delivery of the intervention (in person, remote, web-based) and the intervention intensity and duration needed to achieve lasting weight loss (2 years is considered a minimum). Available data suggest that the degree of weight loss seen with intensive lifestyle interventions will result in changes in potential biologic mediators that could yield clinically relevant improvements in breast cancer outcomes. For example, a weight loss of 10 % has been associated with a reduction in insulin of 20–22 %; (Mason et al. 2011) if this proportionately reversed the reported association of insulin with breast cancer outcome (Goodwin et al. 2002) a clinically important 24 % reduction in relative risk of distant recurrence (HR 0.76) could be seen.

It is essential that weight loss intervention trials powered to examine effects on breast cancer outcomes include measurement of a full range of tumor characteristics including breast cancer subtype and evidence of activation of signaling pathways that may be targets of the altered physiology resulting from a weight loss intervention (e.g. PI3K pathway activation may reflect high insulin levels that can be reduced by weight loss) as well as obesity associated physiologic mediators. The resulting information would greatly enhance our understanding of the obesity—prognosis relationship. It might also facilitate the development of targeted therapies. Metformin is one such therapy that is being tested in the breast cancer adjuvant setting (Goodwin et al. 2011), based in part on its ability to lower insulin and other components of the insulin resistance syndrome that have been associated with poor breast cancer outcomes.

Despite the many challenges, it is essential that these trials be conducted in order to obtain high quality evidence for (or against) the benefits of weight loss in breast cancer patients that will lead to clear recommendations for breast cancer survivors and, ideally, to funding of effective lifestyle interventions by third party payers.

Obesity: Breast Cancer Research Priorities

Major research priorities include a range of observational, interventional, translational and preclinical research studies that would ideally be conducted in parallel, with the primary goal being to develop strategies that will improve breast cancer outcomes (see Table 12.3). The available evidence is sufficiently strong that the

Table 12.3 Obesity and breast cancer outcomes: five top research priorities

1. Association of obesity with prognosis across breast cancer subtypes/treatments
a. Modern prospective population/registry based studies that include subjects regardless of metabolic health—adequately powered across subtypes, with full data on key co-variates (tumor, treatment including BMI used for dosing, objectively measured height and weight), reliable data on outcomes (locoregional, distant recurrence, death including cause) and potential to examine associations over time post-diagnosis
b. Investigation of impact of RCT entry criteria related to cardiac disease, diabetes on metabolic profiles of selected individuals
2. Relative contributions of obesity and physical activity to breast cancer prognosis
a. Prospective prognostic studies including (i) serial, objective measurement of BMI, diet and physical activity (e.g. using accelerometers) in patients recruited at breast cancer diagnosis, (ii) full co-variate, treatment and outcome data (see #1) and (iii) inclusion of translational research into mediators/predictors of associations (collection of tumour tissue and serial blood samples)
b. Intervention research to examine effects of weight loss (diet with or without physical activity) versus physical activity alone (overall, aerobic, resistance) on potential prognostic mediators in the presence/absence of standard breast cancer therapies
3. Definitive RCT of impact of an optimal weight loss intervention on breast cancer outcome
a. Adequately powered to identify clinically relevant HR, rigorous weight loss intervention using optimal weight loss approaches
b. Serial measurement of changes in weight, diet, physical activity
c. Embedded correlative research—serial blood specimens, tumor tissue designed to elucidate biologic processes and to identify predictors of weight loss benefit
4. Identification of biomarkers of obesity—prognosis association
a. Host markers—blood and adipose tissue factors associated with obesity that may mediate prognostic associations (e.g. insulin, glucose, HOMA, adipokines, inflammatory factors), DNA methylation patterns; focus on joint/interacting effects
b. Tumor markers—pathways that may be impacted by prognostic mediators, traditional breast cancer characteristics
5. Pre-clinical investigation of obesity-breast cancer association
a. Development of clinically relevant models of host and cellular metabolism that include the range of breast cancer subtypes
b. Identification of potential host and tumor markers of prognostic effects, including evaluation of potential differences across racial/ethnic groups
c. In vivo modelling of weight loss, physical activity and dietary interventions

Abbreviations: BMI = body mass index; RCT = randomized controlled trial; HOMA = Homeostasis Model Assessment

initiation of definitive RCTs testing the impact of weight loss interventions is high priority; such trials should not be delayed while other research priorities are addressed. These RCTs are expected to contribute key data that will inform the questions raised in other research priorities.

Key priorities include (1) exploration of the association with obesity with prognosis across breast cancer subtypes, including an examination of the impact of selection criteria on the representativeness of women enrolled onto systemic therapy trials, (2) investigation of the relative contributions of obesity and physical activity to outcomes, (3) conduct of adequately powered RCTs (that include a full spectrum of embedded correlative research to identify predictors of benefit) using an effective weight loss intervention to directly test the impact of weight loss on breast cancer outcomes, (4) identification of host and tissue biomarkers of the obesity-prognosis association (some of these may prove useful as intermediate end-points in small trials of specific interventions, prior to testing in full scale trials) and (5) a range of preclinical research that builds on correlative research in clinical settings and includes the development of clinically relevant models of the breast cancer-obesity association and in vivo modelling of the effects of weight loss, physical activity and dietary interventions on breast cancer biology.

This is an ambitious interdisciplinary research agenda that will be costly and time-consuming, however, the benefits will be large if it results in clinically relevant improvements in breast cancer outcomes. Care is needed to prioritize research to focus on areas of potentially greatest impact.

Alcohol

Although there is clear evidence that alcohol intake, even at modest levels, is associated with increased breast cancer risk (Seitz et al. 2012), there is little evidence that intake post diagnosis is associated with risk of breast cancer recurrence or death. Concerns have been raised that alcohol intake after breast cancer diagnosis may increase risk of a new breast primary, however, results of published studies have been inconsistent (Demark-Wahnefried and Goodwin 2013; Newcomb et al. 2013; Kwan et al. 2010). Given these observations, and the recognized benefits of modest alcohol intake on risk of cardiovascular disease (a major source of mortality in breast cancer survivors beyond 10 years post diagnosis), adherence to population based recommendations for alcohol intake appears reasonable in breast cancer populations.

Tobacco

There is growing evidence that tobacco exposure may be associated with a modest increased risk of mainly premenopausal breast cancer, particularly in those with slow acetylation N-acetyl transferase 2 genotypes (Johnson et al. 2011; Land et al. 2011, 2014). There are no data available regarding the association of continued tobacco exposure post-diagnosis and breast cancer outcomes. However, tobacco use post-diagnosis may increase risk of lung and esophageal cancer (as well as other tobacco associated cancers), both of which have been reported to occur with increased frequency in breast cancer survivors. Concerns have been raised that tobacco exposure may alter tamoxifen metabolism in individuals with certain CYP2D6 polymorphisms; it is not clear whether this impacts clinical outcomes in breast cancer patients receiving tamoxifen (Fujita 2006). Because of the well recognized general adverse health effects of smoking, and the excellent long-term outcomes of breast cancer, avoidance of tobacco exposure is recommended for all breast cancer survivors.

The Future

A wealth of primarily observational research over the past 35 years has identified important associations of lifestyle with outcome in breast cancer survivors. This research has led to the testable hypothesis that adoption of a healthier lifestyle, through changes in diet and physical activity, will improve breast cancer outcomes. It has also identified biologically plausible mediators of this association. Well-designed and conducted, adequately powered RCTs, with strong embedded correlative components designed to identify important biologic mediators and predictors of benefit, are needed to provide definitive information regarding the benefits of lifestyle change. Such RCTs may identify benefits that are comparable in magnitude to those seen with drug therapies. They should be assigned a high research priority by funders and breast cancer researchers.

References

Abbenhardt C, McTiernan A, Alfano CM et al (2013) Effects of individual and combined dietary weight loss and exercise interventions in postmenopausal women on adiponectin and leptin levels. J Intern Med 274:163–175

Abe R, Kumagai N, Kimura M et al (1976) Biological characteristics of breast cancer in obesity. Tohoku J Exp Med 120:351–359

Alberti KG, Eckel RH, Grundy SM et al (2009) Harmonizing the metabolic syndrome: a joint interim statement of the International Diabetes Federation Task Force on Epidemiology and Prevention; National Heart, Lung, and Blood Institute; American Heart Association; World Heart Federation; International Atherosclerosis Society; and International Association for the Study of Obesity. Circulation 120:1640–1645

Ballard-Barbash R, Friedenreich CM, Courneya KS et al (2012) Physical activity, biomarkers, and disease outcomes in cancer survivors: a systematic review. J Natl Cancer Inst 104:815–840

Campbell KL, Foster-Schubert KE, Alfano CM et al (2012) Reduced-calorie dietary weight loss, exercise, and sex hormones in postmenopausal women: randomized controlled trial. J Clin Oncol 30:2314–2326

Cecchini R, Swain S, Costantino J et al (2013) Body mass index at diagnosis and breast cancer survival prognosis among clinical trial populations: results from NSABP B-30, B-31, B-34, and B-38. Cancer Res 73(Suppl 24):Abstract nr PD2-1

Chan DS, Vieira AR, Aune D et al (2014) Body mass index and survival in women with breast cancer-systematic literature review and meta-analysis of 82 follow-up studies. Ann Oncol. doi:10.1093/annonc/mdu042

Chlebowski RT, Rose D, Buzzard IM et al (1992) Adjuvant dietary fat intake reduction in postmenopausal breast cancer patient management. The women's intervention nutrition study (WINS). Breast Cancer Res Treat 20:73–84

Crozier JA, Moreno-Aspitia A et al (2013) Effect of body mass index on tumor characteristics and disease-free survival in patients from the HER2-positive adjuvant trastuzumab trial N9831. Cancer 119:2447–2454

Demark-Wahnefried W, Goodwin PJ (2013) To your health: how does the latest research on alcohol and breast cancer inform clinical practice? J Clin Oncol 31:1917–1919

Demark-Wahnefried W, Aziz NM, Rowland JH et al (2005) Riding the crest of the teachable moment: promoting long-term health after the diagnosis of cancer. J Clin Oncol 23:5814–5830

Ewertz M, Gray KP, Regan MM et al (2012) Obesity and risk of recurrence or death after adjuvant endocrine therapy with letrozole or tamoxifen in the breast international group 1-98 trial. J Clin Oncol 30:3967–3975

Fontanella C, von Minckwitz G, Mergler B et al (2013) Body mass index (BMI) and treatment outcome of breast cancer patients receiving neoadjuvant therapy (NACT). Cancer Res 73(Suppl 24):Abstract nr PD2-2

Fujita K (2006) Cytochrome P450 and anticancer drugs. Curr Drug Metab 7:23–37

George SM, Ballard-Barbash R, Shikany JM et al (2014) Better postdiagnosis diet quality is associated with reduced risk of death among postmenopausal women with invasive breast cancer in the women's health initiative. Cancer Epidemiol Biomarkers Prev 23:575–583

Gilbert CA, Slingerland JM (2013) Cytokines, obesity, and cancer: new insights on mechanisms linking obesity to cancer risk and progression. Ann Rev Med 64:45–57

Goodwin P, Stambolic V (2015) Impact of the obesity epidemic on cancer. Ann Rev Med 66:281–296

Goodwin PJ, Ennis M, Pritchard KI et al (2002) Fasting insulin and outcome in early-stage breast cancer: results of a prospective cohort study. J Clin Oncol 20:42–51

Goodwin PJ, Stambolic V, Lemieux J et al (2011) Evaluation of metformin in early breast cancer: a modification of the traditional paradigm for clinical testing of anti-cancer agents. Breast Cancer Res Treat 126:215–220

Goodwin PJ, Ennis M, Pritchard KI et al (2012) Insulin- and obesity-related variables in early-stage breast cancer: correlations and time course of prognostic associations. J Clin Oncol 30:164–171

Goodwin PJ, Segal RJ, Vallis M et al (2014) Randomized trial of a telephone-based weight loss intervention in postmenopausal women with breast cancer receiving letrozole: the LISA trial. J Clin Oncol 32:2231–2239

Imayama I, Ulrich CM, Alfano CM et al (2012) Effects of a caloric restriction weight loss diet and exercise on inflammatory biomarkers in overweight/obese postmenopausal women: a randomized controlled trial. Cancer Res 72:2314–2326

Johnson KC, Miller AB, Collishaw NE et al (2011) Active smoking and secondhand smoke increase breast cancer risk: the report of the Canadian expert panel on tobacco smoke and breast cancer risk (2009). Tob Control 20:e2

Kampman E, Vrieling A, van Duijnhoven FJ et al (2012) Impact of diet, body mass index, and physical activity on cancer survival. Curr Nutr Rep 1:30–36

Kramer CK, Zinman B, Retnakaran R (2013) Are metabolically healthy overweight and obesity benign conditions?: A systematic review and meta-analysis. Ann Intern Med 159:758–769

Kwan ML, Kushi LH, Weltzien E et al (2010) Alcohol consumption and breast cancer recurrence and survival among women with early-stage breast cancer: the life after cancer epidemiology study. J Clin Oncol 28:4410–4416

Land SR, Cronin WM, Wickerham DL et al (2011) Cigarette smoking, obesity, physical activity, and alcohol use as predictors of chemoprevention adherence in the national surgical adjuvant breast and bowel project P-1 breast cancer prevention trial. Cancer Prev Res (Phila) 4:1393–1400

Land SR, Liu Q, Wickerham DL et al (2014) Cigarette smoking, physical activity, and alcohol consumption as predictors of cancer incidence among women at high risk of breast cancer in the NSABP P-1 trial. Cancer Epidemiol Biomarkers Prev 23:823–832

Lof M, Bergstrom K, Weiderpass E (2012) Physical activity and biomarkers in breast cancer survivors: a systematic review. Maturitas 73:134–142

Lyman GH, Sparreboom A (2013) Chemotherapy dosing in overweight and obese patients with cancer. Nat Rev Clin Oncol 10:451–459

Mason C, Foster-Schubert KE, Imayama I et al (2011) Dietary weight loss and exercise effects on insulin resistance in postmenopausal women. Am J Prev Med 41:366–375

Mazzarella L, Disalvatore D, Bagnardi V et al (2013) Obesity increases the incidence of distant metastases in oestrogen receptor-negative human epidermal growth factor receptor 2-positive breast cancer patients. Eur J Cancer 49:3588–3597

Newcomb PA, Kampman E, Trentham-Dietz A et al (2013) Alcohol consumption before and after breast cancer diagnosis: associations with survival from breast cancer, cardiovascular disease, and other causes. J Clin Oncol 31:1939–1946

Niraula S, Ocana A, Ennis M et al (2012) Body size and breast cancer prognosis in relation to hormone receptor and menopausal status: a meta-analysis. Breast Cancer Res Treat 134:769–781

Pajares B, Pollan M, Martin M et al (2013) Obesity and survival in operable breast cancer patients treated with adjuvant anthracyclines and taxanes according to pathological subtypes: a pooled analysis. Breast Cancer Res 15:R105

Pan H, Gray RR, on behalf of the Early Breast Cancer Trialists' Collaborative Group (2014) Effect of obesity in premenopausal ER+ early breast cancer: EBCTCG data on 80,000 patients in 70 trials. J Clin Oncol 32(Suppl 15):503

Pierce JP, Natarajan L, Caan BJ et al (2007) Influence of a diet very high in vegetables, fruit, and fiber and low in fat on prognosis following treatment for breast cancer: the women's healthy eating and living (WHEL) randomized trial. JAMA 298:289–298

Pi-Sunyer X, Blackburn G, Brancati FL et al (2007) Reduction in weight and cardiovascular disease risk factors in individuals with type 2 diabetes: one-year results of the look AHEAD trial. Diabetes Care 30:1374–1383

Protani M, Coory M, Martin JH (2010) Effect of obesity on survival of women with breast cancer: systematic review and meta-analysis. Breast Cancer Res Treat 123:627–635

Rack B, Andergassen U, Neugebauer J et al (2010) The German SUCCESS C study – the first European lifestyle study on breast cancer. Breast Care (Basel) 5:395–400

Reeves MM, Terranova CO, Eakin EG et al (2014) Weight loss intervention trials in women with breast cancer: a systematic review. Obes Rev. doi:10.1111/obr.12190

Rock CL, Byers TE, Colditz GA et al (2013) Reducing breast cancer recurrence with weight loss, a vanguard trial: the exercise and nutrition to enhance recovery and good health for you (ENERGY) trial. Contemp Clin Trials 34:282–295

Seitz HK, Pelucchi C, Bagnardi V et al (2012) Epidemiology and pathophysiology of alcohol and breast cancer: update 2012. Alcohol Alcohol 47:204–212

Sestak I, Distler W, Forbes JF et al (2010) Effect of body mass index on recurrences in tamoxifen and anastrozole treated women: an exploratory analysis from the ATAC trial. J Clin Oncol 28:3411–3415

Sparano JA, Wang M, Zhao F et al (2012) Obesity at diagnosis is associated with inferior outcomes in hormone receptor-positive operable breast cancer. Cancer 118:5937–5946

Suissa S, Pollak M, Spitzer WO et al (1989) Body size and breast cancer prognosis: a statistical explanation of the discrepancies. Cancer Res 49:3113–3116

Turkoz FP, Solak M, Petekkaya I et al (2013) The prognostic impact of obesity on molecular subtypes of breast cancer in premenopausal women. J BUON 18:335–341

Villarini A, Pasanisi P, Traina A et al (2012) Lifestyle and breast cancer recurrences: the DIANA-5 trial. Tumori 98:1–18

Chapter 13
Risk Reduction from Weight Management and Physical Activity Interventions

Melinda L. Irwin, Carol Fabian, and Anne McTiernan

Abstract Obesity and low levels of physical activity are associated with a higher risk of breast cancer recurrence and mortality. Currently, over 65 % of breast cancer survivors are overweight or obese, and fewer than 30 % engage in recommended levels of physical activity. The reason for low adherence to lifestyle guidelines is likely multifactorial. Given the continuing trend of increased obesity and physical inactivity in the United States, worldwide and in breast cancer survivors, more research showing the direct effect of weight loss and/or exercise on breast cancer recurrence and mortality is needed. Many exercise interventions have examined the impact of increasing exercise on changes in quality of life, with most studies showing a favorable effect of exercise on quality of life. Smaller Phase II randomized trials using biomarkers as surrogate endpoints is likely appropriate to answer questions regarding mechanisms of action, exercise type, volume, and intensity, yet a definitive trial of weight loss and exercise on disease-free survival is critical for moving the field forward. Research is also necessary on how to disseminate lifestyle interventions into the clinic and community that lead to clinically meaningful weight losses of at least 5 % that are maintained over time, and favorable sustained changes in physical activity levels. Changes in referrals, access, and reimbursement of lifestyle programs may lead to favorable changes in the prevalence of obesity and physical activity in breast cancer survivors and in turn rates of breast cancer recurrence and mortality.

Keywords Obesity • Weight • Physical activity • Exercise • Interventions • Breast cancer

M.L. Irwin (✉)
Chronic Disease Epidemiology, Yale School of Public Health, New Haven, CT, USA
e-mail: melinda.irwin@yale.edu

C. Fabian
Cancer Prevention, University of Kansas Cancer Center, Kansas, USA
e-mail: cfabian@kumc.edu

A. McTiernan
Cancer Epidemiology, Fred Hutchinson Cancer Research Center, Seatle, WA, USA
e-mail: amctiern@fhcrc.org

© Breast Cancer Research Foundation 2015
P.A. Ganz (ed.), *Improving Outcomes for Breast Cancer Survivors*,
Advances in Experimental Medicine and Biology 862,
DOI 10.1007/978-3-319-16366-6_13

Introduction

Obesity and low levels of physical activity are associated with a higher risk of breast cancer recurrence and mortality (Chan et al. 2014; Ballard-Barbash et al. 2009). Post-diagnosis weight gain has also been associated with a higher risk of recurrence and mortality (Caan 2012; Bradshaw et al. 2012). Obesity, weight gain and physical inactivity are also risk factors for cardiovascular mortality which is higher in breast cancer survivors than those without breast cancer (Darby et al. 2005, 2013).

For achieving and maintaining a healthy weight, the American Cancer Society recommends following a dietary pattern that is high in vegetables, fruits, and whole grains, 150 min per week of aerobic exercise and at least two sessions of strength training exercise per week for cancer survivors, and avoiding physical inactivity (Rock et al. 2012). This is similar to the US Department of Health and Human Resources Physical Activity Guidelines for healthy adults and the American College of Sports Medicine recommendation for healthy adults which suggest 150 min per week of moderate-intensity aerobic physical activity or 75 min/week of vigorous-intensity aerobic physical activity plus two sessions of strength training per week (DHHS 2008; Schmitz et al. 2010a, b). Despite these lifestyle recommendations, over 65 % of breast cancer survivors are overweight or obese, and fewer than 30 % engage in recommended levels of physical activity (Jiralerspong et al. 2013; Mason et al. 2013a, b).

The reason for low adherence to lifestyle guidelines is likely multifactorial and related to the difficulty in making lifestyle changes; lack of access and reimbursement to structured weight management and exercise programs; and lack of evidence from large-scale randomized trials of weight loss and/or exercise as to the amount of weight which needs to be lost and/or exercise that needs to be performed to reduce breast cancer recurrence and mortality. Given the continuing trend of increased obesity and physical inactivity in the United States, worldwide and in breast cancer survivors, more research showing the direct effect of weight loss and/or exercise on breast cancer recurrence and breast cancer, cardiovascular and all-cause mortality is needed. In this chapter we will outline research priorities for energy balance interventions, with a specific focus on physical activity and weight loss interventions in breast cancer survivors including the need for information on: (1) Dose, type, volume and intensity of exercise which will result in improved health outcomes for breast cancer survivors; (2) Amount and duration of weight loss likely to result in reduced breast cancer recurrence; (3) Objective yet cost effective methods for delivering energy balance interventions to general as well as targeted populations which have been historically difficult to reach such as minorities, rural women, and those with physical disabilities or a very limited budget; and (4) Surrogate markers strongly associated with breast cancer recurrence and cardiovascular health which might be substituted for recurrence and cardiac events and used in smaller trials particularly to answer questions of dose, volume intensity of exercise, and amount of weight loss.

Physical Activity Interventions in Breast Cancer Survivors

In the last three decades, observational studies of physical activity have suggested that physical activity is a modifiable health behavior that can play a key role in both reduction of risk and improvement of prognosis in breast cancer (Ballard-Barbash et al. 2009). However, fewer than 30 % of breast cancer survivors attain the recommended 150 min of moderate-intensity aerobic physical activity plus two sessions of strength training per week when exercise is measured by self-report (Mason et al. 2013a, b). Recent accelerometer data from the National Health and Nutrition Examination Survey showed a smaller proportion of cancer survivors met physical activity guidelines when physical activity was measured objectively, with only 13 % of cancer survivors exercising for 150 min or more each week (Loprinzi et al. 2013). Further, the percentage of women meeting exercise guidelines decreases with increasing time since diagnosis such that at 5 or 10 years post-diagnosis, less than 10 % of survivors are meeting guidelines (Mason et al. 2013a, b). A high proportion of physically inactive survivors are also overweight or obese and poorly fit. A number of questions exist about the amount (volume), type, and intensity of exercise that is safe but effective in improving breast cancer specific and overall health outcomes after a diagnosis of breast cancer.

Duration, Intensity and Type of Physical Activity

While most observational research shows a dose-response of more exercise being better for lowering breast cancer risk, recurrence and mortality, we do not know if a threshold level exists or if vigorous-intensity physical activity is beneficial or detrimental. Currently, trials are in progress examining the effect of different durations and intensities of exercise on breast cancer biomarkers in healthy women and breast cancer survivors (clinicaltrial.gov NCT01435005 and NCT01186367). Also of importance is the impact of reducing sedentary time on breast cancer outcomes. A growing number of studies have assessed sedentary behavior and breast cancer-specific and all cause-mortality, with most studies not observing a significant association when adjusting for physical activity levels (George et al. 2013; Kim et al. 2013; Basterra-Gortari et al. 2014).

Future research should examine different types of exercise on cancer outcomes. Trials are in progress examining the impact of resistance training vs. muscle relaxation training on fatigue, quality of life, body composition, fitness and inflammatory biomarkers in breast cancer survivors undergoing chemotherapy or radiation therapy (Potthoff et al. 2013). Recently, Courneya and colleagues showed that recommended amounts of 150 min/week of aerobic exercise had similar effects on physical functioning in breast cancer survivors as did a higher dose of 300 min/week of aerobic exercise or a combined 300 min/week of aerobic exercise and resistance training, but that the higher dose and combined exercise may be more beneficial than lower amounts of aerobic exercise on endocrine symptoms and other QOL endpoints (Courneya et al. 2013).

Different types of exercise have different physiologic effects, with aerobic exercise enhancing cardiorespiratory function to a greater degree than resistance exercise, and resistance training enhancing muscular function to a greater degree than aerobic exercise (DHHS 1996). Additionally, aerobic and resistance exercise impart different effects on body composition, with aerobic exercise leading to larger losses in fat mass, and resistance exercise to larger increases in lean body mass (DHHS 1996). Given these differences, it is likely that different types of exercise impact metabolic and inflammatory biomarkers linked to breast cancer risk and prognosis in different ways, and that these effects could differ based on individual patient characteristics such as age, BMI and menopausal status. Future exercise trials need to carefully specify the type, volume, and intensity of the exercise to allow these characterizations to be made.

Physical Activity, Quality of Life and Side Effects of Breast Surgery and Treatments

Many exercise interventions have examined the impact of increasing exercise on changes in quality of life, with most studies showing a favorable effect of exercise on quality of life (Schmitz et al. 2010a, b). Exercise does prevent weight gain (DHHS 2008), and a recent Cochrane review suggests exercise improves sleep, pain, fatigue, body image, sexuality, anxiety, and global quality of life measures in breast cancer survivors (Mishra et al. 2012). Exercise has also been shown to prevent or improve breast cancer-related lymphedema (Schmitz et al. 2010a, b). However, the effect of exercise on cognition are not clear. A recent randomized trial has shown that higher volumes and intensity of exercise during chemotherapy is safe and associated with improved endocrine symptoms and bodily pain (Irwin et al. 2014). Irwin and colleagues recently conducted the Hormones and Physical Exercise (HOPE) randomized trial, which enrolled 121 breast cancer survivors taking an aromatase inhibitor (AI) and experiencing AI-associated joint pain to either a year of aerobic and resistance training exercise or usual care group. The yearlong exercise program led to a statistically significant 29 % decrease in arthralgia severity among women randomized to exercise vs. an increase among women randomized to usual. Exercise was also associated with an improvement in endocrine-related quality of life in this sample of breast cancer survivors taking AIs and experiencing joint pain. Evaluating type, duration and intensity of exercise on cognition and specific quality of life domains, especially in breast cancer survivors at higher risk of treatment-related side effects, needs to be a priority in the future. Future research should also possible adverse effects of exercise on cancer outcomes (Schmitz et al. 2010a, b). Jones et al. recently reported that patients with cancer randomized to supervised exercise vs. usual care had a higher incidence of cardiovascular mortality and or hospitalization for cardiac events with aerobic exercise than usual care (Jones et al. 2014).

Improving Uptake of Exercise in Cancer Survivors

Currently, the proportion of breast cancer survivors that participate in recommended levels of exercise is very low; and many women decrease physical activity levels further after cancer diagnosis (Mason et al. 2013a, b). These low rates of participation in physical activity have been shown to be a strong risk factor for post-diagnosis weight gain, which is also associated with a higher risk of breast cancer recurrence and mortality. The reasons underlying this low uptake of exercise guidelines are probably multifactorial but there is little third-party reimbursement for exercise programs in breast cancer survivors, and many oncologists do not address these issues with patients. Research on the best, most cost-effective, approach for increasing physical activity levels in breast cancer survivors is necessary; however studies have shown in-person, telephone and use of mailed interventions have all have been associated with increased physical activity levels (Irwin et al. 2009a, b; Cadmus et al. 2009; Demark-Wahnefried et al. 2000). Furthermore, a number of community-based exercise programs are increasingly available to cancer survivors, such as the LIVESTRONG® at the YMCA program, which offers free 12-week exercise programs to cancer survivors at participating YMCAs across the United States. The effectiveness of the LIVESTRONG® at the YMCA program has been evaluated only in Western Washington YMCAs (Rajotte et al. 2012), however a study is underway evaluating the LIVESTRONG® at the YMCAs in MA and CT (clinicaltrials.gov number NCT02112149). Evaluation of exercise interventions in the cooperative group setting was evaluated by Ligibel et al., and showed promise as a strategy towards increases exercise particularly in breast cancer patients treated at community practices (Ligibel et al. 2012).

Future Physical Activity Research Needs

Despite a growing body of observational evidence suggesting a strong link between physical activity and outcomes (especially survival) following breast cancer, there is still the potential for unknown or poorly characterized factors to confound these associations. Women who participate in higher levels of physical activity may engage in many other healthy behaviors that contribute to reduced risk, or they may have higher levels of adherence with their cancer treatments. Thus, a randomized controlled trial testing the effects of a prescribed level of physical activity on breast cancer recurrence and mortality outcomes would, if positive, likely impact the number of oncologists recommending exercise, as well as third-party reimbursement for exercise programs. Although a randomized trial of exercise vs. usual care with primary outcomes of disease-free and overall survival would be ideal in terms of establishing exercise as a treatment for breast cancer survivors and thus reimbursable, such a trial would require significant resources, a challenge in the current funding environment, yet clinically significant. Smaller Phase II randomized trials using biomarkers as surrogate endpoints is likely appropriate to answer questions regarding mechanisms of action, exercise type, volume, and intensity. These smaller studies should include biomarkers for both cardiovascular disease and breast cancer recurrence. Also of great need are studies examining physical activity as a strategy towards increasing medication adherence in breast cancer survivors, as well as randomized trials of exercise vs. novel therapies for breast cancer (e.g., metformin). In summary, physical activity may improve breast cancer and overall survival via favorable changes in biomarkers, body composition, and/or medication adherence. Yet, the impact of physical activity on favorable changes in quality of life, fatigue, and depression may be considered most important by breast cancer survivors, especially in those survivors experiencing common treatment side effects. Research in all of these areas is needed (see Table 13.1) to ultimately improve access to and reimbursement of exercise programs by third party payers, and in turn, more survivors initiating and adhering to physical activity guidelines.

Table 13.1 Top research priorities in physical activity and weight management interventions in breast cancer survivors

Physical activity
1. Trials comparing types, intensity, and dose of exercise (including sedentary activity) on patient-reported outcomes, biomarkers, recurrence and mortality
2. Evaluating impact of exercise on cognition and specific quality of life domains in high risk groups based on diagnosis and/or treatment prescribed
3. Examining if there are adverse effects of exercise in breast cancer survivors
4. Trials of exercise on biomarkers for both cardiovascular disease and breast cancer recurrence
5. Studies examining physical activity as a strategy towards increasing medication adherence in breast cancer survivors, as well as randomized trials of exercise vs. novel therapies for breast cancer (e.g., metformin)
6. Research on the best, most cost-effective, approach for increasing physical activity levels in breast cancer survivors
Weight management
1. Trials of weight loss on recurrence and mortality
2. Studies of weight loss medications or surgeries on breast cancer prognosis
3. Studies comparing diet alone, exercise alone, and combined diet plus exercise interventions on health outcomes in cancer survivors
4. Examining if there are adverse effects of weight loss or dietary change interventions in breast cancer survivors
5. Research on how to disseminate weight management interventions into the clinic and community
6. Novel interventions approaches that are cost-effective strategies (including reimbursement) towards losing and maintaining weight loss
7. Research on what is the most efficient way to lose weight and keep it off particularly in underserved populations (minorities, rural Americans)
8. Research on understudied breast tissue and blood biomarkers include DNA methylation of breast cancer genes and small molecule metabolite levels

Weight Management

Obese breast cancer survivors have a poorer overall and breast cancer specific survival compared with normal-weight breast cancer survivors. A recent systematic review and meta-analysis of 79 cohort studies including over 210,000 women with 41,477 deaths estimated that compared with normal-weight women (BMI 18.5–24.9 kg/m²), those who were overweight (BMI 25.0–29.9 kg/m²) or obese ($\geq$30.0 kg/m²) before diagnosis had statistically significant 11 % and 35 % increased risks for breast-cancer-specific mortality, respectively (Chan et al. 2014). Similar results were observed for BMI after diagnosis. A J-shaped curve of risk was also observed: women who were underweight (BMI < 18.5 kg/m²) within 12 months after diagnosis had a statistically significant 53 % increased risk of breast-cancer-specific mortality (Caan et al. 2008). A similar pattern of risks was observed for overall mortality. Little is known about weight change and prognosis, which has led experts to propose testing weight loss interventions on prognosis in randomized controlled trials before making firm recommendations for weight loss in overweight or obese survivors (Ballard-Barbash et al. 2009). No such trial has been conducted, however. This section reviews the status of research on weight loss and diet interventions in breast cancer survivors, with particular focus on interventions that included caloric reduction as part of the intervention because reducing caloric intake is integral to substantial weight loss. There have been no studies of weight loss medications or surgeries on breast cancer prognosis, so no conclusions of effects of these interventions in this population can be made.

Weight Loss and Diet Interventions

Early suggestions of an association between dietary fat and breast carcinogenesis, with evidence strongest in animal models (Rose 1997), led to the design of several small and two large-scale randomized controlled trials focused on the effect of a diet change intervention on intermediate or prognosis-related outcomes in breast cancer patients (Demark-Wahnefried et al. 2012; Chlebowski et al. 2006; Pierce et al. 2007). The diet change interventions have included reduced fat (typically a goal of less than 20 % of daily calories from fat), increased vegetables and fruits, increased fiber, or various combinations of these components. Durations have ranged from a few months to several years, but most have been of 6 or 12 months' duration. Reporting of effect size varied among studies, with some showing absolute change in weight, others reporting relative change, and a smaller number providing data on other body composition variables such as waist circumference or image-derived body fat. Biological endpoints have included insulin and insulin resistance markers, inflammation-related biomarkers, sex hormones (estrogens, androgens, sex hormone binding proteins), and various adipokines (Scott et al. 2013). Few trials have examined the effect of weight loss on important quality-of-life endpoints in breast cancer survivors.

Two full-scale randomized clinical trials evaluated dietary change in the adjuvant breast cancer setting (Chlebowski et al. 2006; Pierce et al. 2007). The WINS and WHEL study enrolled different populations and studied different dietary patterns, but both aimed to reduce dietary fat intake. Neither targeted weight loss nor physical activity. In the WINS trial, while weight loss was not a specific intervention target, there was a statistically significant ($P=0.005$), 6-pound lower mean body weight in the intervention group at 5 years. There were more recurrence events in the control (181 of 1,462, 12.4 %) compared to the intervention group (96 of 975, 9.8 %, hazard ratio (HR) 0.76, 95 % CI 0.60–0.98, p=0.034). The WINS results suggest that a lifestyle intervention reducing dietary fat intake and associated with modest weight loss may improve outcome of breast cancer patients receiving conventional cancer management.

Following the observations that overweight and obesity adversely affect prognosis, a number of randomized controlled trials have tested the effect of weight loss on various health factors in women with breast cancer. None, however, have been specifically designed or sufficiently powered to test the effect of weight loss on survival. Several diet or diet plus exercise intervention trials have tested weight loss interventions on health factors other than survival. Earlier studies used individual in-person counseling to deliver guidance on caloric-restriction, while more recently, group-based or telephone support have been used (Goodwin et al. 2014).

The Lifestyle Intervention Study in Adjuvant Treatment of Early Breast Cancer (LISA) Weight Loss randomized controlled trial enrolled 338 women with early stage estrogen receptor positive breast cancer to either a telephone-based weight loss intervention or educational control group (Goodwin et al. 2014). The initial aim was to assess weight loss effect on disease-free survival but the trial was stopped due to lack of funding. Eligibility included diagnosis of Stage I-III breast cancer, BMI ≥ 24 kg/m^2, and treatment with letrozole. The weight loss intervention, based on the Diabetes Prevention Program lifestyle change intervention (DPP 2002a, b), focused on weight reduction through calorie restriction and increased physical activity. The weight loss intervention arm lost significantly more weight than the control arm, with mean reductions of 5.3 vs. 0.7 % at 6 months (p<0.001) and 3.6 vs. 0.4 % at 24 months (p<0.001).

A 12-month trial with 48 obese stage I-II breast cancer patients, produced weight losses of <1 % in controls, 8.4 % with individualized counseling, and 9.8 % with individualized counseling paired with Weight Watchers® group classes (Djuric et al. 2002). Two other group-based randomized clinical trials in breast cancer survivors, i.e., the Healthy Weight Management Study (n=85) (Mefferd et al. 2007), and the Survivors Health And Physical Exercise (SHAPE) trial (n=258) tested the effect of a cognitive-behavioral weight loss program plus telephone counseling vs. wait-list controls (Taylor et al. 2010). The Healthy Weight Management intervention produced an 8 % weight loss at 12 months, while the SHAPE intervention yielded a 4.5 % weight loss at 18 months. The weight loss interventions were also associated with favorable changes in self-esteem, depression and serum concentrations of sex hormone binding globulin, estradiol, bioavailable estradiol, insulin, leptin and total and LDL cholesterol.

The ongoing Exercise and Nutrition to Enhance Recovery and Good Health for You (ENERGY) Trial, is a multi-site randomized controlled trial designed to promote and sustain a 7 % weight loss over a 2-year period in 693 overweight or obese women who have been diagnosed with early stage breast cancer (Rock et al. 2013a, b). Secondary aims are to evaluate weight loss at 24 months according to time since diagnosis and type of tumor and therapy; to assess the impact of the intervention on quality of life; and to prospectively collect biological samples for future biomarker studies to help explain the mechanism and probable differential response across subgroups. The group-class weight loss intervention addresses breast cancer specific issues and promotes an energy-restricted diet, plus increased physical activity, behavioral strategies, cognitive restructuring, skills to facilitate and maintain good choices, social support, self-nurturing, and body image and self-acceptance.

As in persons without cancer (Butryn et al. 2011; DPP 2002a, b), randomized trials in breast cancer survivors indicate that optimal weight loss effects result from multicomponent behavior change interventions that target dietary calorie reduction to reach a deficit of 500–1,000 kcal/day, moderate or greater intensity physical activity for at least 150 min/week, and behavior change principles including goal setting, self-monitoring, and stimulus control. Interventions that include group behavior change sessions have produced results equal to or greater than one-on-one counseling, although optimal results provide for some individual contact with a counselor/case-worker (Befort et al. 2014).

The considerable costs of delivering in-person individual or group interventions, and the difficulties accruing participants who live at some distance from research centers, has led to several trials testing home interventions with remote contacts with case-workers. For cancer survivors, these remote contacts have primarily been via telephone. Befort et al. delivered a group behavioral weight loss intervention by conference call to obese breast cancer survivors living in remote rural locations after first recruiting them in person with the assistance of their local caregivers (Befort et al. 2012). The intervention included a reduced calorie diet incorporating prepackaged entrees and low calorie high protein shakes, advice on physical activity which was gradually increased to 225 min/week of moderate intensity exercise, and weekly group phone sessions which included education about breast cancer as well as advice on how manage life on a diet. Adherence was excellent with a loss of 13.9 % of baseline weight and significant reductions in leptin and insulin. A follow-up randomized study of usual care vs. a structured weight loss and maintenance intervention patterned on the above has completed accrual.

Irwin et al. 2015a, b recently completed a 6-month diet- and exercise-induced randomized weight loss trial in overweight and obese breast cancer survivors who had completed adjuvant treatment, entitled the Lifestyle, Exercise and Nutrition (LEAN) Study (Irwin et al. 2014). The LEAN Study randomized 100 women to one of three arms: an 11-session weight loss counseling program occurring over 6 months delivered in-person (Arm 1) vs. 11-session weight loss counseling over 6 months delivered via telephone (Arm 2) vs. usual care group where women received AICR pamphlets on healthy eating and exercise (Arm 3). The weight loss counseling was adapted from the 2010 U.S. Dietary Guidelines, the Diabetes Prevention

Program, and American Cancer Society and AICR publications. They found statistically significant decreases in body weight among women randomized to in-person (−6.2 % weight loss) and telephone (−5.8 % weight loss) counseling compared to usual care, as well as significant decreases in several biomarkers related to breast cancer including C-reactive protein, insulin, and leptin levels. In addition to being of potential beneficial for breast cancer survivors, the changes seen in these biomarkers could predict reduced risk of diabetes and heart disease for those in the weight loss groups.

Possible Adverse Effects of Purposeful Weight Loss in Cancer Survivors

Most of the previously reported randomized clinical trials of weight loss used diet change interventions for weight loss, without addition of an exercise program. While diet change to reduce calories and fat has been shown to be highly efficacious in inducing relatively long-term weight loss (Foster-Schubert et al. 2012), it does so at the expense of muscle loss (Mason et al. 2013a, b). This is a significant issue for cancer survivors, who have a high prevalence of sarcopenia, among both obese and non-obese survivors, and sarcopenia has been associated with poorer prognosis (Villasenor et al. 2012). In non-cancer populations, exercise aids with weight loss maintenance (Miller et al. 2013), and somewhat with weight loss efficacy (Foster-Schubert et al. 2012). Yet, there are no controlled clinical trial data comparing effects of diet alone, exercise alone, and combined diet plus exercise interventions on health outcomes in cancer survivors. Given the findings in non-cancer populations, more recent weight loss trials in cancer survivors should include an exercise component.

Other adverse effects of weight loss through caloric reduction have been observed in populations without cancer, including reduced white blood cell and neutrophil counts (Imayama et al. 2012a, b), but this have been largely unexplored in weight loss trials in breast cancer survivors. Weight loss programs that include exercise interventions could carry risk for musculoskeletal injuries or cardiovascular events (Campbell et al. 2012a, b; Dahabreh and Paulus 2011). These, too, have not been part of outcomes reporting for most weight loss trials in breast cancer survivors.

Future Weight Loss Research Needs

Ideally, resources would be available to determine effects of various weight loss, diet, and physical activity interventions on breast cancer prognosis. An alternative would be to launch a full-scale randomized controlled trial testing the effect of a weight loss intervention on overall and breast-cancer-specific survival with an intervention known to maximize weight loss while having high acceptability to survivors and a favorable risk profile. The same trial could also test mediating biomarkers that could then be used as endpoints in future trials of other weight loss interventions. Effects on health and quality of life factors relevant to breast cancer survivors should be assessed, including lymphedema, bone density, diabetes, cardiovascular disease, arthralgias, cognitive function, fatigue, anxiety, depression, and adverse effects should be enumerated. Such a trial has been proposed, although resources have not been available (Ballard-Barbash et al. 2009). While these definitive trials of weight loss and exercise on disease-free survival are critical for moving the field forward, dissemination and implementation of evidence-based lifestyle interventions needs to occur. Research is necessary on how to disseminate lifestyle interventions into the clinic and community that lead to clinically meaningful weight losses of at least 5 % that are maintained over time. Whether these interventions are more effective when implemented in cancer hospital survivorship clinics/centers or when implemented via referrals to community-based programs needs to be examined. In summary, a growing number of observational studies have consistently shown obesity to be associated with a higher risk of breast cancer and all-cause mortality, yet no randomized controlled trial of weight loss on disease-free survival has been conducted (see Table 13.1 for future research needs). A growing number of randomized weight loss trials on biomarkers or quality of life have been conducted, yet it is unknown if these findings will lead to implementation and reimbursement of weight management programs in the clinic or community. If so, then we could expect to see decreases in obesity in breast cancer survivors, as well as prevention of weight gain in women newly diagnosed with breast cancer.

Surrogate Endpoints for Exercise and Weight Loss Trials for Breast Cancer Recurrence and Mortality

Increased concentrations of several obesity- and physical inactivity-related blood proteins have been associated with increased breast-cancer-specific and all-cause mortality in breast cancer survivors, including insulin, c-peptide, C-reactive protein, and estrogens, making these markers ideal surrogate markers of breast cancer risk, recurrence and mortality when those definitive endpoints cannot be assessed (Duggan et al. 2011; Irwin et al. 2011; Goodwin et al. 2002; Pierce et al. 2009; Villaseñor et al. 2014). Some of these endpoints are also related to risk for cardiovascular disease, although associations of these biomarkers with cardiovascular mortality in breast cancer survivors have not been adequately studied. Given these associations, it is prudent to identify interventions that can favorably change these surrogate biomarkers. While this will not prove cause-and-effect (Fleming and Powers 2012), it can point to types of interventions that could have biological effects, and which would be most advantageous to test in a randomized clinical trial with survival and recurrence endpoints.

Surrogate endpoints obtained from blood that likely impact both risk for breast cancer and cardiovascular outcomes include: (1) inflammatory cytokines such as TNF-α, Interleukin 1, 6, 8, 10, macrophage chemoattractant protein (MCP-1), and

C-reactive protein (CRP). CRP is often assessed as a general marker of inflammation as hepatic production of CRP is increased in response to IL6, and TNF-α (Kasapis and Thompson 2005); (2) adipokines such as adiponectin and leptin; (3) bioavailable hormones especially estrogen; (4) insulin sensitivity; (5) markers of angiogenesis and tissue invasion such as VEGF, PAI-1, PEDF, and metalloproteinases; and (6) leukocyte telomere length. Many of these markers are profoundly affected by weight, body fat, time interval since last food intake, medications, and recent vigorous exercise. Consequently, it is important to select a relatively homogenous group and perform the biomarker assessments under controlled conditions. For example several of the plasma inflammatory markers including TNF-α, IL6, IL10, and CRP exhibit large increases after vigorous exercise. If blood is sampled prior to an appropriate interval after exercise, spurious increases in these cytokines could occur, particularly in small studies (Mishra et al. 2012).

Interventional trials of exercise and diet-induced weight loss on breast cancer outcomes have also differed by cohort characteristics in terms of initiation of intervention during adjuvant chemotherapy, or later post-adjuvant treatment, homogeneity of the cohort in terms of BMI and physical activity levels, receipt of endocrine therapy or anti-inflammatory drugs, type and intensity of physical activity during the intervention, type of intervention for the control group, whether exercise was supervised, biomarkers assessed, and specified interval since last exercise session when biomarkers were drawn.

Estrogens

One of the most plausible mechanisms of how exercise may reduce breast cancer risk, recurrence and mortality is by lowering estrogen concentrations through reduction in body fat and decreased estrogen production from aromatization of androgens. Two randomized controlled exercise trials, conducted in healthy women have shown an increase in sex hormone binding globulin and an ~10 % decrease in bioavailable estrogen and testosterone primarily in those women who lost body fat (McTiernan et al. 2004; Friedenreich et al. 2010). In a 4-arm randomized controlled trial, a far greater reduction in serum estradiol was observed with weight reduction through caloric restriction, with or without exercise, compared with controls or with an exercise-only intervention (Campbell et al. 2012a, b). The greater effect of dietary weight loss on serum estrogens compared with exercise alone is not surprising, since caloric reduction of about 500–1,000 kcal/day typically produces 10 % weight loss over 6–12 months, while exercise alone produces 1–2 % loss (DHHS 1996). The effect of weight loss on blood estrogens in women with breast cancer has been little studied, likely because of the potential for confounding effects of some treatments such as aromatase inhibitors and tamoxifen. One study in 220 survivors enrolled in a weight loss intervention found that postmenopausal women who lost $\geq$5 % of body weight at 6 months had lower estrone (P=0.02), estradiol (P=0.002), and bioavailable estradiol (P=0.001) concentrations than women who did not lose at least 5 % of body weight (Rock et al. 2013a, b).

Insulin Sensitivity

Elevated insulin levels have been linked to an increased risk of breast cancer, and several reports have demonstrated that women with higher levels of insulin at the time of breast cancer diagnosis are at increased risk of cancer recurrence and death (Duggan et al. 2011; Irwin et al. 2011; Goodwin et al. 2002). These findings showed that a lowering of insulin levels by 25 % may be associated with a 5 % absolute improvement in breast cancer mortality, and this strong association between fasting insulin levels and breast cancer mortality has led a number of oncologists and scientists to consider the targeting of insulin as a therapeutic modality in breast cancer.

A number of exercise and weight loss interventions have been shown to impact insulin in healthy women. One recent trial, conducted by Dr. McTiernan, randomized 439 overweight/obese, sedentary postmenopausal women to one of three energy balance interventions (dietary weight loss alone, exercise alone or dietary weight loss plus exercise) or to control and demonstrated that the weight loss groups experienced the most significant changes in insulin (−22.3 % in the dietary weight loss alone and −24 % in the combined diet and exercise group vs. −7.8 % in the exercise alone group and −1.9 % in the control group) (Mason et al. 2011).

There are fewer data regarding the impact of energy balance interventions upon insulin in breast cancer survivors. One study looked at the impact of three different dietary weight loss interventions (Weight Watchers, an individualized weight loss program or a combination of the two) vs. control on fasting insulin in 48 breast cancer survivors and demonstrated an average 12 % reduction in insulin levels in the three dietary intervention groups. Another study looked at the impact of a diet and exercise weight loss program on insulin levels in 35 rural breast cancer survivors and demonstrated a 17 % reduction in fasting insulin levels. Finally a few small studies have looked at the impact of exercise-only interventions upon insulin levels in breast cancer survivors. One exercise study demonstrated a 28 % reduction in fasting insulin levels in 101 inactive, overweight breast cancer survivors participating in a mixed strength and aerobic exercise intervention ($p = 0.07$) (Ligibel et al. 2008). The other exercise study looked at the impact of a moderate-intensity aerobic exercise intervention in 68 sedentary, overweight breast cancer survivors, and demonstrated an 8 % decrease in insulin levels in exercisers and a 20 % between group difference ($p = 0.089$) (Irwin et al. 2009a, b). Thus there is preliminary evidence in healthy populations that weight loss may be the most important factor in reducing insulin, but data are limited in breast cancer survivors. Metformin reduces insulin levels by 22 % in non-diabetic breast cancer survivors (Palmirotta et al. 2009), and a randomized trial of metformin vs. placebo is being tested in the adjuvant setting (clinicaltrials.gov NCT01101438), as well as trials of metformin alone or with exercise or with weight loss are being tested in the NCI-funded Transdisciplinary Research on Energetics and Cancer studies (clinicaltrials.gov NCT01340300 and NCT01302379). These findings will move the field forward in regards to the role of lifestyle factors compared to medication upon lowering insulin levels in breast cancer survivors.

Inflammatory Cytokines

Exercise training seems to lower both resting and post exercise inflammatory cytokine levels through reduction of circulating monocyte as well as tissue macrophage production and release (Kasapis and Thompson 2005). Preclinical studies suggest that exercise can have a profound effect on macrophage infiltration into adipose and muscle tissue with reduction in M1 macrophage concentration associated with cytokine production and chronic inflammation particularly in diet induced obesity (Kawanishi et al. 2010). Most moderate volume and intensity exercise intervention studies in the general population have found no significant change in inflammatory biomarkers (Marcell et al. 2005; Hammett et al. 2006; Arsenault et al. 2009). Those studies in which inflammatory markers particularly TNF-α, IL6, and/or CRP were favorably modulated with exercise tended to be those in which: (a) individuals were obese at baseline and thus had higher baseline levels of inflammatory cytokines (Kasapis and Thompson 2005; Christiansen et al. 2009; Arikawa et al. 2011; Phillips et al. 2012); (b) exercise volume and intensity were high enough to result in loss of weight and/or body fat (Christiansen et al. 2009); and/or (c) where cytokine production (TNF-α or IL6) was stimulated with lipopolysaccharide exposure (Phillips et al. 2012). Loss of 5–10 % of baseline weight through caloric reduction with or without an exercise program has been shown to reduce inflammation-related biomarkers such as CRP and IL-6 by 20–40 % (Imayama et al. 2012a, b). These effects far exceed those seen with exercise interventions in the absence of significant weight loss. A systematic review concluded that across lifestyle and surgical weight loss interventions, for each 1 kg of weight loss, the mean change in CRP level was −0.13 mg/L (with a weighted Pearson correlation of r=0.85) (Selvin et al. 2007). Although future research in this area is definitely warranted, investigating more sensitive circulating as well as breast and adipose tissue based immune parameters is warranted.

Surrogate Biomarker Summary

In summary, although an exercise or weight loss threshold for reduction in risk for breast cancer development, recurrence or mortality has yet to be defined, biomarker studies to date in largely sedentary women suggest approximately 2.5–3.0 h per week of moderate-intensity exercise, and weight losses of 5 % or more, are sufficient to observe changes in insulin sensitivity. Changes in many inflammatory, hormonal, and angiogenic markers may be more dependent on both decreases in fat mass and weight than exercise alone, although chronic exercise may reduce both resting cytokine output in response to various stressors.

Other newer potential mechanisms of action and biomarkers from breast tissue are largely unexplored in trials of exercise or weight loss and may help define the optimum exercise and/or weight loss prescription. Assessing changes in proliferation or cytomorphology in benign breast tissue is not likely to be helpful since the majority of breast cancer survivors are peri or postmenopausal and on prolonged endocrine therapy. Under these conditions ductal tissue is largely replaced by fat with very low if any Ki-67 (Woolcott et al. 2010). Mammographic breast density is likely to be increased not decreased with exercise particularly if there is a reduction in fat mass (Woolcott et al. 2010). However, assessment of methylation, gene changes at the mRNA level including microRNA, tissue cytokine changes, or changes in key proteins in pathways such as MAP kinase and mTOR can now be performed on very small amounts obtained inexpensively by the minimally invasive technique of random peri-areolar fine needle aspiration (RPFNA) (Fabian et al. 2005). Fabian et al. have performed RPFNA on women undergoing combined caloric restriction and exercise and showed changes in a variety of blood and tissue biomarkers for women losing 10 % or more of their initial weight (Fabian et al. 2013). Irwin et al. are currently performing needle core biopsies (which may be more appropriate for studying macrophage infiltration, aromatase activity and miRNAs) in overweight breast cancer survivors enrolled into a healthy eating and exercise (weight loss) trial (clinicaltrials.gov NCT02110641). Some studies are exploring breast tumor tissue biomarkers. Specifically, a study of exercise between diagnosis and surgery on breast tumor markers (e.g., Ki-67) is being conducted (clinicaltrials.gov NCT01516190). Other novel, understudied biomarkers include DNA methylation of breast cancer genes and small molecule metabolite levels.

Whatever the biomarker used as a surrogate endpoint, it is important that the subject population for these translational trials be relatively homogenous with meticulous detail paid to other medications, sample acquisition, processing and assessment for meaningful answers to be obtained. Sufficient funds should be allocated for bio-specimen screening with the acknowledgement that the majority of potential subjects screened may not be medically eligible or because the primary biomarker of interest may not be measurable to advance onto the intervention.

Summary and Future Directions

Physical activity and weight management have not traditionally been a part of cancer treatment/survivorship programs. Given, physical activity and weight management programs carry tremendous potential to affect length and quality of survival in a positive manner and prevent or control morbidity associated with breast cancer or its treatment, oncologists and primary care physicians should be encouraged to counsel cancer survivors proactively about exercise and weight management. There are, clearly, many questions to be answered concerning who would benefit, and what type of intervention, duration and intensity of exercise would be most beneficial. A better understanding of the effect of exercise and/or weight loss upon pathways linked to breast cancer risk and prognosis could lead to lifestyle prescriptions better targeted to impact these pathways and thus more likely to improve breast cancer prognosis. Personalized lifestyle prescriptions based on patient and treatment characteristics may also lead to better compliance, given the stronger biologic rationale for potential benefit and the parallels to modern adjuvant therapy paradigms focusing on host and tumor biology. This may be especially true in patients for whom current therapies are less effective, such as those with triple-negative breast cancer.

Given weight loss and exercise are associated with reductions in risk for a number of diseases (including breast cancer, cardiovascular disease, diabetes, osteoporosis, and mental health) and treatment side effects (including fatigue, lymphedema, and arthralgia), knowing that weight loss and exercise could benefit many health outcomes may have a positive effect on making favorable behavioral changes. Future research needs to also focus on novel interventions approaches that are cost-effective strategies (including reimbursement) towards losing and maintaining weight loss and increasing exercise, as well as how to incorporate weight management and exercise counseling into the clinic (and when, i.e., during or post-treatment) (see Table 13.2). Additional research on novel measurement techniques of body composition, exercise and sedentary behavior are also encouraged. Lastly, research on what is the most efficient way to lose weight and keep it off particularly in underserved populations (minorities, rural Americans) is necessary, as well as how weight loss medications and/or bariatric surgery can best be studied in morbidly obese breast cancer survivors, while also including exercise interventions?

In summary, obesity and low levels of physical activity are risk factors for poor breast cancer outcomes, but we do not know how much weight loss or how much exercise is necessary, and for how long, to change breast cancer outcomes. It is unclear if being overweight or even in the lower BMI levels of obesity is a risk factor for poor breast cancer outcomes in women who are physically fit or physically active. Biomarker studies can help with some of these questions, as can large epidemiological observational studies, but ultimately it is likely that large-scale randomized trials of weight loss and exercise on breast cancer recurrence, breast cancer mortality and all-cause mortality will be necessary to lead to significant changes in referrals, access, and reimbursement of lifestyle programs, which in turn may lead to favorable changes in the prevalence of obesity and physical activity in breast cancer survivors and in turn rates of breast cancer recurrence and mortality.

Table 13.2 Approaches for improving nutrition and physical activity after a breast cancer diagnosis

• Oncologists should discuss weight management, physical activity, and healthy eating with their patients and refer them to exercise and nutrition programs
• Cancer survivors and providers can consult
– The American College of Sports Medicine's website (http://members.acsm.org/source/custom/Online_locator/OnlineLocator.cfm) using the "Profinder" feature to locate a ACSM/ACS certified cancer exercise trainer in their community
– The Academy of Nutrition and Dietetics website (www.eatright.org), using the "Find a registered dietitian" feature and clicking "Cancer/Oncology Nutrition" in the expertise tab to find a dietitian in their community
• Cancer survivors should contact their health insurance company to find out if post-treatment care is covered, and if so, what lifestyle programs are covered, e.g., health club membership, certified personal trainer, dietitian
• Cancer survivors should keep a daily diary of their nutrition and physical activity practices to discuss with their oncologist, nutritionist, and certified cancer exercise trainer

References

Arikawa AY, Thomas W, Schmitz KH, Kurzer MS (2011) Sixteen weeks of exercise reduces C-reactive protein levels in young women. Med Sci Sports Exerc 43(6):1002–1009

Arsenault BJ, Côté M, Cartier A, Lemieux I, Després JP, Ross R, Earnest CP, Blair SN, Church TS (2009) Effect of exercise training on cardiometabolic risk markers among sedentary, but metabolically healthy overweight or obese post-menopausal women with elevated blood pressure. Atherosclerosis 207(2):530–533

Ballard-Barbash R et al (2009) Physical activity, weight control, and breast cancer risk and survival: clinical trial rationale and design considerations. J Natl Cancer Inst 101(9):630–643

Basterra-Gortari FJ, Bes-Rastrollo M, Gea A et al (2014) Television viewing, computer use, time driving and all-cause mortality. J Am Heart Assoc 3(3):e000864

Befort CA, Klemp JR, Austin HL, Perri MG, Schmitz KH, Sullivan DK, Fabian CJ (2012) Outcomes of a weight loss intervention among rural breast cancer survivors. Breast Cancer Res Treat 132(2):631–639

Befort CA, Klemp JR, Fabian C et al (2014) Protocol and recruitment results from a randomized controlled trial comparing group phone-based versus newsletter interventions for weight loss maintenance among rural breast cancer survivors. Contemp Clin Trials 37(2):261–271

Bradshaw et al (2012) Epidemiology 23(2):320–327

Butryn ML, Webb V, Wadden TA (2011) Behavioral treatment of obesity. Psychiatr Clin North Am 34(4):841–859

Caan BJ (2012) Weight change and survival after breast cancer in the after breast cancer pooling project. Cancer Epidemiol Biomarkers Prev 21(8):1260–1271

Caan BJ et al (2008) Pre-diagnosis body mass index, post-diagnosis weight change, and prognosis among women with early stage breast cancer. Cancer Causes Control 19(10):1319–1328

Cadmus L, Salovey P, Yu H, Chung G, Kasl S, Irwin ML (2009) Exercise and quality of life during and after breast cancer treatment: results from two randomized controlled exercise trials. Psychooncology 18(4):343–352

Campbell K et al (2012a) Injuries in sedentary individuals enrolled in a 12-month, randomized, controlled, exercise trial. J Phys Act Health 9(2):198–207

Campbell KL, Foster-Schubert KE, Alfano CM, Wang C-C, Wang C-Y, Duggan CR, Mason C, Imayama I, Kong A, Bain CE, Blackburn GL, Stanczyk FZ, McTiernan A (2012b) Independent and combined effects of dietary weight loss and exercise on sex hormones in overweight and obese postmenopausal women: a randomized controlled trial. J Clin Oncol 30(19):2314–2326 (Epub 2012 May 21)

Chan DS et al (2014) Body mass index and survival in women with breast cancer – systematic literature review and meta-analysis of 82 follow-up studies. Ann Oncol 25:1901–1914

Chlebowski RT et al (2006) Dietary fat reduction and breast cancer outcome: interim efficacy results from the women's intervention nutrition study. J Natl Cancer Inst 98(24):1767–1776

Christiansen T et al (2009) A yearlong exercise intervention decreased CRP among obese postmenopausal women. Med Sci Sports Exerc 41(8):1533–1539

Courneya KS, McKenzie DC, Mackey JR et al (2013) Effects of exercise dose and type during breast cancer chemotherapy: multicenter randomized trial. J Natl Cancer Inst 105(23):1821–1832

Dahabreh IJ, Paulus JK (2011) Association of episodic physical and sexual activity with triggering of acute cardiac events: systematic review and meta-analysis. JAMA 305(12):1225–1233

Darby SC, McGale P, Taylor CW, Peto R (2005) Long-term mortality from heart disease and lung cancer after radiotherapy for early breast cancer: prospective cohort study of about 300,000 women in US SEER cancer registries. Lancet Oncol 6(8):557–565

Darby SC, Ewertz M, McGale P et al (2013) Risk of ischemic heart disease in women after radiotherapy for breast cancer. N Engl J Med 368(11):987–998

Demark-Wahnefried W et al (2000) Current health behaviors and readiness to pursue life-style changes among men and women diagnosed with early stage prostate and breast carcinomas. Cancer 88(3):674–684

Demark-Wahnefried W, Campbell KL, Hayes SC (2012) Weight management and its role in breast cancer rehabilitation. Cancer 118(Suppl 8):2277–2287

Diabetes Prevention Program Research Group (2002a) Reduction in the incidence of type 2 diabetes with lifestyle intervention or metformin. N Engl J Med 346:393–403

Diabetes Prevention Program Research Group (2002b) The diabetes prevention program (DPP): description of lifestyle intervention. Diabetes Care 25(12):2165–2171

Djuric Z et al (2002) Combining weight-loss counseling with the weight watchers plan for obese breast cancer survivors. Obes Res 10(7):657–665

Duggan C, Irwin ML, Xiao L et al (2011) Associations of insulin resistance and adiponectin with mortality in women with breast cancer. J Clin Oncol 29(1):32–39

Fabian CJ, Kimler BF, Mayo MS, Khan SA (2005) Breast tissue sampling for risk assessment and prevention. Endocr Relat Cancer 12:185–213

Fabian CJ, Kimler BF, Donnelly JE, Sullivan DK, Klemp JR, Petroff BK, Phillips TA, Metheny T, Aversman S, Yeh HW, Zalles CM, Mills GB, Hursting SD (2013) Favorable modulation of benign breast tissue and serum risk biomarkers is associated with >10 % weight loss in postmenopausal women. Breast Cancer Res Treat 142(1):119–132

Fleming TR, Powers JH (2012) Biomarkers and surrogate endpoints in clinical trials. Stat Med 31(25):2973–2984

Foster-Schubert KE et al (2012) Effect of diet and exercise, alone or combined, on weight and body composition in overweight-to-obese postmenopausal women. Obesity 20(8):1628–1638

Friedenreich CM, Woolcott CG, McTiernan A, Ballard-Barbash R, Brant RF, Stanczyk FZ, Terry T, Boyd NF, Yaffe MJ, Irwin ML, Jones CA, Yasui Y, Campbell KL, McNeely ML, Karvinen KH, Wang Q, Courneya KS (2010) Alberta physical activity and breast cancer prevention trial: sex hormone changes in a year-long exercise intervention among postmenopausal women. J Clin Oncol 28(9):1458–1466

George SM, Smith AW, Alfano CM, Bowles HR, Irwin ML, McTiernan A, Bernstein L, Baumgartner KB, Ballard-Barbash R (2013) The association between television watching time and all-cause mortality after breast cancer. J Cancer Surviv 7(2):247–252

Goodwin PJ, Ennis M, Pritchard KI, Trudeau ME et al (2002) Insulin- and obesity-related variables in early-stage breast cancer: correlations and time course of prognostic associations. J Clin Oncol 10(30):164–171

Goodwin PJ, Segal RJ, Vallis M et al (2014) Randomized trial of a telephone-based weight loss intervention in postmenopausal women with breast cancer receiving letrozole: the LISA trial. J Clin Oncol 32:2231–2239

Hammett CJK, Prapavessis H, Baldi JC, Varo N, Schoenbeck U, Ameratunga R, French JK, White HD, Stewart RAH (2006) Effects of exercise training on 5 inflammatory markers associated with cardiovascular risk. Am Heart J 151:367.e7–367.e16

Imayama I et al (2012a) Effects of a caloric restriction weight loss diet and exercise on inflammatory biomarkers in overweight/obese postmenopausal women: a randomized controlled trial. Cancer Res 72(9):2314–2326

Imayama I, Ulrich CM, Alfano CM et al (2012b) Effects of dietary weight loss and exercise on inflammation in postmenopausal women: a randomized controlled trial. Cancer Res 72(9):2314–2326

Irwin ML, Alvarez-Reeves M, Cadmus L et al (2009a) Randomized controlled exercise trial on body fat, lean mass, and bone mineral density in breast cancer survivors: the Yale exercise and survivorship study. Obesity 17(8):1534–1541

Irwin ML, Varma K, Alvarez-Reeves et al (2009b) Randomized controlled exercise trial on insulin and IGFs in breast cancer survivors: the Yale exercise and survivorship study. Cancer Epidemiol Biomarker Prev 18(1):306–313

Irwin ML, Duggan C, Smith AW et al (2011) Fasting C-peptide levels and death due to all causes and breast cancer: the health eating activity and lifestyle (HEAL) study. J Clin Oncol 29(1):47–53

Irwin ML et al (2014) Randomized exercise trial of aromatase inhibitor-induced arthralgia in breast cancer survivors. J Clin Oncol. pii: JCO.2014.57.1547. Epub ahead of print

Irwin ML et al (2015a) Effect of exercise on aromatase inhibitor-associated arthralgias in breast cancer survivors. J Clin Oncol

Irwin ML et al (2015b) The effect of an in-person vs. telephone weight loss intervention on changes in body weight in breast cancer survivors

Jiralerspong S, Kim ES, Dong W et al (2013) Obesity, diabetes, and survival outcomes in a large cohort of early-stage breast cancer patients. Ann Oncol 24:2506–2514

Jones LW, Douglas PS, Khouri MG et al (2014) Safety and efficacy of aerobic training in patients with cancer who have heart failure: an analysis of the HF-ACTION randomized trial. J Clin Oncol 32:2496–2502

Kasapis C, Thompson PD (2005) The effects of physical activity on serum C-reactive protein and inflammatory markers: a systematic review. J Am Coll Cardiol 45(10):1563–1569 (Epub 2005 Apr 25)

Kawanishi N, Yano H, Yokogawa Y, Suzuki K (2010) Exercise training inhibits inflammation in adipose tissue via both suppression of macrophage infiltration and acceleration of phenotypic switching from M1 to M2 macrophages in high-fat-diet-induced obese mice. Exerc Immunol Rev 16:105–118

Kim RB, Phillips A, Herrick K et al (2013) Physical activity and sedentary behavior of cancer survivors and non-cancer individuals. PLoS ONE 8(3):e57598

Ligibel JA, Campbell N, Partridge A, Chen WY, Salinardi T, Chen H, Adloff K, Keshaviah A, Winer EP (2008) Impact of a mixed strength and endurance exercise intervention on insulin levels in breast cancer survivors. J Clin Oncol 26(6):907–912

Ligibel JA, Meyerhardt J, Pierce JP et al (2012) Impact of a telephone-based physical activity intervention upon exercise behaviors and fitness in cancer survivors enrolled in a cooperative group setting. Breast Cancer Res Treat 132(1):205–213

Loprinzi P, Lee H, Cardinal B (2013) Objectively measured physical activity among US cancer survivors: considerations by weight status. J Cancer Surviv 7:493–499

Marcell TJ, McAuley KA, Traustadóttir T (2005) Reaven PD Exercise training is not associated with improved levels of C-reactive protein or adiponectin. Metabolism 54(4):533–541

Mason C, Foster-Schubert KE, Imayama I, Kong A, Xiao L, Bain C, Campbell KL, Wang CY, Duggan CR, Ulrich CM, Alfano CM, Blackburn GL, McTiernan A (2011) Dietary weight loss and exercise effects on insulin resistance in postmenopausal women. Am J Prev Med 41(4):366–375

Mason C, Alfano CM, Smith AW et al (2013a) A long-term physical activity trends in breast cancer survivors. Cancer Epidemiol Biomarkers Prev 22(6):1153–1161

Mason C et al (2013b) Influence of diet, exercise, and serum vitamin D on sarcopenia in postmenopausal women. Med Sci Sports Exerc 45(4):607–614

McTiernan A, Tworoger SS, Ulrich CM et al (2004) Effect of exercise on serum estrogens in postmenopausal women: a 12-month randomized clinical trial. Cancer Res 64(8):2923–2928

Mefferd K et al (2007) A cognitive behavioral therapy intervention to promote weight loss improves body composition and blood lipid profiles among overweight breast cancer survivors. Breast Cancer Res Treat 104(2):145–152

Miller CT et al (2013) The effects of exercise training in addition to energy restriction on functional capacities and body composition in obese adults during weight loss: a systematic review. PLoS ONE 8(11):e81692

Mishra SI, Scherer RW, Geigle PM et al (2012) Exercise interventions on health-related quality of life for cancer survivors. Cochrane Database Syst Rev 8, CD007566

Palmirotta R, Ferroni P, Savonarola A et al (2009) Prognostic value of pre-surgical plasma PAI-1 (plasminogen activator inhibitor-1) levels in breast cancer. Thromb Res 124(4):403–408

Phillips MD, Patrizi RM, Cheek DJ, Wooten JS, Barbee JJ, Mitchell JB (2012) Resistance training reduces subclinical inflammation in obese, postmenopausal women. Med Sci Sports Exerc 44(11):2099–2110

Physical Activity Guidelines Advisory Committee (2008) Physical activity guidelines advisory committee report, 2008. U.S. Department of Health and Human Services, Washington, DC

Pierce JP et al (2007) Influence of a diet very high in vegetables, fruit, and fiber and low in fat on prognosis following treatment for breast cancer: the women's healthy eating and living (WHEL) randomized trial. JAMA 298(3):289–298

Pierce BL, Ballard-Barbash R, Bernstein L, Baumgartner RN, Neuhouser ML, Wener MH, Baumgartner KB, Gilliland FD, Sorensen BE, McTiernan A, Ulrich CM (2009) Elevated bio-markers of inflammation are associated with reduced survival among breast cancer patients. J Clin Oncol 27(21):3437–3444

Potthoff K, Schmidt ME, Wiskemann J, Hof H, Klassen O, Habermann N, Beckhove P, Debus J, Ulrich CM, Steindorf K (2013) Randomized controlled trial to evaluate the effects of progres-sive resistance training compared to progressive muscle relaxation in breast cancer patients undergoing adjuvant radiotherapy: the BEST study. BMC Cancer 13:162

Rajotte EJ et al (2012) Community-based exercise program effectiveness and safety for cancer survivors. J Cancer Surviv 6:219–228

Rock C et al (2012) Nutrition and physical activity guidelines for cancer survivors. CA Cancer J Clin 62(4):243–274

Rock CL et al (2013a) Reducing breast cancer recurrence with weight loss, a vanguard trial: the exercise and nutrition to enhance recovery and good health for you (ENERGY) trial. Contemp Clin Trials 34(2):282–295

Rock CL, Pande C, Flatt SW, Ying C, Pakiz B, Parker BA, Williams K, Bardwell WA, Heath DD, Nichols JF (2013b) Favorable changes in serum estrogens and other biologic factors after weight loss in breast cancer survivors who are overweight or obese. Clin Breast Cancer 13(3):188–195

Rose DP (1997) Dietary fatty acids and prevention of hormone-responsive cancer. Proc Soc Exp Biol Med 216(2):224–233

Schmitz KH et al (2010) American college of sports medicine roundtable on exercise guidelines for cancer survivors. Med Sci Sports Exerc 42(7):1409–1426

Schmitz KH, Ahmed RL, Troxel AB et al (2010b) Weight lifting for women at risk for breast cancer-related lymphedema: a randomized trial. JAMA 304(24):2699–2705

Scott E et al (2013) Effects of an exercise and hypocaloric healthy eating program on biomarkers associated with long-term prognosis after early-stage breast cancer: a randomized controlled trial. Cancer Causes Control 24(1):181–191

Selvin E, Paynter NP, Erlinger TP (2007) The effect of weight loss on C-reactive protein: a system-atic review. Arch Intern Med 167(1):31–39

Taylor DL et al (2010) Relationships between cardiorespiratory fitness, physical activity, and psy-chosocial variables in overweight and obese breast cancer survivors. Int J Behav Med 17(4):264–270

United States Public Health Service, Office of the Surgeon General, National Center for Chronic Disease Prevention and Health Promotion, President's Council on Physical Fitness and Sports (1996) Physical activity and health: a report of the Surgeon General. U.S. Department of Health and Human Services, Centers for Disease Control and Prevention, National Center for Chronic Disease Prevention and Health Promotion; President's Council on Physical Fitness and Sports, Atlanta, GA

Villasenor A et al (2012) Prevalence and prognostic effect of sarcopenia in breast cancer survivors: the HEAL study. J Cancer Surviv 6(4):398–406

Villaseñor A, Flatt SW, Marinac C, Natarajan L, Pierce JP, Patterson RE (2014) Postdiagnosis C-reactive protein and breast cancer survivorship: findings from the WHEL study. Cancer Epidemiol Biomarkers Prev 23(1):189–199

Woolcott CG, Courneya KS, Boyd NF, Yaffe MJ, Terry T, McTiernan A, Brant R, Ballard-Barbash R, Irwin ML, Jones CA, Brar S, Campbell KL, McNeely ML, Karvinen KH, Friedenreich CM (2010) Mammographic density change with 1 year of aerobic exercise among postmenopausal women: a randomized controlled trial. Cancer Epidemiol Biomarkers Prev 19(4):1112–1121

Chapter 14
Prevention and Treatment of Cardiac Dysfunction in Breast Cancer Survivors

Carol Fabian

Abstract As recurrence free survival following a breast cancer diagnosis continues to improve, cardiovascular morbidity and mortality will assume greater importance in the breast cancer survivorship research agenda particularly for women receiving potentially cardiotoxic therapy. Development of (1) tools to readily identify pre-diagnostic risk factors for cardiac dysfunction, (2) well-tolerated prophylactic treatments to reduce the risk of cardiac injury, and (3) sensitive and affordable monitoring techniques which can identify subclinical toxicity prior to a drop in left ventricular ejection fraction are or should be focus areas of cardio-oncology research. Since weight as well as cardiorespiratory fitness generally decline after a breast cancer diagnosis, behavioral approaches which can improve energy balance and fitness are important to optimize cardiovascular health in all breast cancer survivors not just those undergoing cardiotoxic therapy. These goals are likely best achieved by partnerships between cardiologists, oncologists and internists such as those initiated with the formation of the International CardiOncology Society (ICOS) and the NCI Community Cardiotoxicity Task Force.

Keyword Risk factors and prevention of cardiac toxicity with breast cancer treatment

Introduction

Cardiovascular disease is the most common cause of death for women with Stage I breast cancer who are 67 years of age or older (van de Water et al. 2012) and the third most common cause of death in women undergoing adjuvant treatment irrespective of age and type of treatment (Schonberg et al. 2011) behind breast cancer

C. Fabian, M.D. (✉)
Director Breast Cancer Prevention and Survivorship Center,
University of Kansas Cancer Center, 2330 Shawnee Mission
Parkway Suite 1102, Westwood, KS 66205, USA
e-mail: cfabian@kumc.edu

© Breast Cancer Research Foundation 2015
P.A. Ganz (ed.), *Improving Outcomes for Breast Cancer Survivors*,
Advances in Experimental Medicine and Biology 862,
DOI 10.1007/978-3-319-16366-6_14

213

recurrence and second primary tumor. Treatment can increase the risk of cardiovascular morbidity and mortality through (1) damage to cardiac myocytes (anthracyclines and HER-2 targeted agents) (Swain et al. 2003; Naumann et al. 2013); (2) damage to blood vessels (radiation) (Darby et al. 2013); (3) induction of hypertension (VEGF inhibitors, platinum) (Steingart et al. 2012; Cameron et al. 2013); (4) reduction in tissue estrogen levels with premature menopause or antihormonal therapies (Rivera et al. 2009; Ewer and Glück 2009); (5) weight gain (Rock et al. 1999); and (6) reduction in cardiorespiratory fitness (Darby et al. 2013; Bowles et al. 2012; Barlow et al. 2012) due to a decrease in physical activity after diagnosis (Irwin et al. 2003; Lakoski et al. 2013). As the proportion of women surviving a breast cancer diagnosis continues to increase, the prevalence of cardiovascular disease and cardiac dysfunction due to the combination of pre-existing risk factors and cancer treatment is also likely to rise (Carver et al. 2007). A major thrust of survivorship research needs to be the identification of those at highest risk for developing cardiac dysfunction and development of pathways and treatment protocols to reduce dysfunction. The National Cancer Institute has formed a work group called the NCI Community Cardiotoxicity Task Force in an effort to standardize terminology and to help refine and prioritize clinical cardio-oncology research. In this chapter we will focus primarily on cardiac dysfunction and heart failure as opposed to, coronary artery and peripheral artery disease although these may be important pre-existing factors or in some cases induced by treatment such as radiation therapy (Darby et al. 2013).

Identification of Pre-existing Risk Factors for Cardiovascular Disease and Cardiac Dysfunction

Risk factors for cardiovascular disease (age, obesity, diabetes, dyslipidemia, hypertension, family history, and poor cardio-respiratory fitness) are so prevalent in our society that as oncologists we give little thought as to whether a patient should avoid potentially cardiotoxic therapy unless the individual has previously suffered a major cardiac event, is of advanced age, or has an abnormal left ventricular ejection fraction (Bowles et al. 2012; Chavez-MacGregor et al. 2013). Left ventricular ejection fraction is the proportion of blood volume in the left ventricle that is pumped out of the heart with each contraction and is normally between 55 and 70 %. We standardly use left ventricular ejection fraction (LVEF) to screen for women who should not have cardiotoxic therapy because cardiac damage or impairment of ventricular muscle strength is already present (Lenihan et al. 2013); but a normal LVEF does not mean normal function. Women with hypertension often have a normal LVEF but other evidence of cardiac dysfunction (Young et al. 2012). Prior to initiating potentially cardiotoxic therapy, women should be screened for hypertension, diabetes, hyperlipidemia, and prolongation of the QT interval, even with a normal LVEF as

Table 14.1 Screening prior to initiation of cardiotoxic therapy

History	Parameter	Action
Age/family history		
Obesity	BMI	Avoid further gain, gradual loss
Diabetes	HbA1C/Fasting glucose	Initiate diabetic therapy
Inactivity	Minutes of recreational physical activity/week	Encourage 150 min or more recreational physical activity per week
Fitness	VO2 peak/6 min walk	Gradual increase with exercise to moderately fit or better
Hypertension	BP	Monitor/correct
Dyslipidemia	Fasting lipid profile	Initiate therapy
Smoking		Smoking cessation aids
Cardiac evaluation	LVEF: Echocardiogram or MUGA	Avoid cardio-toxic drugs if abnormal Referral to cardiologist
Cardiac evaluation	EKG/QT interval	Avoid cardio-toxic drugs if abnormal Referral to cardiologist

measured by multi-gated acquisition (MUGA) scan or 2D echocardiogram. Treatment should be initiated to correct risk factors prior to chemotherapy where possible (Ewer and Glück 2009; Lenihan et al. 2013; Mosca et al. 2012). All women should be encouraged to implement a healthy lifestyle including smoking cessation, a balanced diet high in fruits and vegetables but low enough in calories to avoid weight gain, and 150 min of physical activity a week (Mosca et al. 2012) (See Table 14.1). The complexity of decision making regarding systemic cancer treatment, tight time frames, and reluctance to intrude on what is generally considered the general internist's or cardiologist's territory often relegates initiation of treatment of mild hypertension, type II diabetes and hyperlipidemia, obesity or poor fitness to the back burner to be dealt with after chemotherapy. There is generally little discussion by oncologists of behavioral approaches to improve the cardiovascular risk profile. On the other hand automatic referrals of women to general internists to have their mild hypertension normalized before instituting chemotherapy can have untoward consequences as decreases in blood pressure and postural hypotension often occur with commonly used chemotherapeutic agents for breast cancer including anthracyclines and taxanes.

Development of simple evidence based oncology guidelines for the optimal screening of asymptomatic women for cardiac risk factors, and timing of initiation of treatment for reversible conditions should have major importance in the survivorship research agenda. This is will take a collaborative effort between Medical Oncologists, Cardiologists and Primary Care Physicians. The International CardiOncology Society (ICOS) was founded to review emerging trial evidence and make recommendations to assess risk and provide treatment recommendations for patients undergoing treatment for a variety of cancers (Lenihan et al. 2010).

Need for Use of Standard Nomenclature to Describe Risk and Severity of Cardiac Dysfunction

The increase in rates of clinical heart failure in pivotal trials of trastuzumab in women with metastatic disease, especially those who were receiving or who had recently received anthracyclines, prompted establishment of the Cardiac Review and Evaluation Committee or CREC. Initial CREC criteria used to describe cardiac dysfunction and subsequently employed in many adjuvant trials were (1) cardiomyopathy characterized by a global decrease in left ventricular ejection fraction (LVEF); (2) signs or symptoms of congestive heart failure (CHF); (3) decline in LVEF of at least 5 % to less than 55 % with signs or symptoms of CHF; or (4) decline in LVEF of at least 10 % to less than 55 % without signs or symptoms of CHF (Seidman et al. 2002). The definition of cardiac dysfunction in oncology trials has differed somewhat from trial to trial making cross trial comparisons somewhat difficult. For example a drop in LVEF by 10 points or more to less than 55 % was considered evidence of cardiac dysfunction in the NSABP B-31 trial but the HERA trial required an absolute drop of 10 points or more to an LVEF of less than 50 % (Tan-Chiu et al. 2005; Piccart-Gebhart et al. 2005). Research in cardiac dysfunction/heart failure in breast cancer survivors would be facilitated by agreement on standard terminology for assessment in clinical trials. Use of American Heart Association criteria for heart failure is appropriate: Stage A risk factors present but no structural damage; Stage B structural damage but no signs or symptoms; Stage C structural damage with current or prior symptoms; and Stage D structural damage with symptoms with any physical activity or at rest (Yancy et al. 2013) (see Table 14.2). Asymptomatic reduction in left

Table 14.2 American Heart Association criteria for heart failure (Yancy et al. 2013) and treatment by stage

AHA heart failure stage	New York Heart Association	Current Treatment Recommendations (Rx)	Research needed
Stage A: High risk but no structural damage	I	Correct risk factors: hypertension, hyperlipidemia, diabetes, obesity. poor fitness, alcohol and smoking	Predictive model of transition A to B Protective Rx to prevent A to B transition Application research
Stage B: Structural damage but no signs or symptoms of heart failure (LVEF < 50 % but usually >40–45 %)	I	Correct risk factors B blockers, ACEI or ARBs as appropriate	Sensitive monitoring tools detect A to B transition Rx to allow cardiotoxic drugs
Stage C: Structural heart disease. prior or current symptoms (LVEF <40 %)	I-IV	Discontinue cardiotoxic drug Heart failure therapy	Rx to allow re-institution of cardiotoxic drugs once compensated
Stage D: Symptoms at rest or any physical activity	IV	Heart failure therapy	N/A

ventricular ejection fraction (LVEF) by 10 or more points to <50 % is generally viewed as representative of the Stage A to Stage B transition and is associated with a significant increase in cardiac mortality (Lenihan et al. 2013). Consequently, an asymptomatic reduction in left ventricular ejection fraction by 10 or more points to <50 % has come to represent a surrogate endpoint for cardiac injury in clinical trials and in the remainder of this manuscript will be referred to as subclinical cardiac toxicity and/or cardiac dysfunction.

Drug Related Cardiac Toxicity

Although many drugs can result in cardiac damage (Yeh et al. 2004; Bovelli et al. 2010), we will focus here on the two most commonly used types of agents with the greatest potential for cardiac dysfunction, namely anthracyclines and HER-2 targeted agents.

Anthracyclines

Anthracyclines increase free radical formation, mitochondrial oxidative stress, disruption of myofibrils, apoptosis of cardiomyocytes, and reduction of the cardiac stem cell pool (Kumar et al. 1999; Zhang et al. 2012; De Angelis et al. 2010). A recent meta-analysis suggests that without regard to dose, treatment with anthracyclines increases clinical cardiac toxicity, usually manifested as heart failure, by approximately fivefold, subclinical toxicity by sixfold, and the risk of cardiac death by fivefold (Smith et al. 2010). The absolute risk of clinical or subclinical cardiac toxicity depends upon the type of anthracycline, the cumulative dose, exposure to additional cardiotoxic agents, patient age, African American race, and other comorbidities (Bowles et al. 2012; Lotrionte et al. 2013; Perez et al. 2004; Bird and Swain 2008). By the time significant changes are noted in LVEF (drop of 10 or more points to <50 %) permanent damage has generally already occurred.

Clinical heart failure is very rare in healthy individuals taking a cumulative doxorubicin dose of 240 mg/m^2 (the average with four cycles of doxorubicin and cyclophosphamide) unless other cardiotoxic agents are being administered concomitantly; but subclinical cardiac toxicity (an asymptomatic decrease in LVEF by 10 or more points to <50 %) was reported in 3.3 % of healthy women with a median age of 52 receiving four cycles of this anthracycline based regimen with short follow-up (Perez et al. 2004). A recent review of 18 studies with over 20,000 women treated with anthracyclines at varying cumulative doses and followed for a median of 9 years, reports an asymptomatic drop in LVEF to <50 % occurred in 18 %; and symptomatic cardiac toxicity, primarily heart failure, occurred in 6 % (Lotrionte et al. 2013). Clinical heart failure in the 40 % of women with breast cancer over 65 treated with anthracyclines is substantially higher due in large part to the underlying presence of asymptomatic heart disease. Using data from a large SEER data base,

38 % of women age 66–70 at the time they took anthracycline-based chemotherapy had developed congestive heart failure 10 years later compared to 32 % of women taking non-anthracycline chemotherapy and 29 % of women not taking any chemotherapy (Pinder et al. 2007).

Epirubicin is ~60 % less likely to result in cardiac toxicity than doxorubicin and liposomal doxorubicin has a 22 % lower risk than doxorubicin. Finally, continuous infusion doxorubicin over several days has approximately one-fourth of the cardiac toxicity as bolus doxorubicin (Smith et al. 2010).

The substantially higher rates of congestive failure in women over 65 taking bolus doxorubicin suggests that most older women should receive either non-anthracycline containing regimens, less toxic forms of anthracyclines, or protective therapy. Continuing research in this are using sensitive biomarkers to predict a drop in left ventricular ejection fraction area the abnormal range with early intervention prior to drop in ejection fraction is warranted (see below).

Inhibition of topo-isomerase II DNA binding appears to be an important factor in both anthracycline induced tumor cell death and cardiomyocyte injury. However, recent evidence suggests that TOP2A may be the primary target for doxorubicin induced tumor cell death whereas TOP2B may be the primary intermediate in cardiac induced injury (Vejpongsa and Yeh 2014). These data suggest that development of TOP2A specific anthracyclines may be an important future area of research (Sawyer 2013).

Trastuzumab and Other HER-2 Targeted Agents

The epidermal growth factor receptors are involved in proliferation and regeneration, metabolism, differentiation and cell survival. HER-2 (ErbB2) is one of four epidermal growth factor receptors expressed on the surface of cardiomyocytes as well as breast cancer cells. Hetero- or homo-dimerization of receptors is necessary for downstream signaling. ErbB2 has no identified natural ligand but is the preferred binding partner for the other ErbB receptors. Dimerization of HER-2 can be induced by an increase in receptor concentration or by ligand binding (EGF, TGF alpha and amphiregulin for ErbB1 and neuregulin for ErbB3/4) with one of the other ErbB receptors. Homo-dimerization of ERbB2 or hetero-dimerization of ErB2 and ErbB3 in HER-2 amplified breast cancer leads to a dramatic increase in proliferative and survival signals primarily through the PI3 kinase pathway (De Keulenaer et al. 2010). ErbB2 is expressed at low levels in the adult heart and is up regulated in response to stress or injury (such as with anthracyclines) (De Keulenaer et al. 2010). Neuregulin is released by endothelial cells and once bound to ErbB4 results in hetero-dimerization with ErbB2 and proliferation of cardiac progenitor cells and possibly de-differentiation and proliferation of differentiated cardiomyocytes (De Keulenaer et al. 2010; Hervent et al. 2012). Trastuzumab binds with ErB2, disrupting the Neuregulin 1β /ErB2/ErbB4 complex which in turn prevents proliferation of cardiac progenitor cells in response to stress (Bersell et al. 2009; Fedele et al. 2012). Investigators are looking at rational designs for HER-2 targeted agents which will not disrupt the neuregulin/ErbB4 complex (Fedele et al. 2012). Use of neuregulin to prevent or treat preclinical cardiac damage is also of interest (Bersell et al. 2009).

Trastuzumab without prior anthracyclines or other underlying cardiac risk factors may be associated with declines in LVEF but generally not irreversible heart failure. However, both asymptomatic cardiac dysfunction and symptomatic heart failure occur more frequently in individuals given trastuzumab after or concomitantly with an anthracycline compared to an anthracycline alone (De Keulenaer et al. 2010; Perez et al. 2008; Gianni et al. 2011; Goldhirsch et al. 2013). Utilizing CREC criteria, trastuzumab with a taxane in women with prior anthracycline exposure had a cardiac dysfunction rate of 13–16 % and a New York Heart Association class III or IV heart failure rate of 2–4 % whereas trastuzumab used concomitantly with anthracyclines was associated with a cardiac dysfunction rate of ~27 % and a New York Heart Association class III or IV heart failure rate of ~16 % in early trials (Seidman et al. 2002). A recent update of the Herceptin Adjuvant or HERA trial in which one or 2 years of trastuzumab was given after adjuvant therapy, cardiac adverse event leading to discontinuation occurred in 9.4 % of women on the 2 years arm vs. 5.2 % of women on the 1 year arm. All but 12–20 % of women with significant LVEF declines recovered with less than 1 % developing symptomatic congestive heart failure (de Azambuja et al. 2014). Risk factors for cardiac dysfunction in addition to anthracyclines for women receiving adjuvant trastuzumab are age >60, a borderline normal left ventricular ejection fraction (50–55 %) at baseline and pre-existing hypertension (Tan-Chiu et al. 2005). Despite theoretical concerns, using two HER-2 targeted agents simultaneously such as pertuzumab and trastuzumab or lapitinib and trastuzumab does not appear to increase cardiac toxicity to a greater extent than trastuzumab alone, although there is limited long term experience (Valachis et al. 2013; Baselga et al. 2012).

Older women are likely to have one or more cardiac risk factors at baseline and were under-represented in clinical trials. An analysis from a Medicare claims data base of women 67 and older with early breast cancer indicates that 32 % had evidence of cardiac dysfunction or heart failure if they took trastuzumab alone, 42 % if they received both trastuzumab and anthracyclines but only 18 % of those receiving no adjuvant therapy (Vaz-Luis et al. 2014). Another population based study of women >65 most of whom took their trastuzumab concomitantly with chemotherapy noted a 3.6 % hospitalization rate for cardiac events during treatment (Chen et al. 2012) Research with cardio-protective regimens coupled with biomarkers of early injury is needed targeting older women receiving trastuzumab or others with baseline risk factors for cardiac dysfunction (Wells and Lenihan 2010).

Physical Activity and Cardiorespiratory Fitness

Although, oncologists are increasingly aware of the potential adverse effects of excessive weight on breast cancer outcomes and mortality, there has not been the same emphasis on physical activity and cardiorespiratory fitness.

Physical activity is associated with lower cardiovascular, all cause and breast cancer mortality (George et al. 2011; Irwin et al. 2011; Dhaliwal et al. 2013). In the Women's Health Initiative 9 MET hours or about 3 h of fast walking per week pre or post diagnosis of breast cancer was enough to see an ~40 % decrease in breast cancer and all-cause mortality compared with sedentary women (Irwin et al. 2011). The important message then for women is to become active even if they were not prior to their diagnosis of breast cancer.

Cardiorespiratory fitness as measured by oxygen consumption at peak exercise ($VO2_{max}$ or $VO2_{peak}$) is correlated with cardiovascular and all-cause mortality (Peel et al. 2009). In a general population increasing fitness by only one metabolic equivalent (1 MET corresponds to 3.5 mL/min/kg of oxygen consumption) is estimated to reduce risk of death by 13 % (Kodama et al. 2009). Individuals with low CRF (<7.9 METs) had a 40 % increase in all-cause mortality and 47 % increase in risk for cardiovascular events compared with those with intermediate CRF (7.9–10.8 METs). Women with low CRF had a 70 % increase in all-cause mortality and 56 % increase in cardiovascular events compared to those with high CRF ($\geq$10.9 METs) (Kodama et al. 2009). Further, fitness may be a more important predictor of mortality than Body Mass Index (BMI) until one reaches the extremes of obesity where serious metabolic abnormalities are prevalent. In a recent meta-analysis, fit overweight and obese women had similar mortality as fit normal weight women, and were generally better off than normal weight unfit women unless the obese fit woman also had a chronic disease (Barry et al. 2014). 150 min of moderate physical activity per week or that sufficient to expend at least 1,000 Kcal per week is likely to allow most women to attain at least the lower bound of the intermediate CRF category (Lee and Skerrett 2001).

Women with breast cancer appear to have lower baseline CR fitness than age-matched individuals without cancer and fitness declines during treatment (Jones et al. 2012; Peel et al. 2014). Low fitness was reported in approximately half of women who had undergone chemotherapy with anthracyclines + taxanes with or without trastuzumab ~2 years after chemotherapy completion despite a normal LVEF in all but 8 % (Jones et al. 2007). These rates were dramatically higher than age-matched controls who had not received chemotherapy (Jones et al. 2007).

Research efforts need to focus on effective interventions which will prevent reduction of physical activity and fitness during and after treatment. Courneya et al. using a supervised aerobic and strength training exercise program have demonstrated that higher volume exercise can be safely delivered during adjuvant treatment, which in turn appears correlated with improved disease free and overall survival (Courneya et al. 2013, 2014). Higher intensity exercise may also favorably modulate pro-inflammatory biomarkers associated with cardiovascular disease risk (Fairey et al. 2005).

Methods to safely increase physical activity and fitness in a more practical, home-based environment following initial in-person training need to be a research priority, particularly for older women and those with a low level of fitness at baseline. Preliminary pilot studies suggest this is possible (Burnett et al. 2013). Further, simplified methods of assessing fitness which can easily be employed in an oncologist's office such as the 6 min step test need to be validated against more complex tools such as VO2$_{max}$ or VO2$_{peak}$ (Hamilton and Haennel 2000; Simonsick et al. 2006).

Risk Prediction Models for Cardiac Toxicity

Prediction models in older women at highest risk for cardiac toxicity have been suggested using variables of age, type of adjuvant therapy, and prior history of hypertension, diabetes, and symptomatic heart disease (Ezaz et al. 2014). Research is needed to develop more sensitive and specific cardiac dysfunction prediction models for women considering potentially cardiotoxic therapy which would include risk biomarkers and historical variables. These prediction models would ideally have the ability to include some of the new very sensitive indicators of left ventricular function (Fallah-Rad et al. 2011), in addition to weighted factor scores for age, BMI, a measure of physical activity or cardiorespiratory fitness, hypertension, diabetes, dyslipidemia, and any prior cardiac event. Ideally the models could also be adapted to include provision for genetic polymorphisms predisposing to cardiac risk such as the common HER-2 Ile655Val allele in the HER-2 gene (Beauclair et al. 2007), and polymorphisms in NADPH oxidase, MDR 1, MDR 2, catalase, superoxide dismutase, NADPH:quinone oxidoreductase, carbonyl reductase 3, and glutathione s-transferase (Wojnowski et al. 2005; Deng and Wojnowski 2007).

Monitoring Cardiac Function During Treatment with Cardiotoxic Agents

Cardiac MRI is a sensitive method for detecting left ventricular remodeling and early subclinical cardiac toxicity and is considered by some to be the gold standard (Fallah-Rad et al. 2011). It is currently being used in the MANTICORE trial to measure left ventricular end diastolic volumes (see below). However, cardiac MRI is expensive and thus not optimal for serial monitoring in the clinical community setting (Bellenger et al. 2000). Longitudinal or global left ventricular strain, which can be calculated from an echocardiogram with the appropriate software, is a measure of cardiac muscle deformability. The greater the negative value the more powerful the contraction. Normal strain values vary with age, sex and the software system used from approximately −15 to −22 (Yingchoncharoen et al. 2013; Cheng et al. 2013), but a value of −19 or more negative is highly unlikely to be associated with cardiac dysfunction or clinical congestive heart failure over the ensuing 3 months of cardiotoxic treatment (Sawaya et al. 2011, 2012). Adding a serum troponin drawn before and immediately after chemotherapy to left ventricular strain is reported to improve both sensitivity and negative predictive value for left ventricular dysfunction after anthracyclines (Fallah-Rad et al. 2011; Cardinale et al. 2010).

Although some studies have suggested additional serum markers such as and high sensitivity c-reactive protein (hsCRP) may aid in predicting cardiac dysfunction, others have not found that the addition of serum biomarkers in addition to troponin to substantially increase sensitivity (Onitilo et al. 2012), in 78 patients receiving both doxorubicin and trastuzumab, found the addition of hsCRP and BNP did not add additional predictive information to ultrasensitive troponin and myeloperoxidase in predicting dysfunction by CREC criteria (Ky et al. 2014). 3D echocardiography may be more sensitive than 2D to declines in left ventricular function (Khouri et al. 2014).

Studies incorporating one or more of these markers into the monitoring process for cardiac toxicity (i.e., PREDICT trial) are currently ongoing. Left ventricular strain has perhaps the greatest potential in that the software is relatively easy to add to an echocardiogram machine and is a non-invasive procedure. Unfortunately, there are variations in the software and interpretations of results such that at present there is not a clear indication as to what constitutes a definitely abnormal strain or the amount of change which should be viewed with alarm.

Trials comparing the relative efficacy of newer sensitive biomarkers of subclinical injury prior to significant decline in 2D echo left ventricular ejection fraction, including high sensitivity troponin and other serum biomarkers, left ventricular strain, and cardiac MRI are ongoing and results are awaited with interest. Translational trials incorporating prophylactic treatment with beta blockers and angiotensin converting enzyme inhibitors at first signs of subclinical dysfunction are warranted.

Treatment of Cardiac Dysfunction

Beta blockers, angiotensin converting enzyme inhibitors (ACEI), and angiotensin receptor blockers (ARBs) are commonly used to treat heart failure regardless of the inciting event. They are recommended in the general cardiovascular setting for asymptomatic women with a drop in left ventricular ejection fraction below 40 % or women with symptomatic congestive heart failure regardless of the amount of decline in LVEF (Yancy et al. 2013). Patients who develop symptomatic cardiac dysfunction while on treatment with a cardiotoxic agent should be treated as would anyone not on chemotherapy (Yeh et al. 2004). For women with early breast cancer, treatment with the cardiotoxic agent should be discontinued and non-cardiotoxic therapy substituted where possible. For women with metastatic HER-2 amplified breast cancer, temporarily discontinuing HER-2 targeted agents, treatment with blockers and ACEIs and then cautious re-introduction of the HER-2 targeted agent is often successful with continued indefinite use of the beta blocker and ACE inhibitor (Vaz-Luis et al. 2014).

What about asymptomatic women with subclinical cardiac toxicity whose LVEF is below 50 % but above 40 %? From the general population experience, it is clear that individuals with an asymptomatic ejection fraction below 50 % have a ~3.5-fold increase in all- cause mortality over the ensuing 9–10 years (Yeboah et al. 2012a). Use of ACEI and beta blockers in women with LVEF <50 %, and appropriate surgical treatment of heart valve problems resulting from radiation or medical or surgical treatment of coronary artery blockage is suggested (Lenihan et al. 2013; Lenihan 2012).

Prophylactic Treatment with Cardioprotective Drugs

An area gaining momentum is the use of prophylactic drugs to reduce the incidence of asymptomatic left ventricular dysfunction (Swain and Vici 2004; van Dalen et al. 2008), particularly if early warning biomarkers can be used to trigger the use of the agent. Prophylactic cardioprotective therapy is not a new concept. A decade ago Swain et al. published a study suggesting doxorubicin induced cardiac toxicity can be reduced ~70 % by also giving the iron chelating agent dexrazoxane (Smith et al. 2010; Swain and Vici 2004). The current recommendation is that dexrazoxane can be given prophylactically once the cumulative doxorubicin dose exceeds 300 mg/m^2 (Yeh et al. 2004). Dexrazoxane is not widely used in clinical practice due to concerns that it may reduce effectiveness of doxorubicin as it binds to both TOPO 2A and TOPO 2B (Sawyer 2013).

Since individuals with a low LVEF, even if asymptomatic, have an increased risk of cardiac events and mortality, prophylactic cardio-preventive treatment trials are ongoing in the adjuvant setting of HER-2 positive breast cancer. Several small trials have shown cardioprotective effects of ACEI or beta blockers, especially when given with anthracyclines (Kalay et al. 2006; Bosch et al. 2011). Adjuvant trials with endpoints of symptomatic heart failure or a 2D echo measured LVEF of <50 % would require a very large number of participants. An alternative approach is to use a more sensitive indicator of early cardiac dysfunction. In the MANTICORE trial (Fig. 14.1) women taking trastuzumab are randomized to prophylactic cardiac protective therapy with beta blockers and/or ACEI but the primary outcome is change in left ventricular end diastolic volume as measured by cardiac MRI (Pituskin et al. 2011). With this endpoint as opposed to 2D echo LVEF, the trial coordinators are predicting that 158 randomized subjects will be adequate. Another approach to assess the benefit of prophylactic therapy is to use the traditional endpoint of LVEF drop by 10 points to <50 % but with a much higher risk group as the cohort, such as women with HER-2 amplified metastatic disease. Since these women have generally been previously treated with cardiotoxic drugs and since survival is dependent on being able to continue to receive HER-2 targeted therapy after first progression, the study question is of practical importance (Extra et al. 2010). Such a trial has been proposed in the Southwest Oncology Group Survivorship Committee in women with first and second line HER-2 amplified metastatic disease on HER targeted therapy with LVEF >50 % at baseline to determine whether prophylactic beta blocker therapy with Carvedilol will reduce cardiac dysfunction (See Fig. 14.2). Other target populations for prophylactic cardio-protective therapy where the event rate is likely to be high in either the metastatic or adjuvant setting are women 70 or over, high coronary artery calcium, and hypertension, or a high score on a CVD risk prediction model (Yeboah et al. 2012b).

MANTICORE Trial of Beta Blocker or ACE Inhibitor for Women Receiving Adjuvant Trastuzumab

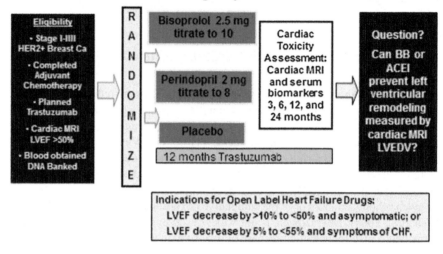

Fig. 14.1 Design of the multidisciplinary approach to novel therapies in cardiology oncology research trial (MANTICORE 101-Breast) (Kalay et al. 2006)

Carvedilol To Prevent Cardiac Toxicity in Women with HER-2 + Metastatic Breast Cancer (SWOG Proposed Concept)

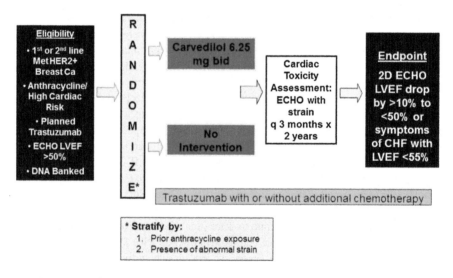

Fig. 14.2 Design of a proposed SWOG trial concept

Looking Forward

Priorites for cardio-oncology research in breast cancer are summarized in Table 14.3. Developing biomarkers and models to predict cardiac dysfunction, developing less cardiotoxic drug regimens and preventive therapy for high risk individuals, more sensitive monitoring techniques for cardiac dysfunction and treatment guidelines which might permit continuation of therapy are all important. This will take a co-ordinated research efforts of oncologists, cardiologists, and internists. An equally pressing issue is once these new treatments and guidelines are established, what type of clinical environment and training will be needed to carry them out all in a cost effective manner. Are we going to cross train oncologists in cardiology and cardiologists in oncology? With a forecast of 40 % shortage of medical oncologists over the next decade, and similar or worse shortages for general internists and cardiologists is this even reasonable? The answer is yes. After all we all started out with training in general internal medicine and most oncologists still carry a stethoscope. Cardiologists with a particular interest in heart failure can receive training in this area through combined disciplinary meetings and seminars. Many oncologists are very interested in prevention and survivorship issues but to date there have been financial disencentives to anything other than administering chemotherapy. This needs change. Older oncologists considering retirement might be persuaded to stay in the field a little longer if their practice could be focused on prevention and survivorship issues, and more emphasis on prevention and survivorship with cross

Table 14.3 Areas of research need and opportunity in cardio-oncology

1. Develop standard nomenclature to describe cardiac dysfunction following treatment
2. Develop Sensitive biomarkers and models which will predict dysfunction (i.e., drop in LVEF or transition from Stage A to B Heart Failure)
3. Develop less cardiotoxic chemotherapy
Develop TOPO 2A specific anthracyclines
Non-anthracycline containing regimens
HER-2 targeted agents which will not disrupt neuregulin/ERβ
4. Develop cardioprotective drug regimens
Establish efficacy and safety
Clinical and biomarker indications for use
5. Develop behavioral interventions for survivors which improve fitness and CV health
Develop safe but effective home-based interventions to increase fitness
Develop interventions to increase exercise uptake and compliance
Simple office-based techniques for serially assessing fitness
6. Guidelines for monitoring cardiac function during and after cardiotoxic treatment
7. Guidelines for treatment of cardiac dysfunction and continuing/re-instituting cancer treatment

disciplinary training needs to become an important part of oncology fellowship training. Guidelines and pathway development will make it easier to incorporate general internists and nurse practioners pre, during and post treatment phases of potentially cardiotoxic treatment.

Conclusion

Development of easy to use tools which will combine clinical factors and biomarkers to identify those individuals at highest risk for development of cardiac dysfunction, sensitive biomarkers of cardiac injury which will detect reversible cardiac structural change and to develop prophylactic treatments to prevent women from developing early stage cardiac dysfunction or progression to a later stage is a challenge for cardio-oncology survivorship research.

References

Barlow CE, Defina LF, Radford NB et al (2012) Cardiorespiratory fitness and long-term survival in "low-risk" adults. J Am Heart Assoc 1(4):e001354

Barry VW, Baruth M, Beets MW et al (2014) Fitness vs. fatness on all-cause mortality: a meta-analysis. Prog Cardiovasc Dis 56(4):382–390

Baselga J, Cortés J, Kim SB et al (2012) Pertuzumab plus trastuzumab plus docetaxel for metastatic breast cancer. N Engl J Med 366(2):109–119

Beauclair S, Formento P, Fischel JL et al (2007) Role of HER2Ille65VAL genetic polymorphism in tumorgenesis and in the risk of trastuzumab-related cardiotoxicity. Ann Oncol 18: 1335–1341

Bellenger NG, Grothues F, Smith GC et al (2000) Quantification of right and left ventricular function by cardiovascular magnetic resonance. Herz 25:392–399

Bersell K, Arab S, Haring B et al (2009) Neuregulin1/ErbB4 signaling induces cardiomyocyte proliferation and repair of heart injury. Cell 138:257–270

Bird BR, Swain SM (2008) Cardiac toxicity in breast cancer survivors: review of potential cardiac problems. Clin Cancer Res 14(1):14–24

Bosch X, Esteve J, Sitges M et al (2011) Prevention of chemotherapy-induced left ventricular dysfunction with enalapril and carvedilol: rationale and design of the OVERCOME trial. J Card Fail 17(8):643–648

Bovelli D, Plataniotis G, Roila F (2010) Cardiotoxicity of chemotherapeutic agents and radiotherapy-related heart disease: ESMO clinical practice guidelines. Ann Oncol 21(Suppl 5):v277–v282

Bowles EJ, Wellman R, Feigelson HS et al (2012) Risk of heart failure in breast cancer patients after anthracycline and trastuzumab treatment: a retrospective cohort study. J Natl Cancer Inst 104(17):1293–1305

Burnett D, Kluding P, Porter C et al (2013) Cardiorespiratory fitness in breast cancer survivors. Springerplus 2(1):68 (Epub 2013 Feb 25)

Cameron D, Brown J, Dent R et al (2013) Adjuvant bevacizumab-containing therapy in triple-negative breast cancer (BEATRICE): primary results of a randomised, phase 3 trial. Lancet Oncol 14(10):933–942

Cardinale D, Colombo A, Torrisi R et al (2010) Trastuzumab-induced cardiotoxicity: clinical and prognostic implications of troponin I evaluation. J Clin Oncol 28(25):3910–3916

Carver JR, Shapiro CL, Ng A et al (2007) American society of clinical oncology clinical evidence review on the ongoing care of adult cancer survivors: cardiac and pulmonary late effects. J Clin Oncol 25:3991–4008

Chavez-MacGregor M, Zhang N, Buchholz TA et al (2013) Trastuzumab-related cardiotoxicity among older patients with breast cancer. J Clin Oncol 31(33):4222–4228

Chen J, Long JB, Hurria A et al (2012) Incidence of heart failure or cardiomyopathy after adjuvant trastuzumab therapy for breast cancer. J Am Coll Cardiol 60(24):2504–2512

Cheng S, Larson MG, McCabe EL et al (2013) Age- and sex-based reference limits and clinical correlates of myocardial strain and synchrony: the Framingham heart study. Circ Cardiovasc Imaging 6(5):692–699

Courneya KS, McKenzie DC, Mackey JR et al (2013) Effects of exercise dose and type during breast cancer chemotherapy: multicenter randomized trial. J Natl Cancer Inst 105(23): 1821–1832

Courneya KS, Segal RJ, McKenzie DC et al (2014) Effects of exercise during adjuvant chemotherapy on breast cancer outcomes. Med Sci Sports Exerc Mar 46(9):1744–1751

Darby SC, Ewertz M, Hall P (2013) Ischemic heart disease after breast cancer radiotherapy. N Engl J Med 368(26):2527

De Angelis A, Piegari E, Cappetta D et al (2010) Anthracycline cardiomyopathy is mediated by depletion of the cardiac stem cell pool and is rescued by restoration of progenitor cell function. Circulation 121(2):276–292

de Azambuja E, Procter MJ, van Veldhuisen DJ, Agbor-Tarh D, Metzger-Filho O, Steinseifer J, Untch M, Smith IE, Gianni L, Baselga J, Jackisch C, Cameron DA, Bell R, Leyland-Jones B, Dowsett M, Gelber RD, Piccart-Gebhart MJ, Suter TM (2014) Trastuzumab-associated cardiac events at 8 years of median follow-up in the herceptin adjuvant trial (BIG 1-01). J Clin Oncol 32(20):2159–2165

De Keulenaer GW, Doggen K, Lemmens K (2010) The vulnerability of the heart as a pluricellular paracrine organ: lessons from unexpected triggers of heart failure in targeted ErbB2 anticancer therapy. Circ Res 106(1):35–46

Deng S, Wojnowski L (2007) Genotyping the risk of anthracycline-induced cardiotoxicity. Cardiovasc Toxicol 7:129–134

Dhaliwal SS, Welborn TA, Howat PA (2013) Recreational physical activity as an independent predictor of multivariable cardiovascular disease risk. PLoS ONE 8(12):e83435

Ewer MS, Glück S (2009) A woman's heart: the impact of adjuvant endocrine therapy on cardiovascular health. Cancer 115(9):1813–1826

Extra JM, Antoine EC, Vincent-Salomon A et al (2010) Efficacy of trastuzumab in routine clinical practice and after progression for metastatic breast cancer patients: the observational Hermine study. Oncologist 15(8):799–809

Ezaz G, Long JB, Gross CP et al (2014) Risk prediction model for heart failure and cardiomyopathy after adjuvant trastuzumab therapy for breast cancer. J Am Heart Assoc 3(1):e000472

Fairey AS, Courneya KS, Field CJ et al (2005) Effect of exercise training on C-reactive protein in postmenopausal breast cancer survivors: a randomized controlled trial. Brain Behav Immun 19(5):381–388

Fallah-Rad N, Walker JR, Wassef A et al (2011) The utility of cardiac biomarkers, tissue velocity and strain imaging, and cardiac magnetic resonance imaging in predicting early left ventricular dysfunction in patients with human epidermal growth factor receptor II-positive breast cancer treated with adjuvant trastuzumab therapy. J Am Coll Cardiol 57:2263–2270

Fedele C, Riccio G, Malara AE et al (2012) Mechanisms of cardiotoxicity associated with ErbB2 inhibitors. Breast Cancer Res Treat 134(2):595–602

George SM, Irwin ML, Smith AW et al (2011) Postdiagnosis diet quality, the combination of diet quality and recreational physical activity, and prognosis after early-stage breast cancer. Cancer Causes Control 22(4):589–598

Gianni L, Dafni U, Gelber RD et al (2011) Treatment with trastuzumab for 1 year after adjuvant chemotherapy in patients with HER2-positive early breast cancer: a 4-year follow-up of a randomized controlled trial. Lancet Oncol 12(3):236–244

Goldhirsch A, Gelber RD, Piccart-Gebhart MJ et al (2013) 2 years versus 1 year of adjuvant trastuzumab for HER2-positive breast cancer (HERA): an open-label, randomised controlled trial. Lancet 382(9897):1021–1028

Hamilton DM, Haennel RG (2000) Validity and reliability of the 6-minute walk test in a cardiac rehabilitation population. J Cardiopulm Rehabil 20(3):156–164

Hervent AS, De Keulenaer GW et al (2012) Molecular mechanisms of cardiotoxicity induced by ErbB receptor inhibitor cancer therapeutics. Int J Mol Sci 13(10):12268–12286

Irwin ML, Crumley D, McTiernan A et al (2003) Physical activity levels before and after a diagnosis of breast carcinoma: the health, eating, activity, and lifestyle (HEAL) study. Cancer 97:1746–1757

Irwin ML, McTiernan A, Manson JE et al (2011) Physical activity and survival in postmenopausal women with breast cancer: results from the women's health initiative. Cancer Prev Res (Phila) 4(4):522–529

Jones LW, Haykowsky M, Peddle CJ et al (2007) Cardiovascular risk profile of patients with HER2/neu-positive breast cancer treated with anthracycline-taxane-containing adjuvant chemotherapy and/or trastuzumab. Cancer Epidemiol Biomarkers Prev 16(5):1026–1031

Jones LW, Courneya KS, Mackey JR et al (2012) Cardiopulmonary function and age-related decline across the breast cancer survivorship continuum. J Clin Oncol 30(20):2530–2537

Kalay N, Basar E, Ozdogru I et al (2006) Protective effects of carvedilol against anthracycline-induced cardiomyopathy. J Am Coll Cardiol 48:2258–2262

Khouri MG, Hornsby WE, Risum N et al (2014) Utility of 3-dimensional echocardiography, global longitudinal strain, and exercise stress echocardiography to detect cardiac dysfunction in breast cancer patients treated with doxorubicin-containing adjuvant therapy. Breast Cancer Res Treat 143(3):531–539

Kodama S, Saito K, Tanaka S et al (2009) Cardiorespiratory fitness as a quantitative predictor of all-cause mortality and cardiovascular events in healthy men and women: a meta-analysis. JAMA 301(19):2024–2035

Kumar D, Kirshenbaum L, Li T et al (1999) Apoptosis in isolated adult cardiomyocytes exposed to adriamycin. Ann NY Acad Sci 874:156–168

Ky B, Putt M, Sawaya H et al (2014) Early increases in multiple biomarkers predict subsequent cardiotoxicity in patients with breast cancer treated with Doxorubicin, taxanes, and trastuzumab. J Am Coll Cardiol 63(8):809–816

Lakoski SG, Barlow CE, Koelwyn GJ et al (2013) The influence of adjuvant therapy on cardiorespiratory fitness in early-stage breast cancer seven years after diagnosis: the Cooper Center Longitudinal Study. Breast Cancer Res Treat 138(3):909–916

Lee IM, Skerrett PJ (2001) Physical activity and all-cause mortality: what is the dose-response relation? Med Sci Sports Exerc 33(6 suppl):S459–S471

Lenihan DJ (2012) Progression of heart failure from AHA/ACC stage A to stage B or even C: can we all agree we should try to prevent this from happening? J Am Coll Cardiol 60:2513–2514

Lenihan DJ, Cardinale D, Cipolla CM (2010) The compelling need for a cardiology and oncology partnership and the birth of the International CardiOncology Society. Prog Cardiovasc Dis 53(2):88–93

Lenihan DJ, Oliva S, Chow EJ et al (2013) Cardiac toxicity in cancer survivors. Cancer 119(Suppl 11):2131–2142

Lotrionte M, Biondi-Zoccai G, Abbate A et al (2013) Review and meta-analysis of incidence and clinical predictors of anthracycline cardiotoxicity. Am J Cardiol 112(12):1980–1984

Mosca L, Benjamin EJ, Berra K et al (2012) Effectiveness-based guidelines for the prevention of cardiovascular disease in women – 2011 update: a guideline from the American Heart Association. J Am Coll Cardiol 57(12):1404–1423

Naumann D, Rusius V, Margiotta C et al (2013) Factors predicting trastuzumab-related cardiotoxicity in a real-world population of women with HER2+ breast cancer. Anticancer Res 33(4):1717–1720

Onitilo AA, Engel JM, Stankowski RV et al (2012) High-sensitivity C-reactive protein (hs-CRP) as a biomarker for trastuzumab-induced cardiotoxicity in HER2-positive early-stage breast cancer: a pilot study. Breast Cancer Res Treat 134(1):291–298

Peel JB, Sui X, Adams SA et al (2009) A prospective study of cardiorespiratory fitness and breast cancer mortality. Med Sci Sports Exerc 41(4):742–748

Peel AB, Thomas SM, Dittus K et al (2014) Cardiorespiratory fitness in breast cancer patients: a call for normative values. J Am Heart Assoc 3(1):e000432

Perez EA, Suman VJ, Davidson NE et al (2004) Effect of doxorubicin plus cyclophosphamide on left ventricular ejection fraction in patients with breast cancer in the North central cancer treatment group N9831 intergroup adjuvant trial. J Clin Oncol 22(18):3700–3704 (Erratum in: (2005) J Clin Oncol 23(7):1594)

Perez EA, Suman VJ, Davidson NE et al (2008) Cardiac safety analysis of doxorubicin and cyclophosphamide followed by paclitaxel with or without trastuzumab in the North central cancer treatment group N9831 adjuvant breast cancer trial. J Clin Oncol 26:1231–1238

Piccart-Gebhart MJ, Procter M, Leyland-Jones B et al (2005) Trastuzumab after adjuvant chemotherapy in HER2-positive breast cancer. N Engl J Med 353(16):1659–1672

Pinder MC, Duan Z, Goodwin JS et al (2007) Congestive heart failure in older women treated with adjuvant anthracycline chemotherapy for breast cancer. J Clin Oncol 25(25):3808–3815

Pituskin E, Haykowsky M, Mackey JR et al (2011) Rationale and design of the multidisciplinary approach to novel therapies in cardiology oncology research trial (MANTICORE 101-breast): a randomized, placebo-controlled trial to determine if conventional heart failure pharmacotherapy can prevent trastuzumab-mediated left ventricular remodeling among patients with HER2+ early breast cancer using cardiac MRI. BMC Cancer 11:318

Rivera CM, Grossardt BR, Rhodes DJ et al (2009) Increased cardiovascular mortality after early bilateral oophorectomy. Menopause 16(1):15–23

Rock CL, Flatt SW, Newman V et al (1999) Factors associated with weight gain in women after diagnosis of breast cancer. Women's healthy eating and living study group. J Am Diet Assoc 99:1212–1221

Sawaya H, Sebag IA, Plana JC et al (2011) Early detection and prediction of cardiotoxicity in chemotherapy-treated patients. Am J Cardiol 107:1375–1380

Sawaya H, Sebag IA, Plana JC et al (2012) Assessment of echocardiography and biomarkers for the extended prediction of cardiotoxicity in patients treated with anthracyclines, taxanes, and trastuzumab. Circ Cardiovasc Imaging 5(5):596–603

Sawyer DB (2013) Anthracyclines and heart failure. N Engl J Med 368(12):1154–1156

Schonberg MA, Marcantonio ER, Ngo L et al (2011) Causes of death and relative survival of older women after a breast cancer diagnosis. J Clin Oncol 29(12):1570–1577

Seidman A, Hudis C, Pierri MK et al (2002) Cardiac dysfunction in the trastuzumab clinical trials experience. J Clin Oncol 20:1215–1221

Simonsick EM, Fan E, Fleg JL (2006) Estimating cardiorespiratory fitness in well-functioning older adults: treadmill validation of the long distance corridor walk. J Am Geriatr Soc 54(1):127–132

Smith LA, Cornelius VR, Plummer CJ et al (2010) Cardiotoxicity of anthracycline agents for the treatment of cancer: systematic review and meta-analysis of randomized controlled trials. BMC Cancer 10:337

Steingart RM, Bakris GL, Chen HX et al (2012) Management of cardiac toxicity in patients receiving vascular endothelial growth factor signaling pathway inhibitors. Am Heart J 163(2):156–163

Swain SM, Vici P (2004) The current and future role of dexrazoxane as a cardioprotectant in anthracycline treatment: expert panel review. J Cancer Res Clin Oncol 130(1):1–7

Swain SM, Whaley FS, Ewer MS (2003) Congestive heart failure in patients treated with doxorubicin: a retrospective analysis of three trials. Cancer 97(11):2869–2879

Tan-Chiu E, Yothers G, Romond E et al (2005) Assessment of cardiac dysfunction in a randomized trial comparing doxorubicin and cyclophosphamide followed by paclitaxel, with or without trastuzumab as adjuvant therapy in node-positive, human epidermal growth factor receptor 2-overexpressing breast cancer: NSABP B-31. J Clin Oncol 23(31):7811–7819

Valachis A, Nearchou A, Polyzos NP et al (2013) Cardiac toxicity in breast cancer patients treated with dual HER2 blockade. Int J Cancer 133(9):2245–2252

van Dalen EC, Caron HN, Dickinson HO et al (2008) Cardioprotective interventions for cancer patients receiving anthracyclines. Cochrane Database Syst Rev 2208(2):CD003917

van de Water W, Markopoulos C, van de Velde CJ et al (2012) Association between age at diagnosis and disease-specific mortality among postmenopausal women with hormone receptor-positive breast cancer. JAMA 307(6):590–597

Vaz-Luis I, Keating NL, Lin NU, Lii H, Winer EP, Freedman RA (2014) Duration and toxicity of adjuvant trastuzumab in older patients with early-stage breast cancer: a population-based study. J Clin Oncol 32(9):927–934

Vejpongsa P, Yeh ET (2014) Topoisomerase 2β: a promising molecular target for primary prevention of anthracycline-induced cardiotoxicity. Clin Pharmacol Ther 95(1):45–52

Wells QS, Lenihan DJ (2010) Reversibility of left ventricular dysfunction resulting from chemotherapy: can this be expected? Prog Cardiovasc Dis 53(2):140–148

Wojnowski L, Kulle B, Schirmer M et al (2005) NADPH oxidase and multidrug resistance protein genetic polymorphisms are associated with doxorubicin-induced cardiotoxicity. Circulation 112:3754–3762

Yancy CW, Jessup M, Bozkurt B et al (2013) 2013 ACCF/AHA guideline for the management of heart failure: a report of the American College of Cardiology Foundation/American Heart Association Task Force on Practice Guidelines. J Am Coll Cardiol 62(16):e147–e239

Yeboah J, Rodriguez CJ, Stacey B et al (2012a) Prognosis of individuals with asymptomatic left ventricular systolic dysfunction in the multi-ethnic study of atherosclerosis (MESA). Circulation 126(23):2713–2719

Yeboah J, McClelland RL, Polonsky TS et al (2012b) Comparison of novel risk markers for improvement in cardiovascular risk assessment in intermediate-risk individuals. JAMA 308(8):788–795

Yeh ET, Tong AT, Lenihan DJ et al (2004) Cardiovascular complications of cancer therapy: diagnosis, pathogenesis, and management. Circulation 109(25):3122–3131

Yingchoncharoen T, Agarwal S, Popović ZB et al (2013) Normal ranges of left ventricular strain: a meta-analysis. J Am Soc Echocardiogr 26(2):185–191

Young MN, Shoemaker MB, Kurtz EG et al (2012) Heart failure with preserved left ventricular function: diagnostic and therapeutic challenges in patients with diastolic heart failure. Am J Med Sci 344(5):399–405

Zhang S, Liu X, Bawa-Khalfe T et al (2012) Identification of the molecular basis of doxorubicin-induced cardiotoxicity. Nat Med 18(11):1639–1642

Chapter 15
Psychological Adjustment in Breast Cancer Survivors

Annette L. Stanton and Julienne E. Bower

Abstract Women living with a diagnosis of breast cancer constitute more than 20 % of the cancer survivor population in the United States. Research on trajectories of psychological adjustment in women recently diagnosed with breast suggests that the largest proportion of women evidences relatively low psychological distress either from the point of diagnosis or after a period of recovery. Substantial heterogeneity exists, however, and some women are at risk for lingering depression, anxiety, fear of cancer recurrence and other long-term psychological effects. Most women diagnosed with breast cancer also report a number of benefits that arise from their experience of cancer. Longitudinal studies have illuminated risk and protective factors for psychological adjustment in breast cancer survivors, which we describe in this chapter. Effective psychosocial interventions, as evidenced in randomized controlled trials, also are available for bolstering breast cancer-related adjustment. We offer directions for research to deepen the understanding of biological, psychological, and social contributors to positive adjustment in the context of breast cancer, as well as suggestions for the development of optimally efficient evidence-based psychosocial interventions for women living with the disease.

Keywords Breast cancer • Psychological distress • Quality of life • Randomized controlled trial • Intervention • Survivorship

Introduction

At the beginning of 2012, the number of women living with a history of breast cancer in the United States was nearly three million, or 22 % of the survivor population. By 2024, the cancer survivor population is projected to approach 19 million (American Cancer Society 2014). In this chapter, we aim to characterize negative

A.L. Stanton (✉) • J.E. Bower
Departments of Psychology and Psychiatry/Biobehavioral Sciences,
Jonsson Comprehensive Cancer Center, University of California, Los Angeles CA, USA
e-mail: astanton@ucla.edu; jbower@ucla.edu

© Breast Cancer Research Foundation 2015
P.A. Ganz (ed.), *Improving Outcomes for Breast Cancer Survivors*,
Advances in Experimental Medicine and Biology 862,
DOI 10.1007/978-3-319-16366-6_15

and positive psychological outcomes in women diagnosed with breast cancer, as well as their contributors. We also address implications for future investigation in this area, including psychosocial intervention research. Although they are important phenomena that certainly have psychological concomitants and consequences, we do not discuss outcomes that are covered in other chapters in this volume (i.e., fatigue, cognitive dysfunction, neuropathy, sexual health). We also do not address the experience of women with metastatic breast cancer, as covered in Chap. 16, or prominent issues for young breast cancer survivors, as described in Chap. 2.

The Nature of Psychological Adjustment in Breast Cancer Survivors

What constitutes "good" psychological adjustment in the breast cancer context? Most research focuses on low or absent symptoms of depression, anxiety, or general or cancer-specific distress (e.g., fear of cancer recurrence, intrusive thoughts and feelings related to cancer) to indicate positive psychological adjustment. Reports of positive quality of life in social, physical, psychological, and spiritual realms, positive mood, and perceptions of cancer-related benefits (e.g., deepened relationships) also are used to signify positive adjustment.

Initially, receiving a breast cancer diagnosis is profoundly stressful for most women. Many feel that cancer is a death sentence and poses an immediate threat to their physical well-being; they may also be concerned about side effects of breast cancer treatments. Indeed, research suggests that symptoms of anxiety and depression are highest at the time of breast cancer diagnosis (Stafford et al. 2013). Patients may experience symptoms of shock, disbelief, denial, or despair as they struggle to accept and incorporate the reality of the diagnosis. This initial stage may be followed by a period of turmoil and distress, characterized by symptoms of anxiety, sadness, ruminative thoughts, irritability, and difficulty sleeping, eating, and concentrating. These symptoms typically stabilize as patients adjust to new information, make decisions about treatment, and resume their normal activities. However, elevations in symptoms may occur during other transition points, including treatment onset, treatment completion (the "re-entry" phase), and cancer recurrence.

Prospective research suggests that a diagnosis of breast cancer also confers risk for compromised longer-term adjustment, although substantial heterogeneity exists. Specifically, population-based longitudinal research documents decrements in quality of life and indicators of psychological and physical functioning that can persist for years among women who receive a breast cancer diagnosis versus those with no incident cancer. For example, 759 women were diagnosed with breast cancer over a 4-year period in the Nurses' Health Study cohort of 48,892 women (Michael et al. 2000). In analyses controlling for multiple covariates, diagnosed women, and particularly those aged 40 and younger (Kroenke et al. 2004), evidenced an increase in pain and declines in physical and social function, vitality, and ability to perform emotional and physical roles, relative to women who did not receive a cancer diagnosis. Problems resolved over time, but significant group differences persisted in four of seven quality of life domains up to 4 years after diagnosis. Of note, mental health (including feelings of anxiety and sadness) was the one domain that did *not* decline following a breast cancer diagnosis, suggesting that initial elevations in these symptoms do not persist for most women.

Although such large-scale studies document the life disruption that accompanies a breast cancer diagnosis, they do not pinpoint specific periods in cancer survivorship during which women are at risk for decrements in psychological and physical health. In addition, studies that examine overall patterns of adjustment may mask individual differences in patient outcomes—for example, do all (or most) women evidence declines in quality of life after breast cancer diagnosis, or are these declines driven by a subgroup of survivors? Over the past decade, studies have begun to examine distinct trajectories of adjustment, which provide insight into the periods that are most distressing and the people who are most at risk for distress. As shown in Fig. 15.1, an investigation in the Netherlands beginning prior to surgery and concluding 6 months after treatment completion indicated four unique trajectories of psychological distress in 171 women diagnosed with breast cancer: 36 % reported no or minimal distress across the five assessment points, 33 % evidenced distress from the point of diagnosis through medical treatment and then a decline in distress (i.e., recovery), 15 % reported heightened distress beginning at treatment completion and through the next 6 months (i.e., re-entry phase), and 15 % experienced high distress throughout the study period (Henselmans et al. 2010).

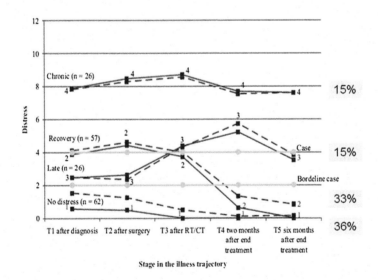

Fig. 15.1 Trajectories of distress in the first year after breast cancer diagnosis (N = 171; Henselmans et al. 2010). Predicted (*solid lines*) and observed (*dashed lines*) levels of distress are displayed. "Case" indicates psychological morbidity (i.e., a score of 4 or greater on the General Health Questionnaire-12)

Another trajectory study that assessed 285 breast cancer patients in China from 5 days to 8 months after surgery also found four trajectories: 66 % reported low distress across the assessment period, 12 % reported elevated distress at 5 days and 1 month that resolved by 3 months after surgery (i.e., recovery pattern), 7 % showed increased distress that recovered by 8 months (delayed recovery), and 15 % experienced high distress across the assessment period (Lam et al. 2010). In a trajectory study with extended follow-up, which began shortly after initiation of chemotherapy and spanned more than 4 years after diagnosis (Helgeson et al. 2004), the largest proportion of the breast cancer patient sample reported quality of life matching or exceeding population norms on both mental (43 %) and physical (55 %) functioning across the 4 years, with other trajectories indicating either recovery or relatively poor and/or declining functioning.

Overall, this research highlights the psychological resilience of women with breast cancer and suggests that the largest proportion of breast cancer survivors can expect generally positive adjustment either from the point of diagnosis and treatment or after a period of recovery. However, heterogeneity is evident, and a notable proportion (approximately 15 %) appears at risk for distress and life disruption from the point of diagnosis onward for months or years (note that this group also likely includes women whose relatively poor psychological adjustment precedes the cancer diagnosis). It also is possible that the most distressed women are more likely to decline participation in research, leading to underestimates of prevalence of distress and life disruption. Furthermore, there is evidence that groups with particular characteristics, such as low-income and Latina women (e.g., Christie et al. 2010; Yanez et al. 2011), experience relatively high distress and low quality of life. Next, we address specific domains of adjustment, with a focus on depression and anxiety, as well as the factors that confer risk for or protection from negative outcomes.

Negative Psychological Outcomes and Their Contributors

Depression

A meta-analysis of 66 studies of interview-diagnosed major depression in cancer survivors in non-palliative care settings, including 24 studies of breast cancer patients alone, demonstrated a 16.3 % prevalence of major depression, with a similar 14.1 % prevalence in breast cancer patients specifically (Mitchell et al. 2011). These proportions contrast with general population norms of 12 % for women aged 40–59 years and 7 % for women 60 years and older (Pratt and Brody, 2014). The risk of depression appears to be most elevated in the first 1–2 years after diagnosis in cancer survivors generally (Krebber et al. 2014; Mitchell et al. 2013) and in breast cancer patients specifically (Avis et al. 2013). Depression contributes to decreases in quality of life and psychosocial and occupational functioning, interferes with treatment adherence, and has been associated with shorter recurrence-free survival (Satin et al. 2009).

Several risk factors for high depressive symptoms in breast cancer survivors have empirical support. Most of the evidence comes from cross-sectional rather than longitudinal studies, however, and reciprocal relationships or reverse causation is likely. Psychosocial factors appear to be the strongest predictors of elevated depressive symptoms, including prior history of depression, occurrence of other stressful life events, use of avoidant coping strategies, loneliness, low social support, and pessimism (Avis et al. 2013; Bardwell et al. 2006; Jaremka et al. 2013; Stanton and Snider 1993). Other risk factors include younger age, fewer financial resources, and presence of physical symptoms. Chemotherapy may be associated with elevated risk for depression (e.g., Torres et al. 2013), but other disease and treatment-related variables are typically not (Bardwell et al. 2006).

Anxiety and Fear of Breast Cancer Recurrence

The experience of breast cancer can trigger general feelings of anxiety, as well as more specific concerns about cancer recurrence. A meta-analysis found that the prevalence of interview-diagnosed anxiety disorders was 10.3 % among cancer patients in non-palliative care settings (Mitchell et al. 2011). This figure is comparable to the 13 % 6-month prevalence of anxiety disorders in the general population of women (Pigott 2003). Whereas depression tends to improve in the year or two after cancer diagnosis, anxiety is more likely to persist in the years after cancer treatment. A meta-analysis comparing depression and anxiety in long-term cancer survivors (i.e., those at least 2 years post-diagnosis) with healthy controls found an elevated prevalence of anxiety in survivors (17.9 %) vs. controls (13.9 %) but no differences in depression (Mitchell et al. 2013). Of note, this review included both interview-diagnosed anxiety and patient-reported scales, which often yield higher prevalence rates.

One of the factors that may maintain anxiety among breast cancer survivors is concern about cancer recurrence. Indeed, worry that breast cancer may return after treatment is among the most commonly experienced psychological sequelae (Koch et al. 2012). In a review in cancer survivors generally, Koch et al. (2012) found that most long-term survivors experience modest to moderate levels of fear of recurrence. Healthcare professionals find fear of recurrence challenging to manage (Thewes et al. 2013).

Fear of breast cancer recurrence can be amplified or reactivated by several triggers, such as follow-up medical visits, the experience of physical symptoms such as new or persistent pain or fatigue, and cancer diagnosis or death of a public figure, friend, or family member (Gil et al. 2004). Heightened fear of recurrence is reported by adult survivors of younger age, lower educational level, fewer significant others, and Hispanic or non-Hispanic white race/ethnicity (Crist and Grunfeld 2013; Phillips et al. 2013). Lower optimism and social support, more family stressors, depressive symptoms, pain, and other physical symptoms also are linked to higher fear (Crist and Grunfeld 2013; Phillips et al. 2013).

Cancer-related post-traumatic stress disorder (PTSD), as assessed via validated interview or questionnaire, typically is found to occur in less than 10 % of cancer survivors after treatment completion and to decline over time (e.g., Kangas et al. 2002). Women at most risk tend to be younger, have more serious disease and aggressive therapy, and be more likely to have experienced PTSD previously (e.g., O'Connor et al. 2011). Symptoms of subthreshold PTSD, however, such as intrusive thoughts and feelings, re-experiencing of cancer-related events, and avoidance of reminders of cancer, are common among survivors in the 2 years after diagnosis. For example, in a nationwide Danish cohort of women receiving surgery for breast cancer, 20.1 % and 14.3 % reported severe posttraumatic stress symptoms at 3 and 15 months after surgery, respectively (O'Connor et al. 2011). There is evidence that African American and Asian American women are more at risk for breast cancer-related post-traumatic stress symptoms than their non-Latina white counterparts (Vin-Raviv et al. 2013).

Positive Psychological Outcomes and Their Contributors

Along with the distress and life disruption attendant upon the experience of breast cancer, many women find benefit in their experience and maintain positive mood and quality of life. Indeed, we have found that more than 80 % of breast cancer survivors report at least one positive change or benefit related to their cancer experience (Sears et al. 2003). Primary self-reported benefits involve strengthened interpersonal relationships, life appreciation and commitment to priorities, spirituality, personal regard, and attention to health behaviors. These changes have also been described as "posttraumatic growth" (Tedeschi and Calhoun 1996). Reports of benefit finding increase from the diagnostic and treatment phase through re-entry and early breast cancer survivorship and level off at approximately 1 year after diagnosis (Danhauer et al. 2013; Manne et al. 2004). Long-term breast cancer survivors also report cancer-related benefits (Mols et al. 2005), although finding benefit may decrease in the long term (Bower et al. 2005).

Although findings are not completely consistent, longitudinal research suggests that greater impact of the breast cancer diagnosis, in the form of higher perceived threat and life disruption, promotes benefit finding. Greater intentional engagement in the cancer experience, as indicated by more problem-focused coping and intentional positive reappraisal, for example, also predicts benefit finding (Danhauer et al. 2013; Sears et al. 2003; Stanton et al. 2006). Younger women typically report higher levels of benefit finding than older women, and the correlates of benefit finding may differ depending on age. Specifically, negative impact seems to be more important for older women, whereas engagement may be more important for younger women in promoting benefit finding. Social support can also enhance the ability to find benefit in the experience of breast cancer (Danhauer et al. 2013; McDonough et al. 2014; Schroevers et al. 2010). Although finding benefit can be valuable in its own right, it also can contribute to improved psychological and health-related outcomes into longer-term survivorship, as demonstrated by longitudinal and experimental research (e.g., Bower et al. 2005; Carver and Antoni 2004; Stanton et al. 2002). Benefit finding has also been linked to neuroendocrine and immune function in women with breast cancer, including steeper diurnal cortisol slope (Diaz et al. 2014), reduced serum cortisol (Cruess et al. 2000), and increased lymphocyte proliferation (McGregor et al. 2004).

Directions for Psychosocial and Biobehavioral Intervention Research

Randomized, controlled trials (RCTs) of interventions to reduce psychological morbidities and enhance well-being in women with breast cancer have accumulated rapidly over the past two decades. See Table 15.1 for examples of the approaches to psychosocial intervention that have been most commonly used. Most of the research has focused on the diagnostic and treatment phase, although RCTs designed to promote adaptive survivorship into the re-entry phase and beyond are accruing (Stanton et al. 2015). Reviews and meta-analyses demonstrate that efficacious cognitive-behavioral and psychoeducational approaches exist for women diagnosed

Table 15.1 Psychosocial interventions for women diagnosed with breast cancer: major approaches, goals, and mediators of effects

Major intervention approaches	Primary intervention goals
Cognitive-behavioral therapy	Identify and challenge unhelpful cognitions and behaviors
Coping skills training	Teach and practice contextually adaptive coping strategies; Promote helpful thoughts and behaviors
Psychoeducation	Provide information about cancer and strategies for adjustment
Supportive-expressive therapy	Express feelings and thoughts in a group supportive context
Problem-solving therapy	Train in constructive set toward problems and problem-solving
Mindfulness-based stress reduction	Cultivate non-judgmental awareness of present experiences
Relaxation training	Teach relaxation skills (e.g., progressive muscle relaxation)
Couples therapy	Enhance disclosure, intimacy, and couple-focused coping skills
Evidence-based classes of mediators of interventions' effects	
Altered cognitions (e.g., expectancies, illness representations)	
Improved self-efficacy for using coping strategies and skills targeted by the intervention	
Improved cancer-related psychological and physical symptoms (e.g., mood disturbance, pain)	
Bolstered psychosocial resources (e.g., self-esteem)	

Note Table content on mediators was based on a review of mediators of 16 psychosocial interventions for cancer survivors that included examination of mediators of the intervention's effects (Stanton et al. 2013)

with breast cancer (Faller et al. 2013; Stanton 2012; Tatrow and Montgomery 2006) with regard to improving both psychological adjustment and symptoms specifically related to cancer treatments (e.g., menopausal symptoms; Mann et al. 2012). Of note, cancer survivors who are more distressed appear to get the most benefit from these interventions (Faller et al. 2013), suggesting that treatments should be targeted to those who are experiencing difficulties with adjustment.

Recent research also documents the efficacy of mind-body and other approaches for improving psychological adjustment. For example, RCTs demonstrate the benefits of yoga on depression and anxiety in breast cancer patients, at least over the short-term and for women in active cancer treatment (Cramer et al. 2012). Furthermore, mindfulness-based stress reduction is promising in its effects on depression and anxiety in survivors of breast cancer (Zainal et al. 2013a. Mindfulness-based interventions have also been shown to reduce fear of recurrence (Lengacher et al. 2009) and improve positive psychological outcomes in breast cancer survivors, including peace and meaning in life (Bower et al. 2014). Physical activity also can enhance quality of life and reduce breast cancer concerns in women with breast cancer (Speck et al. 2010; Vallance et al. 2007).

Continued development of efficient interventions for women and their loved ones, extension to diverse groups, and dissemination research are needed. Designing interventions for dissemination remains a significant challenge (Glasgow et al. 2012). Effectiveness and efficiency of interventions will be promoted through several lines of research. First, research to identify key mechanisms for interventions' effects will promote incorporating and strengthening those mechanisms to increase intervention efficacy (Stanton et al. 2013). Second, in light of the evidence that a substantial proportion of women adjust well psychologically in their own environments, research is warranted to develop and test stepped-care interventions consistent with breast cancer survivors' psychosocial needs and to target women most in need of psychosocial care (see American Society of Clinical Oncology guidelines for screening, assessment and care of symptoms of depression and anxiety in adults with cancer; Andersen et al. 2014). Such research will increase efficiency and accessibility of interventions, as will research to create broad reach of interventions through advanced technologies. Third, comparative effectiveness research to identify approaches that reduce both cancer-related psychological morbidities and medical costs (e.g., emergency room visits, interim physician appointments, medical treatment nonadherence) will help justify weaving them into the fabric of standard care.

Research Challenges and Opportunities

Substantial progress over the past few decades is evident in the specification of psychosocial and behavioral concomitants of breast cancer, identification of associated risk and protective factors, and development of evidence-based interventions to improve psychosocial adjustment. Going forward, inter-professional collaborations promise to develop the research base further. Translation of empirical findings into increasingly effective and efficient strategies to prevent and treat psychosocial morbidities are needed. In addition, evidence-based approaches to enhance well-being and health require further development.

Continued investigation is vital to identifying biopsychosocial etiologies of specific problems (and symptom clusters), such as depression, fatigue, and pain. Intensive longitudinal and experimental research is needed to assess biomarkers, psychological processes, and social contexts that promote or impede positive psychosocial outcomes in samples of breast cancer survivors. Examination of cohorts of breast cancer survivors followed over time and compared to their disease-free counterparts are necessary to understand the distinct influence that the cancer experience has on psychosocial and biobehavioral outcomes. Research with existing large population cohorts [e.g., Hispanic Community Health Study/Study of Latinos (SOL)] would allow prospective examination of adults from prior to cancer diagnosis through periods of survivorship with respect to psychological and physical health outcomes. Use of brief, valid self-report instruments, administered over time, can provide efficient assessment of progress and deterioration on those outcomes for both research and clinical use (Andersen et al. 2014; Basch et al. 2012; Vodermaier et al. 2009).

Although relevant evidence is accruing, the existing psychosocial knowledge base largely derives from studies of white, middle class, early-stage breast cancer survivors treated at large cancer centers. Additional study is needed of women with metastatic disease, fewer financial resources, and diverse backgrounds. Research suggests that quality of life is compromised in ethnic/racial minorities diagnosed with breast cancer relative to their majority group counterparts (e.g., Janz et al. 2008; Yanez et al. 2011). Although socioeconomic disparities account for some of the difference in psychological outcomes, other factors clearly are at play in influencing adjustment, and these warrant study. Research and intervention development are needed with regard to lack of access to survivorship resources, the role of specific culturally grounded beliefs (e.g., fatalism) to psychosocial outcomes, and barriers to effective communication with the medical team.

Nearly a decade has passed since the Institute of Medicine (IOM 2006, 2008) urged comprehensive survivorship care after medical treatments are completed, including provision of psychosocial care. As the mandate grows to integrate psychosocial care into routine medical treatment over the survivorship trajectory (Jacobsen and Wagner 2012), inter-professional collaborations in research and clinical care will be essential (IOM 2013). Although much work remains, equipped with the science at hand, we are well positioned to contribute to the next generation of research and evidence-based practice to promote the well-being and health of the millions of adults who are living beyond a breast cancer diagnosis.

References

American Cancer Society (2014) Cancer treatment and survivorship facts and figures 2014–2015. American Cancer Society, Atlanta. Andersen BL, Anderson

Andersen BL, DeRubeis RJ, Berman BS, Gruman J, Champion VL, Massie MJ, Holland JC, Partridge AH, Bak K, Somerfield MR, Rowland JH (2014) Screening, assessment and care of anxiety and depressive symptoms in adults with cancer: an American society of clinical oncology guideline adaptation. J Clin Oncol 32:1605–1619

Avis NE, Levine B, Naughton MJ, Case LD, Naftalis E, Van Zee KJ (2013) Age-related longitudinal changes in depressive symptoms following breast cancer diagnosis and treatment. Breast Cancer Res Treat 139:199–206

Basch E, Abernethy AP, Mullins CD, Reeve BB, Smith ML, Coons SJ, Sloan J, Wenzel K, Chauhan C, Eppard W, Frank ES, Lipscomb J, Raymond SA, Spencer M, Tunis S (2012) Recommendations for incorporating patient-reported outcomes into clinical comparative effectiveness research in adult oncology. J Clin Oncol 30:4249–4255

Bardwell WA, Natarajan L, Dimsdale JE, Rock CL, Mortimer JE, Hollenbach K, Pierce JP (2006) Objective cancer-related variables are not associated with depressive symptoms in women treated for early-stage breast cancer. J Clin Oncol 24:2420–2427

Bower JE, Meyerowitz BE, Desmond KA, Bernaards CA, Rowland JH, Ganz PA (2005) Perceptions of positive meaning and vulnerability following breast cancer: predictors and outcomes among long-term breast cancer survivors. Ann Behav Med 29:236–245

Bower JE, Ganz PA, Crosswell AD, Crespi CM, Stanton AL, Winston D, Cole SW (2014) Effects of mindfulness meditation on stress and inflammation in breast cancer survivors: a randomized controlled trial. Paper presented at the annual meeting of the American psychosomatic society, San Francisco, CA, March 2014

Carver CS, Antoni MH (2004) Finding benefit in breast cancer during the year after diagnosis predicts better adjustment 5 to 8 years after diagnosis. Health Psychol 23:595–598

Christie KM, Meyerowitz BE, Maly RC (2010) Depression and sexual adjustment following breast cancer in low-income Hispanic and non-Hispanic white women. Psycho-Oncology 19: 1069–1077

Cramer H, Lange S, Klose P, Paul A, Dobos G (2012) Yoga for breast cancer patients and survivors: a systematic review and meta-analysis. BMC Cancer 18:412. doi:10.1186/1471-2407-12-412

Crist JV, Grunfeld EA (2013) Factors reported to influence fear of recurrence in cancer patients: a systematic review. Psycho-Oncology 22: 978–986

Cruess DG, Antoni MH, McGregor BA, Kilbourn KM, Boyers AE, Alferi SM, Carver CS, Kumar M (2000) Cognitive-behavioral stress management reduces serum cortisol by enhancing benefit finding among women being treated for early stage breast cancer. Psychosom Medicine, 62:304–308

Danhauer SC, Case LD, Tedeschi R, Russell G, Vishnevsky T, Triplett K, Ip EG, Avis NE (2013) Predictors of posttraumatic growth in women with breast cancer. Psycho-Oncology 22: 2676–2683

Diaz M, Aldridge-Gerry A, Spiegel D (2014) Posttraumatic growth and diurnal cortisol slope among women with metastatic breast cancer. Psychoneuroendocrinology. 44:83–87

Faller H, Schuler M, Richard M, Heckl U, Weis J, Küffner R (2013) Effects of psycho-oncologic interventions on emotional distress and quality of life in adult patients with cancer: systematic review and meta-analysis. J Clin Oncol 31:782–793

Gil KM, Mishel M, Bleyea M, Germino B, Porter LS, LaNey IC, Stewart J (2004) Triggers of uncertainty about recurrence and long-term treatment side effects in older African American and Caucasian breast cancer survivors. Oncol Nurs Forum 31:633–639

Glasgow RE, Vinson C, Chambers D, Khoury MJ, Kaplan RM, Hunter C (2012) National institutes of health approaches to dissemination and implementation science: current and future directions. Am J Public Health 102:1274–1281

Helgeson VS, Snyder P, Seltman H (2004) Psychological and physical adjustment to breast cancer over 4 years: identifying distinct trajectories of change. Health Psychol 23:3–15

Henselmans I, Helgeson VS, Seltman H, de Vries J, Sanderman R, Ranchor AV (2010) Identification and prediction of distress trajectories in the first year after a breast cancer diagnosis. Health Psychol 29:160–168

Institute of Medicine, Committee on Cancer Survivorship: Improving Care and Quality of Life, Hewitt M, Greenfield S, Stovall E (eds) (2006) From cancer patient to cancer survivor: lost in transition. National Academies Press, Washington, DC

Institute of Medicine, Committee on Psychosocial Services to Cancer Patients/Families in a Community Setting, Adler NE, Page AEK (eds) (2008) Cancer care for the whole patient: meeting psychosocial health needs. National Academies Press, Washington, DC

Institute of Medicine, Committee on Improving the Quality of Cancer Care: Addressing the Challenges of an Aging Population, Levit LA, Balogh EP, Nass SJ, Ganz PA (eds) (2013) Delivering high quality cancer care: charting a new course for a system in crisis. National Academies Press, Washington, DC

Jacobsen PB, Wagner LI (2012) A new quality standard: the integration of psychosocial care into routine cancer care. J Clin Oncol 30:1154–1159

Janz NK, Mujahid MS, Hawley ST, Griggs JJ, Hamilton AS, Katz SJ (2008) Racial-ethnic differences in adequacy of information and support for women with breast cancer. Cancer 113:1058–1067

Jaremka LM, Andridge RR, Fagundes CP, Alfano CM, Povoski SP, Lipari AM, Kiecolt-Glaser JK (2013) Pain, depression, and fatigue: loneliness as a longitudinal risk factor. Health Psychol 33:948–957

Kangas M, Henry JL, Bryant RA (2002) Posttraumatic stress disorder following cancer: a conceptual and empirical review. Clin Psychol Rev 22:499–524

Koch L, Jansen L, Brenner H, Arndt V (2012) Fear of recurrence and disease progression in long-term ($\geq$5 years) cancer survivors-a systematic review of quantitative studies. Psycho-Oncology 22:1–11

Krebber AMH, Buffart LM, Kleijn G, Riepma IC, de Bree R, Leemans CR, Leeuw IMV (2014) Prevalence of depression in cancer patients: a meta-analysis of diagnostic interviews and self-report instruments. Psycho-Oncology 23:121–130

Kroenke CH, Rosner B, Chen WY, Kawachi I, Colditz GA, Holmes MD (2004) Functional impact of breast cancer by age at diagnosis. J Clin Oncol 22:1849–1856

Lam WW, Bonanno GA, Mancini AD, Ho S, Chan M, Hung WK, Or A, Fielding, R. (2010) Trajectories of psychological distress among Chinese women diagnosed with breast cancer. Psycho-Oncology 19:1044–1051

Lengacher CA, Johnson-Mallard V, Post-White J, Moscoso MS, Jacobsen, PB, Klein TW, ... Kip KE (2009) Randomized controlled trial of mindfulness-based stress reduction (MBSR) for survivors of breast cancer. Psycho-Oncology 18:1261–1272

Mann E, Smith MJ, Hellier J, Balabanovic JA, Hamed H, Grunfeld EA, Hunter MS (2012) Cognitive behavioural treatment for women who have menopausal symptoms after breast cancer treatment (MENOS1): a randomized controlled trial. Lancet Oncol 13:309–318

McGregor BA, Antoni MH, Boyers A, Alferi SM, Blomberg BB, Carver CS (2004) Cognitive–behavioral stress management increases benefit finding and immune function among women with early-stage breast cancer. J Psychosom Research 56:1–8

Manne S, Ostroff J, Winkel G, Goldstein L, Fox K, Grana G (2004) Posttraumatic growth after breast cancer: patient, partner, and couple perspectives. Psychosom Med 66:442–454

Michael YL, Kawachi I, Berkman LF, Holmes MD, Colditz GA (2000) The persistent impact of breast carcinoma on functional health status. Cancer 89:2176–2186

Mitchell AJ, Chan M, Bhatti H, Halton M, Grassi L, Johansen C, Meader N (2011) Prevalence of depression, anxiety, and adjustment disorder in oncological, haematological, and palliative-care settings: a meta-analysis of 94 interview-based studies. Lancet Oncol 12:160–174

Mitchell AJ, Ferguson DW, Gill J, Paul J, Symonds P (2013) Depression and anxiety in long-term cancer survivors compared with spouses and healthy controls: a systematic review and meta-analysis. Lancet Oncol 14:721–732

Mols F, Vingerhoets AJJM, Coebergh JW, van de Poll-Franse LV (2005) Quality of life among long-term breast cancer survivors: a systematic review. Eur J Cancer 14:2613–2619

O'Connor M, Christensen S, Jensen AB, Møller S, Zachariae R (2011) How traumatic is breast cancer? Post-traumatic stress symptoms (PTSS) and risk factors for severe PTSS at 3 and 15 months after surgery in a nationwide cohort of Danish women treated for primary breast cancer. British J Cancer 104:419–426

Phillips KM, McGinty HL, Gonzalez BD, Jim HSL, Small BJ, Minton S, Jacobsen PB (2013) Factors associated with breast cancer worry 3 years after completion of adjuvant treatment. Psycho-Oncology 22:936–939

Pigott TA (2003) Anxiety disorders in women. Psychiatr Clin N Am 26:621–672

Pratt LA, Brody DJ. Depression in the U.S. household population, 2009–2012. NCHS data brief, no 172. Hyattsville, MD: National Center for Health Statistics. 2014

Satin JR, Linden W, Phillips MJ (2009) Depression as a predictor of disease progression and mortality in cancer patients. Cancer 115:5349–5361

Schroevers MJ, Helgeson VS, Sanderman R, Ranchor AV (2010) Type of social support matters for prediction of posttraumatic growth among cancer survivors. Psycho-Oncology 19:46–53

Sears SR, Stanton AL, Danoff-Burg S (2003) The yellow brick road and the emerald city: benefit finding, positive reappraisal coping and posttraumatic growth in women with early-stage breast cancer. Health Psychol 22:487–497

Speck RM, Courneya KS, Mâsse LC, Duval S, Schmitz KH (2010) An update of controlled physical activity trials in cancer survivors: a systematic review and meta-analysis. J Cancer Surviv 4:87–100

Stafford L, Judd F, Gibson P, Komiti A, Mann GB, Quinn M (2013) Screening for depression and anxiety in women with breast and gynaecologic cancer: course and prevalence of morbidity over 12 months. Psycho-Oncology 22:2071–2078

Stanton AL, Snider PR (1993) Coping with a breast cancer diagnosis: A prospective study. Health Psychol 12:16–23

Stanton AL (2012) What happens now? Psychosocial care for cancer survivors after medical treatment completion. J Clin Oncol 30:1215–1220

Stanton AL, Danoff-Burg S, Sworowski LA, Collins CA, Branstetter AD, Rodriguez-Hanley A, Austenfeld JL (2002) Randomized, controlled trial of written emotional expression and benefit-finding in breast cancer patients. J Clin Oncol 20:4160–4168

Stanton AL, Bower JE, Low CA (2006) Posttraumatic growth after cancer. In: Calhoun LG, Tedeschi RG (eds) Handbook of posttraumatic growth: research and practice. Erlbaum, Mahwah, NJ, pp 138–175

Stanton AL, Rowland JH, Ganz PA (2015) Life after diagnosis and treatment of cancer in adulthood: contributions from research in psychosocial oncology. Am Psychol 70:159–174

Stanton AL, Luecken LJ, MacKinnon DP, Thompson EH (2013) Mechanisms in psychosocial interventions for adults living with cancer: opportunity for integration of theory, research, and practice. J Consulting Clinical Psychol 81:318–335

Tatrow K, Montgomery GH (2006) Cognitive behavioral therapy techniques for distress and pain in breast cancer patients: a meta-analysis. J Behavioral Medicine 29:17–27

Tedeschi RG, Calhoun LG (1996) The posttraumatic growth inventory: measuring the positive legacy of trauma. J Trauma Stress 9:455–471

Thewes B, Brebach R, Dzidowska M, Rhodes P, Sharpe L, Butow P (2013) Current approaches to managing fear of recurrence: a descriptive survey of psychosocial and clinical health professionals. Psycho-Oncology 23:390–396

Torres MA, Pace TW, Liu T, Felger JC, Mister D, Doho GH, Kohn JN, Barsevick AM, Long Q, Miller AH (2013) Predictors of depression in breast cancer patients treated with radiation: role of prior chemotherapy and nuclear factor kappa B. Cancer 119:1951–1959

Vallance JKH, Courneya KS, Plotnikoff RC, Yasui Y, Mackey JR (2007) Randomized controlled trial of the effects of print materials and step pedometers on physical activity and quality of life in breast cancer survivors. J Clin Oncol 25:2352–2359

Vin-Raviv N, Hillyer GC, Hershman DL, Galea S, Leoce N, Bovbjerg DH, Neugut AI (2013) Racial disparities in posttraumatic stress after diagnosis of localized breast cancer: the BQUAL study. J Natl Cancer Inst 105:563–572

Vodermaier A, Linden C, Siu C (2009) Screening for emotional distress in cancer patients: a systematic review of assessment instruments. J Natl Cancer Inst 101:1464–1488

Yanez B, Thompson EH, Stanton AL (2011) Quality of life among Latina breast cancer patients: a systematic review of the literature. J Cancer Surviv 5:191–207

Zainal NZ, Booth S, Huppert FA (2013) The efficacy of mindfulness-based stress reduction on mental health of breast cancer patients: a meta-analysis. Psycho-Oncology 22:1457–1465

Chapter 16
Living with Metastatic Breast Cancer

Patricia A. Ganz and Annette L. Stanton

Abstract Although prevalence estimates are imprecise, growing numbers of women in the United States are living longer with metastatic breast cancer, attributable at least in part to the availability of effective targeted therapies. Women living with metastatic disease are understudied, however, and substantial heterogeneity exists in both the clinical characteristics of metastatic tumors and the physical and psychological experience of patients living with the disease. Survivorship issues are complex for patients who are living with metastatic disease over extended periods of time, from years to decades. Newly diagnosed patients with stage IV disease are confronting cancer for the first time, while others have metastatic disease as a result of breast cancer recurrence. Many patients are able to live for years on stable medical regimens, and yet others live with a moving target of aggressive disease with arduous treatments and uneven response. The psychological common denominator is the experience of profound life threat and the accompanying uncertainty, for both the affected woman and her loved ones. Maintaining life balance in the face of metastatic disease, as well as managing pain, fatigue, and other physical and psychological symptoms are major challenges. Increasingly, the clinical approach to metastatic disease reflects the consensus that palliative and supportive care are essential from the point of diagnosis. To remedy the paucity of systematic research on women living with metastatic breast cancer for extended periods, we offer directions for research to understand the experience of metastatic breast cancer and to provide evidence-based inter-professional care.

Keywords Metastatic breast cancer • Advanced cancer • Psychological distress • Quality of life

P.A. Ganz (✉)
UCLA Schools of Medicine and Public Health, Jonsson Comprehensive
Cancer Center, Los Angeles, CA, USA
e-mail: pganz@mednet.ucla.edu

A.L. Stanton
Departments of Psychology and Psychiatry/Biobehavioral Sciences,
Jonsson Comprehensive Cancer Center, University of California,
Los Angeles, CA, USA
e-mail: astanton@ucla.edu

© Breast Cancer Research Foundation 2015
P.A. Ganz (ed.), *Improving Outcomes for Breast Cancer Survivors*,
Advances in Experimental Medicine and Biology 862,
DOI 10.1007/978-3-319-16366-6_16

243

Introduction

With all of the attention given to early breast cancer detection and the highly favorable outcomes for so many breast cancer patients (Desantis et al. 2014), the small number of women with stage IV disease at diagnosis or who are living for extended periods of time with metastatic disease as a result of breast cancer recurrence are relatively neglected. Now, growing numbers of women and men live for extended periods of time with metastatic disease, some with long durable remissions and others moving from one treatment to the next. This change is attributable to the increased numbers of targeted therapies, especially for hormone sensitive and HER-2 positive disease. Some patients, particularly those with stage IV disease at diagnosis, may enjoy complete remissions or long-lasting control of their disease for extended periods. Others, who experience recurrence of breast cancer after an initial disease-free interval, usually have a more varied course both physically and emotionally. In this chapter, we address the prevalence and clinical heterogeneity of metastatic breast cancer, the physical and psychological consequences of long-term cancer-directed therapy, the experience of women living with metastatic disease, ideally how care should be delivered to these survivors, and the research challenges and opportunities related to studying this growing population of breast cancer survivors.

The Nature of Metastatic Breast Cancer Today

Of the more than 232,000 cases of female breast cancer in 2014, only 5 % of white women and 8 % of African American women are expected to be diagnosed initially with stage IV breast cancer (Siegel et al. 2014). For many of these women metastatic disease at presentation is occult and is identified due to aggressive staging, although a substantial number have clinically apparent and symptomatic disease. Very little attention has been devoted to newly diagnosed stage IV patients in terms of their presentation characteristics and psychosocial needs. An interesting and provocative analysis by Johnson et al. (2013) suggested that while the incidence pattern of stage IV disease at diagnosis has been stable among women older than 40 years, it has steadily increased among younger women, with estrogen receptor positive disease accounting for much of the increase. Approximately 12,000 newly diagnosed women enter the ranks of those living with metastatic breast cancer each year.

In contrast, it is exceedingly difficult to find data on the number of women who are living with metastatic cancer as a result of recurrence—that is, how many are newly recurrent each year for the first time (incidence) and the prevalence of women living with recurrent metastatic disease. As one breast cancer advocate for patients with metastatic breast cancer commented to us, "If we are not counted, we do not exist." The nature of metastatic disease varies substantially, with local recurrences on the chest wall or skin that may seem limited, but can be a potential harbinger of more distant disease. More often, recurrences are in regional or distant sites, and are usually identified due to symptoms. Patterns of recurrence vary depending on the initial tumor characteristics. Hormone receptor positive tumors can have very late recurrences, often decades later. Thus the period of risk for recurrence can be lengthy, especially in younger women for whom competing causes of death are less frequent; for younger women, breast cancer is most often the cause of death, in contrast to older women (Early Breast Cancer Trialists' Collaborative Group 2005). Thus, women living with metastatic breast cancer for long periods of time may have a higher representation of younger women than for incident breast cancer. With these two sources of women living with metastatic cancer (incident stage IV and recurrent breast cancer), some have estimated that there may be as many as 160,000 women and men living with metastatic disease (http://mbcn.org/education/category/most-commonly-used-statistics-for-mbc), but this estimate is uncertain.

Just as we now recognize multiple genomic subtypes of breast cancer at diagnosis, these subtypes can play out in different patterns of metastatic disease (e.g., early vs. late recurrence; soft tissue vs. visceral disease; bone dominant). The options for therapy will depend not only on the site and pattern of disease, but the disease-free interval, what prior therapy has been given, and whether or not endocrine or HER 2-directed therapies are appropriate and available. Unlike the situation several decades ago, we now have many additional endocrine therapies, and the ability to use several sequential HER2-directed therapies has completely transformed what was a rapidly fatal form of breast cancer. In addition, women with isolated ipsilateral local recurrence that is excised have a survival benefit from the reintroduction of chemotherapy, particularly in the setting of hormone receptor positive disease (Aebi et al. 2014). Thus, the treatments and outlook for women living with metastatic breast cancer today are varied, with some subsets of women living for extended periods of time with stable, well controlled disease, and others requiring continuous and serial therapies, with only modest responses. It is therefore difficult to generalize about the medical aspects of living with metastatic breast cancer.

While this chapter could focus on the important issues associated with end-of-life care for women with advanced metastatic breast cancer, we have chosen instead to address the complexities of survivorship for breast cancer patients who are living with disease over extended periods of time from years to decades. As recently recognized in the Institute of Medicine report on the Delivery of High-Quality Cancer Care (Institute of Medicine 2013), palliative and psychosocial care services should be delivered to all patients with advanced cancer, as part of cancer care. We will assume that we will strive toward this goal in all women who are living with metastatic breast cancer, and in the sections below, focus on the consequences of enduring ongoing disease-directed therapy in this setting.

The Metastatic Disease Experience and Consequences of Long-Term Therapy

Just as the medical presentation of metastatic breast cancer is heterogeneous, so too is the psychosocial experience for women living with the disease. Some women are confronting cancer for the first time, others with recurrent disease are able to live for many years on stable, well-tolerated medical regimens, and yet others live with a moving target of more aggressive disease with arduous treatments and variable response. The psychological common denominator is the experience of profound life threat and concomitant uncertainty, for both the affected woman and her loved ones. Maintaining a balance of attending to threatening and difficult thoughts, feelings, and requisite medical demands while pursuing a meaningful and rewarding life, is a major task of living with metastatic disease. Another common psychological experience includes the need to alter major life goals as the cancer and its treatment impinge on the ability to function in central roles or as one pursues specific cherished life priorities while at the same time contending with limited energy.

Interpersonal challenges include garnering effective support and dealing with concerns for the well-being of close family, children, and friends. In qualitative interviews of women with recurrent breast or gynecologic cancer, most women reported receiving emotional support from family and friends. Erosion of social support also was evident, however, in perceptions of intentional distancing by some close others, others' lack of understanding that recurrent cancer indicates a chronic illness, and women's curtailing their requests for support so as not to burden others (Thornton et al. 2014).

These and other challenges of living with metastatic disease are summarized in Table 16.1. Some of the tasks overlap with those encountered by women managing early-stage disease, but often are intensified in women with metastatic breast cancer (e.g., fatigue), and others are unique to the experience of metastasized disease, such as accepting stable disease as a desirable outcome of treatment. Particularly frequent or severe problems are addressed in this section.

Pain and fatigue are the two most common symptoms experienced by women living with metastatic breast cancer. Pain is often the first symptom of recurrent breast cancer; in women with stage IV disease at diagnosis, it may also be a presenting symptom. Pain can result from the after effects of initial breast cancer surgery and radiation, as well as in association with local recurrence and/or lymphedema. The latter may produce both psychological consequences and physical sequelae, such as arm heaviness and pain. Bone metastases and skeletal events (e.g., fractures) have become less frequent with bisphosphonate therapy; however, women still may suffer from severe pain and limitation of function as a result of bone metastases and nerve entrapment syndromes. Fortunately, skeletal metastases are often very responsive to radiation as well as analgesics, but the chronic and ongoing nature of pain when metastatic disease is in the bones can be burdensome. Similarly, visceral disease (e.g., liver, intra-abdominal or thoracic) can be responsible for substantial pain that is often more challenging to control. Cumulative toxicities from chemotherapy and radiation therapy can also contribute to pain syndromes, such as post-taxane neuropathy and radiation fibrosis and nerve entrapment. Scar tissue can lead to functional limitations and associated pain.

Among the challenges of pain management in women living with metastatic disease is their desire to be alert and functional, and not be dragged down by the sedation of narcotics. Many women continue to work and actively manage their households, and their reluctance to take analgesics on a regular basis may reduce the quality of their pain control. Complementary and alternative medicine (CAM)

Table 16.1 Adaptive tasks faced by women with metastatic breast cancer[a]

Physical and medical challenges
Managing physical symptoms and side effects (e.g., pain, fatigue)
Dealing with constant or changing treatment schedules
Accepting stable disease as a desirable outcome of treatment
Maintaining adequate communication with the medical treatment team
Fearing abandonment by the medical team
Deciding to end curative treatment and accepting palliative care
Psychological challenges
Coping with uncertainty and unpredictability
Perceiving a lack of control
Fearing dependency on others
Progressively losing functional ability
Maintaining valued life goals
Fearing death and suffering
Balancing hope with realistic preparations for the future
Managing complex emotions
Having unmet informational needs
Interpersonal challenges
Communicating with friends and family about illness and death
Feeling socially isolation and lacking emotional or instrumental support
Having concerns for loved ones
Spiritual and existential challenges
Making sense of and accepting the cancer diagnosis in the context of spiritual beliefs
Finding meaning in one's life and death
Practical concerns
Knowing when and how to seek home help, transportation assistance, or other services
Managing financial and legal affairs

[a]Adapted from Low et al. (2007) with permission

approaches are used by many women, although systematic and evidence-based data are lacking. Cancer-directed therapies will often relieve pain, e.g., radiation, chemotherapy. CAM therapies may help with management of treatment side effects as well. Because women living with metastatic breast cancer are hopeful for treatment responses, they are highly motivated to find a therapy that will relieve pain as well as prolong life. Some women move through serial treatments and look for experimental opportunities.

Fatigue, which is another serious problem for women living with metastatic breast cancer, is multi-factorial; contributors include the disease itself, treatments, and probably deconditioning from the physical symptoms associated with the disease. Proinflammatory cytokines, frequently elevated in advanced cancer (de Raaf et al. 2012), may be responsible for cancer-related fatigue that can seem out of proportion to the tumor burden. In addition, chemotherapy, radiation, and many of the newer targeted therapies (e.g., everolimus) can contribute to ongoing fatigue (Baselga et al. 2012). Although physical activity may be effective in relieving cancer-related fatigue in patients with less tumor burden, in patients with metastatic disease, some balance of energy conservation and physical activity may be the most appropriate strategy (Howell et al. 2013). CAM therapies such as yoga and Tai chi may be effective, but may have to be done cautiously in the setting of bone metastases.

Table 16.2 Factors associated with poor psychological adjustment in the context of metastatic breast cancer[a]

Severe physical symptoms (especially pain) and poor functional status
Younger age
Low dispositional optimism
Low perceived social support
Suppression of emotional experience or expression
High coping through avoidance and low coping through approach-oriented strategies

[a]Adapted from Low et al. (2007) with permission

Clinically significant depression, anxiety, and adjustment disorders are prevalent in adults with advanced cancer (Miovic and Block 2007) and in women with recurrent or metastatic breast cancer specifically (Burgess et al. 2005; Okamura et al. 2000). For example, in a 5-year study of women diagnosed with early-stage breast cancer within 5 months of study entry (Burgess et al. 2005), depression and anxiety diagnosed via interview using standard diagnostic criteria were more prevalent (45 %) in the 3 months following diagnosis of recurrent cancer than after initial breast cancer diagnosis (36 %). Cancer-related distress, in the form of intrusive thoughts and feelings about the disease, also is elevated after diagnosis of recurrent breast cancer (Andersen et al. 2005; Oh et al. 2004). Whereas cancer-specific distress and general quality of life improve over the year after diagnosis, problems with physical symptoms and functioning persist (Yang et al. 2008b). Although very few longitudinal studies are available, attributes associated with poorer psychological adjustment in women with recurrent and metastatic disease (see Table 16.2) include such factors as younger adult age, more severe physical symptoms (e.g., pain, fatigue), low social support, and more coping with the cancer experience through avoidance and less approach-oriented coping (e.g., planning, positive reappraisal; Yang et al. 2008a).

Certainly, a diagnosis of metastatic breast cancer generates psychological, interpersonal, and physical demands. It appears, however, that most women maintain or recover generally positive psychological health. In addition, adults with advanced cancer report that benefits such as enhanced relationships, deepened spirituality, and strengthened life appreciation and priorities can accompany the experience (Moreno and Stanton 2013).

Care of Women with Metastatic Disease

Women living with metastatic breast cancer have frequent and ongoing contact with the oncology care system. Initial treatment planning should be multidisciplinary, as is recommended for initial diagnosis and treatment (Cardoso et al. 2012). Even when disease is controlled and stable, as with responsive endocrine sensitive cancer, regular visits to the oncologist will occur at least every 2–3 months. Monitoring of disease status will often focus on tumor markers and specific scans, and patients may have need for symptomatic management of disease-related or treatment-related symptoms. Often, women will be able to continue working and do other meaningful activities, but some may have serious fatigue, cognitive difficulties or pain that may make activities difficult.

Living with the uncertainty of how long a specific treatment regimen will provide benefit is one of the critical challenges that the patient and her physician must face. The tempo of the disease recurrence as well as the burden of metastatic disease sites (a few or many; soft tissue vs. visceral) will provide some indication of whether or not complex multi-agent therapy is recommended or single agent serial treatments are appropriate. Increasingly, the approach to metastatic disease (Cardoso et al. 2012) reflects the consensus that palliative and supportive care are essential, and that the patient's preferences need to be taken into consideration (Table 16.3 from Cardoso). In addition, a recent consensus panel outlined specific strategies for addressing the supportive and palliative care needs of women living with metastatic disease, from a global perspective, with organ-specific approaches (Cleary et al. 2013). However, most of these recommendations are consensus based, with few randomized studies available.

Table 16.3 Guideline statement for management of advanced breast cancer (ABC)[a]

(1) The management of ABC is complex and, therefore, involvement of all appropriate specialties in a multidisciplinary team (including but not restricted to medical, radiation, surgical oncologists, imaging experts, pathologists, gynecologists, psycho-oncologists, social workers, nurses, and palliative care specialists), is crucial
(2) From the time of diagnosis of ABC, patients should be offered appropriate psychosocial care, supportive care, and symptom-related interventions as a routine part of their care. The approach must be personalized to meet the needs of the individual patient
(3) Following a thorough assessment and confirmation of MBC, the potential treatment goals of care should be discussed. Patients should be told that MBC is incurable but treatable, and women can live with MBC for extended periods of time (many years in some circumstances). This conversation should be conducted in accessible language, respecting patient privacy and cultural differences, and whenever possible, written information should be provided
(4) Patients (and their families, caregivers or support network, if the patient agrees) should be invited to participate in the decision-making process at all times. When possible, patients should be encouraged to be accompanied by persons who can support them and share treatment decisions (e.g. family members, caregivers, support network)
(5) There are few proven standards of care in ABC management. After appropriate informed consent, inclusion of patients in well-designed, prospective, randomized trials must be a priority whenever such trials are available and the patient is willing to participate
(6) The medical community is aware of the problems raised by the cost of ABC treatment. Balanced decisions should be made in all instances; patients' well being, length of life and patient's preference should always guide decisions
(7) Validated patient reported outcome measures provide useful information about symptom severity and the burden and the impact of these symptoms on overall quality of life. Systematic collection of such data should be integrated with other clinical assessments and form part of the decision-making about treatment and care

[a]Adapted from Cardoso et al. (2012) with permission. MBC is metastatic breast cancer

Compared with efficacious psychosocial interventions tested in randomized controlled trials (RCTs) for adults with early-stage cancer (e.g., Faller et al. 2013), the number of trials for women with metastatic disease is small. Women with metastatic breast cancer often are not included or included in such small numbers in those trials that reliable subgroup analyses are not possible. A recent review and meta-analysis of ten psychological RCTs with 1,378 women diagnosed with metastatic breast cancer included three trials of distinct individual approaches and seven group psychotherapy trials (four supportive-expressive therapy trials and three cognitive-behavioral trials) (Mustafa et al. 2013). Although some trials produced psychological benefit, the meta-analysis did not yield a clear pattern of psychological effects, given that a wide variety of outcome measures and follow-up durations were used. Across three trials, however, supportive-expressive group therapy produced a significant reduction in pain compared to usual care. In addition, there was some evidence of a survival benefit associated with intervention participation at 1 year (six trials) but not at 5 years (four trials) after the interventions.

Research Challenges and Opportunities

The most pressing challenge today is the lack of systematic research on women living with metastatic breast cancer for lengthy periods of time. Although many women have a relatively rapid progressive course from inception of metastatic recurrence to end-of-life care, there are both intermediate and long-term survivors for whom we have little information about their disease trajectory and experience of living with ongoing therapy that includes disease-related symptoms and treatment toxicity. For example, at one extreme, women who experience an ipsilateral breast cancer recurrence may have a variable course, with a continuous risk of recurrence after tumor excision that can be improved with the addition of adjuvant chemotherapy, especially in patients with estrogen receptor negative tumors in the CALOR trial (Aebi et al. 2014). Five year disease-free survival in those treated with chemotherapy was 69 vs. 57 % in those who did not receive chemotherapy. When multiple site metastatic recurrence occurs, the outcomes are less favorable, although durable periods of remission may occur for those with limited soft-tissue and bone-dominant disease that is hormone sensitive, as well as with patients for whom both endocrine and HER 2 targeted therapies are available. The major challenge for researchers is to be able to identify these patients and engage them in trials. The CALOR trial took many years to accrue and closed without meeting its initial accrual goal. In our own experience in a major metropolitan area, it also is difficult to recruit women living with metastatic disease for studies of psychosocial outcomes. Why do we have such a limited database? What are the issues we should study?

Adequate assessment of quality of life, cancer- and treatment-related symptoms and side effects, health behaviors, and psychosocial status is essential in women with metastatic disease. Patient-reported outcomes, such as quality of life and symptoms (e.g., fatigue, pain), are important targets of intervention as well as indicators of prognosis in metastatic disease (Gotay et al. 2008; Quinten et al. 2011). Especially in the context of metastatic disease, in which energy to complete assessments might be limited, development of measures that are brief, reliable, and valid is vital. For example, the Patient-Reported Outcomes Measurement Information System (PROMIS) contains a number of pertinent measures (e.g., fatigue, pain, depressive symptoms, anxiety; Alonso et al. 2013) for use in research and clinical practice. Psychometrically sound and valid assessments of experiences specific to women with metastatic disease also are needed.

One of the most important opportunities and challenges we face in management of metastatic breast cancer is the integration of palliative care into standard disease management. Because treatment for metastatic breast cancer often involves both medical and radiation oncologists, those specialists are looked to as the managers of care. Many women resist consideration of pain and symptom management while they are undergoing active treatment, such that referral to palliative care specialists does not occur until late in the treatment of metastatic disease. Breast cancer patients living with metastatic cancer are often interested in exploring experimental therapies and may perceive referral to palliative care as an indication of the oncology care team giving up on their cancer-directed care. To the extent that palliative care is integrated into cancer-directed treatment from the time of metastatic recurrence, symptom management and psychological concerns can be effectively co-managed without a sense of abandonment or change in course (Smith et al. 2012; Von Roenn 2013) (see Fig. 16.1).

Other major concerns for patients living with metastatic disease involve how best to live with the disease. Should they continue working? Can they afford their medical care? On whom do they rely for social support, especially as their health declines? Do they have an aging spouse or young children who require care?

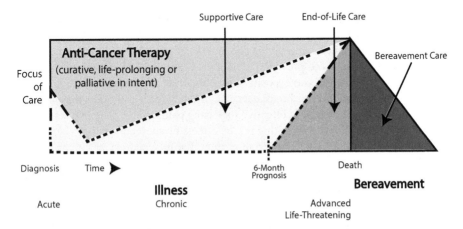

Fig. 16.1 Comprehensive cancer care [Adapted from National Cancer Institute. EPEC™-O. Education in palliative and end-of-life care for oncology. Available at : http://www.cancer.gov/cancertopics/cancerlibrary/epeco. Accessed 20 Sept 2014]

Table 16.4 Key elements of individualized care for patients with advanced cancer[a]

1. Patients should be well informed about their prognosis and treatment options, ensuring that they have opportunities to make their preferences and concerns regarding treatment and supportive care known
2. Anticancer therapy should be discussed and offered when evidence supports a reasonable chance of providing meaningful clinical benefit
3. Options to prioritize and enhance patients' quality of life, should be discussed at the time advanced cancer is diagnosed and throughout the course of illness along with development of a treatment plan that includes goals of therapy
4. Conversations about anticancer interventions should include information on likelihood of response, the nature of response, and the adverse effects and risks of any therapy. Direct costs to the patient in terms of time, toxicity, loss of alternatives, or financial impacts that can be anticipated should also be discussed to allow patients to make informed choices
5. Whenever possible, patients with advanced cancer should be given the opportunity to participate in clinical trials or other forms of research that may improve their outcomes or improve the care of future patients
6. When disease-directed options are exhausted, patients should be encouraged to transition to symptom-directed palliative care alone with the goal of minimizing physical and emotional suffering and ensuring that patients with advanced cancer are given the opportunity to die with dignity and peace of mind

[a]Adapted from Peppercorn (2011)

Unfortunately, all the resources that have been brought to bear for breast cancer survivors, that is, patients diagnosed with early stage disease and treated with curative intent who are living disease-free, do not seem to be suitable for women who are living with chronic and active cancer. Advance care planning is especially important for women living with metastatic breast cancer, yet it can remain unaddressed, primarily because of the slower trajectory of advancing disease, and the serial effective therapies that are available and offered to these patients (Peppercorn et al. 2011). Essential elements of that care are described in Table 16.4. Much more research is needed in women living with advanced breast cancer to determine how best they can maximize physical, emotional and spiritual well-being, while addressing their advance care planning needs.

Effective approaches to prevent and address cancer-related symptoms and side effects, as well as to promote positive psychosocial adjustment, are crucial for women living with metastatic breast cancer. Current evidence suggests that supportive expressive group therapy is effective for easing pain in this group (Mustafa et al. 2013), but strong evidence is lacking for the effects of interventions on other symptoms and psychosocial outcomes. To the extent that they address problems experienced across the cancer trajectory, efficacious psychosocial interventions (Faller et al. 2013) might generalize to women with advanced disease. Women with metastatic breast cancer can face distinct or more severe problems (e.g., life goal adjustment, progressive loss of function), however. Therefore, unique intervention approaches for women with metastatic cancer require development. In addition, disseminable approaches are needed which are readily accessible for women who might be experiencing physical compromise as a result of metastasized cancer and its treatment and therefore cannot attend in-person treatment regularly. For example, we recently found that, compared to standard care, an intervention (Project Connect Online) designed to facilitate personal website development and use to communicate with friends and family about the breast cancer experience produced improvements in depressive symptoms, positive mood, and life appreciation. Effects of this online intervention were particularly evident for breast cancer patients in active medical treatment, most of whom had metastatic disease (Stanton et al. 2013). Clearly, much work remains to promote quantity and quality of life and health for women who live with metastatic breast cancer.

References

Aebi S, Gelber S, Anderson SJ, Láng I, Robidoux A, Martín M, Nortier JWR, Paterson AHG, Rimawi MF, Cañada JMB, Thürlimann B, Murray E, Mamounas EP, Geyer CE Jr, Price KN, Coates AS, Gelber RD, Rastogi P, Wolmark N, Wapnir IL (2014) Chemotherapy for isolated locoregional recurrence of breast cancer (CALOR): a randomised trial. Lancet Oncol 15: 156–163

Alonso J, Bartlett SJ, Rose M, Aaronson NK, Chaplin JE, Efficace F, Leplege A, Lu A, Tulsky DS, Raat H, Ravens-Sieberer U, Revicki D, Terwee CB, Valderas JM, Cella D, Forrest CB (2013) The case for an international patient-reported outcomes measurement information system (PROMIS®) initiative. Health Qual Life Outcomes 11:210

Andersen BL, Shapiro CL, Farrar WB, Crespin T, Wells-Digregorio S (2005) Psychological responses to cancer recurrence. Cancer 104:1540–1547

Baselga J, Campone M, Piccart M, Burris HA III, Rugo HS, Sahmoud T, Noguchi S, Gnant M, Pritchard KI, Lebrun F, Beck JT, Ito Y, Yardley D, Deleu I, Perez A, Bachelot T, Vittori L, Xu Z, Mukhopadhyay P, Lebwohl D, Hortobagyi GN (2012) Everolimus in postmenopausal hormone-receptor-positive advanced breast cancer. N Engl J Med 366:520–529

Burgess C, Cornelius V, Love S, Graham J, Richards M, Ramirez A (2005) Depression and anxiety in women with early breast cancer: five year observational cohort study. BMJ 330:702

Cardoso F, Costa A, Norton L, Cameron D, Cufer T, Fallowfield L, Francis P, Gligorov J, Kyriakides S, Lin N, Pagani O, Senkus E, Thomssen C, Aapro M, Bergh J, Di LA, El SN, Ganz PA, Gelmon K, Goldhirsch A, Harbeck N, Houssami N, Hudis C, Kaufman B, Leadbeater M, Mayer M, Rodger A, Rugo H, Sacchini V, Sledge G, Van't Veer L, Viale G, Krop I, Winer E (2012) 1st international consensus guidelines for advanced breast cancer (ABC 1). Breast 21:242–252

Cleary J, Ddungu H, Distelhorst SR, Ripamonti C, Rodin GM, Bushnaq MA, Clegg-Lamptey JN, Connor SR, Diwani MB, Eniu A, Harford JB, Kumar S, Rajagopal MR, Thompson B, Gralow JR, Anderson BO (2013) Supportive and palliative care for metastatic breast cancer: resource allocations in low- and middle-income countries. A breast health global initiative 2013 consensus statement. Breast 22:616–627

de Raaf PJ, Sleijfer S, Lamers CH, Jager A, Gratama JW, van der Rijt CC (2012) Inflammation and fatigue dimensions in advanced cancer patients and cancer survivors: an explorative study. Cancer 118:6005–6011

Desantis C, Ma J, Bryan L, Jemal A (2014) Breast cancer statistics, 2013. CA Cancer J Clin 64: 52–62

Early Breast Cancer Trialists' Collaborative Group (2005) Effects of chemotherapy and hormonal therapy for early breast cancer on recurrence and 15-year survival: an overview of the randomised trials. Lancet 365:1687–1717

Faller H, Schuler M, Richard M, Heckl U, Weis J, Kuffner R (2013) Effects of psycho-oncologic interventions on emotional distress and quality of life in adult patients with cancer: systematic review and meta-analysis. J Clin Oncol 31:782–793

Gotay CC, Kawamoto CT, Bottomley A, Efficace F (2008) The prognostic significance of patient-reported outcomes in cancer clinical trials. J Clin Oncol 26:1355–1363

Howell D, Keller-Olaman S, Oliver TK, Hack TF, Broadfield L, Biggs K, Chung J, Gravelle D, Green E, Hamel M, Harth T, Johnston P, McLeod D, Swinton N, Syme A, Olson K (2013) A pan-Canadian practice guideline and algorithm: screening, assessment, and supportive care of adults with cancer-related fatigue. Curr Oncol 20:e233–e246

Institute of Medicine (2013) Delivering high-quality cancer care: charting a new course for a system in crisis. The National Academies Press, Washington, DC

Johnson RH, Chien FL, Bleyer A (2013) Incidence of breast cancer with distant involvement among women in the United States, 1976 to 2009. JAMA 309:800–805

Low CA, Beran T, Stanton AL. (2007) Adaptation in the Face of Advanced Cancer. In Feuerstein M (ed) Handbook of Cancer Survivorship. pp 211–228, Springer

Miovic M, Block S (2007) Psychiatric disorders in advanced cancer. Cancer 110:1665–1676

Moreno PI, Stanton AL (2013) Personal growth during the experience of advanced cancer: a systematic review. Cancer J 19:421–430

Mustafa M, Carson-Stevens A, Gillespie D, Edwards AG (2013) Psychological interventions for women with metastatic breast cancer. Cochrane Database Syst Rev 6:CD004253

Oh S, Heflin L, Meyerowitz B, Desmond K, Rowland J, Ganz P (2004) Quality of life of breast cancer survivors after a recurrence: a follow-up study. Breast Cancer Res Treat 87:45–57

Okamura H, Watanabe T, Narabayashi M, Katsumata N, Ando M, Adachi I, Akechi T, Uchitomi Y (2000) Psychological distress following first recurrence of disease in patients with breast cancer: prevalence and risk factors. Breast Cancer Res Treat 61:131–137

Peppercorn JM, Smith TJ, Helft PR, Debono DJ, Berry SR, Wollins DS, Hayes DM, Von Roenn JH, Schnipper LE (2011) American society of clinical oncology statement: toward individualized care for patients with advanced cancer. J Clin Oncol 29:755–760

Quinten C, Maringwa J, Gotay CC, Martinelli F, Coens C, Reeve BB, Flechtner H, Greimel E, King M, Osoba D, Cleeland C, Ringash J, Schmucker-Von KJ, Taphoorn MJ, Weis J, Bottomley A (2011) Patient self-reports of symptoms and clinician ratings as predictors of overall cancer survival. J Natl Cancer Inst 103:1851–1858

Siegel R, Ma J, Zou Z, Jemal A (2014) Cancer statistics, 2014. CA Cancer J Clin 64:9–29

Smith TJ, Temin S, Alesi ER, Abernethy AP, Balboni TA, Basch EM, Ferrell BR, Loscalzo M, Meier DE, Paice JA, Peppercorn JM, Somerfield M, Stovall E, Von Roenn JH (2012) American society of clinical oncology provisional clinical opinion: the integration of palliative care into standard oncology care. J Clin Oncol 30:880–887

Stanton AL, Thompson EH, Crespi CM, Link JS, Waisman JR (2013) Project connect online: randomized trial of an internet-based program to chronicle the cancer experience and facilitate communication. J Clin Oncol 31:3411–3417

Thornton LM, Levin AO, Dorfman CS, Godiwala N, Heitzmann C, Andersen BL (2014) Emotions and social relationships for breast and gynecologic patients: a qualitative study of coping with recurrence. Psychooncology 23:382–389

Von Roenn JH (2013) Optimal cancer care: concurrent oncology and palliative care. J Natl Compr Canc Netw 11(Suppl 1):S1–S2

Yang HC, Brothers BM, Andersen BL (2008a) Stress and quality of life in breast cancer recurrence: moderation or mediation of coping? Ann Behav Med 35:188–197

Yang HC, Thornton LM, Shapiro CL, Andersen BL (2008b) Surviving recurrence: psychological and quality-of-life recovery. Cancer 112:1178–1187

Chapter 17
Quality of Care, Including Survivorship Care Plans

Dawn L. Hershman and Patricia A. Ganz

Abstract With the expectation of prolonged survival in the vast majority of women diagnosed with breast cancer, making initial treatment decisions that minimize or prevent late complications, and maximize the quality as well as quantity of life, is absolutely critical. Unfortunately, such care is not uniformly delivered. Patient, provider, and system barriers contribute to delays in cancer care, lower quality of care, and poorer outcomes in vulnerable populations, including low income, underinsured, and racial/ethnic minority populations. Covering the costs of cancer care is a major concern for many cancer survivors, and as a result, a major challenge will be to provide cost-effective follow-up care by reducing overuse of unnecessary tests and procedures so that access to effective medications can be preserved. One of the recently promoted means of improving the coordination of care for breast cancer survivors has been the use of survivorship care planning, as coordination of care will be absolutely essential to deliver high-quality care. Patient navigation is another approach to help overcome healthcare system barriers and facilitate timely access to quality medical care. Understanding the challenges and opportunities in delivering high-quality cancer care is one of the most critical issues of the day. With the large numbers of breast cancer patients and the tremendous advances in our understanding of the disease and treatments (leading to large numbers of survivors), breast cancer will likely be the focus of new models for the delivery of better and more efficient cancer care.

Keywords Breast cancer survivorship • Quality of care • Cost • Disparities

D.L. Hershman (✉)
Associate Professor of Medicine and Epidemiology, Herbert Irving Comprehensive
Cancer Center Columbia University, 161 Fort Washington, 1068, New York, NY 10032, USA
e-mail: dlh23@cumc.columbia.edu

P.A. Ganz
UCLA Schools of Medicine and Public Health, Jonsson Comprehensive
Cancer Center, Los Angeles, CA, USA
e-mail: pganz@mednet.ucla.edu

© Breast Cancer Research Foundation 2015
P.A. Ganz (ed.), *Improving Outcomes for Breast Cancer Survivors*,
Advances in Experimental Medicine and Biology 862,
DOI 10.1007/978-3-319-16366-6_17

Current Challenges in the Delivery of Quality Care to Breast Cancer Survivors

Definition of Cancer Survivor

Among all of the common epithelial cancers, breast cancer has evidenced one of the most substantial improvements in survival over the past three decades (Siegel et al. 2012). This has occurred through the introduction of population wide screening mammography, as well as the application of adjuvant chemotherapy, adjuvant endocrine therapy, and the two combined in almost all women with breast cancer (Berry et al. 2005). The establishment and dissemination of standards of care for breast cancer treatment have been facilitated by the regular meta-analytic synthesis of clinical trials data by the Early Breast Cancer Clinical Trialists Group who have come together regularly at Oxford University for over two decades (Early Breast Cancer Trialists' Collaborative Group 2005). Their findings have been rapidly translated into clinical guidelines promoted by the American Society of Clinical Oncology (ASCO), as well as by other professional and governmental organizations.

At the time of the 2000 NIH consensus conference on the adjuvant therapy of breast cancer (National Institutes of Health 2001), all women with tumors larger than a centimeter were advised to receive chemotherapy, with the addition of endocrine therapy (tamoxifen) for 5 years if the tumor was positive for hormone receptors. Since that time, we have seen the development of new endocrine therapies (e.g., aromatase inhibitors), the emergence of different and longer endocrine treatment strategies, as well as an explosion in new knowledge about the different genomic subtypes of breast cancer (Perou et al. 2000; Sorlie et al. 2001). These subtypes of breast cancer are now treated with therapies that offer the best chance for cure (e.g., HER2 positive breast cancer) (Romond et al. 2005), and in many cases, toxic chemotherapy can be avoided in women with a very low risk of recurrence (Paik et al. 2004, 2006). Today, most women are diagnosed with stage I breast cancer, and can expect survival outcomes that differ very little from other women their age (DeSantis et al. 2014). However, there is a human and financial cost to these outcomes, given the extended and sometimes complex treatments these women receive.

Conceptualizing when breast cancer survivorship begins is challenging. Historically, one was not considered a cancer survivor until 5 years after diagnosis, and even then, patients with breast cancer were known to experience late recurrences, especially in the setting of hormone receptor positive tumors. However, with the cancer survivorship movement that began in the mid-1980s (Mullan 1985), the founding of the National Coalition for Cancer Survivorship (NCCS) in 1986 led to the first definition of a cancer survivorship as "being from the time of diagnosis through the balance of life," including family, friends and caregivers as part of that journey and as co-survivors (http://www.canceradvocacy.org/about-us/our-history/). This broad definition obviously includes many individuals who may not survive for extended periods of time. However, in the case of breast cancer, this definition is central to delivery of high quality care. With the expectation of prolonged survival in the vast majority of women diagnosed with breast cancer, making initial treatment decisions that minimize or prevent late complications, and maximize the quality as well as quantity of life, is absolutely critical. Unfortunately, such care is not uniformly delivered (Institute of Medicine 2013), and we discuss these issues in this chapter.

For newly diagnosed breast cancer patients, the following issues are relevant to minimizing the long term or persistent effects of treatment, as well as rare late effects. Women of childbearing age who wish to preserve their fertility should be informed about whether the planned breast cancer treatment will have an effect on this, and should be afforded the opportunity to discuss fertility preservation options with a reproductive endocrinologist (Loren et al. 2013). Based on the literature, this is not consistently done even in medical oncology practices that are focused on improving the quality of care (Neuss et al. 2013). While cost may be an important barrier, patients have told us that even if they choose not to take action, the fact that this is discussed with them is deemed very important (see earlier Chap. 9 on reproductive outcomes). In addition, women need to be informed of the potential for many of the long term toxicities of contemporary treatments, including lymphedema, neuropathy, cardiac dysfunction, cognitive dysfunction, and fatigue (see earlier Chaps. 5, 6, 7, 8, 14), many of which are associated with particular local or systemic treatment regimens. To the extent there is flexibility in the exact primary treatment plan, concerns and preferences of the patient should be taken into account, as well as pre-existing risk factors that might increase the likelihood of one of these late effects (Fig. 17.1). Premature menopause is extremely common in women over age 40 years

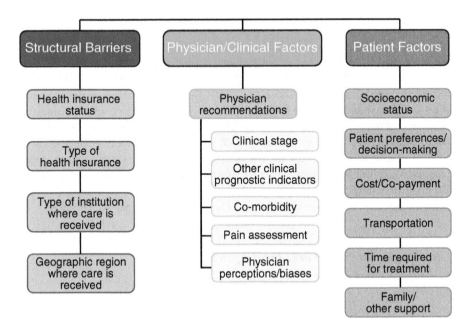

Fig. 17.1 Conceptual framework for receipt of optimal cancer care (Adapted from Shavers and Brown, JNCI 2002 with permission)

who receive chemotherapy (Ganz et al. 2011b), and women need to be made aware of this likely occurrence, as well as be reassured that their symptoms will be appropriately and effectively managed. Being prepared for what to expect during and after treatment, is part of good survivorship care and starts at the time of diagnosis with initial treatment planning (Ganz et al. 1998, 2006, 2011a; Wyatt et al. 1998).

After the initial treatment decisions are made, and treatments are underway, many women want to know what is coming next, and that is where formal survivorship care planning for the post-treatment period has emerged as a major gap in quality care (Hewitt et al. 2006; Ganz and Hahn 2008; Ganz et al. 2008). For almost a decade since the Institute of Medicine (IOM) report on adult cancer survivorship care (Hewitt et al. 2006), various organizations have worked diligently to improve the post-treatment communication and coordination of care, specifically at the transition between active treatment and follow-up care. In breast cancer patients, this usually occurs at the end of adjuvant chemotherapy and/or radiation therapy. For many women, extended adjuvant endocrine therapy will be prescribed; this is a critical and lifesaving component of treatment and not all women understand the importance of this therapy. Non-adherence to oral endocrine therapy is very common and results in poorer breast cancer outcomes (Hershman et al. 2010, 2011). Non-adherence can occur because of uncontrolled and bothersome symptoms, as well as concerns about the financial cost of treatment. Failure to adhere to this treatment is an important quality of care issue, and lack of communication and trust in physicians doing the follow-up care can contribute to this (Kahn et al. 2007).

Breast cancer survivorship does not occur in a vacuum. As discussed elsewhere in this volume, although the average age of breast cancer incidence is 61 years, about 25 % of incident cases are in women younger than 50 years and the majority are over 65 years of age. Life stage, partnership status, financial and other resources, including the generosity of health insurance plans, may contribute substantially to the quality of the survivor's life after cancer. In addition, continuing symptoms (e.g., menopause related, sexuality and intimacy concerns, fatigue, and depression) can disrupt relationships and the ability to work and care for children. The human cost of breast cancer is substantial. Finally, as described in Chap. 16 in this volume on living with metastatic breast cancer, there are more than a 100,000 women living for extended periods of time on cancer directed therapy for whom active disease and its consequences (e.g., pain, physical limitations, treatment toxicities) further complicate the quality of life. We hope these introductory remarks set the stage for a more detailed discussion of the challenges of delivering high quality care to breast cancer patients and survivors.

Challenges for Survivors: Dealing with the Costs of Cancer Care

Covering the costs of cancer care is a major concern for many cancer survivors. Cancer-related medical costs have accelerated at a rate beyond those of other medical treatments (Vanchieri 2005). It is projected that US health care spending will reach \$4.3 trillion and account for 19 % of the national gross domestic product by 2019 (Schnipper et al. 2012). This increase has been driven by a dramatic rise in both the cost of therapy and the extent of care, especially in the last few months of life. Physicians directly or indirectly control or influence the majority of cancer care costs, including the use and choice of drugs, the types of supportive care, the frequency of imaging and the number and the extent of hospitalizations (Smith and Hillner 2011). In addition there are numerous unmeasured costs associated with loss of work and subsequent loss of insurance. Given the long life expectancy of patients with breast cancer, it is not surprising that total costs of breast cancer care in both the metastatic and non-metastatic setting can be higher than other cancers.

Patients are most directly affected by out-of-pocket costs, which have increased as more therapies have switched from intravenous to oral therapies. It is estimated that more than one quarter of the 400 antineoplastic agents now in the pipeline are oral drugs. Oral cancer therapies are often advertised as being more convenient than parenteral therapies as they can reduce patient travel, eliminate time spent in the infusion center, and avoid issues related to intravenous access. However there are a number of concerns about oral therapies that have arisen. As with other new cancer therapies, they are accompanied by increased costs and financial burdens for patients (Vanchieri 2005; Benson et al. 1998). Total prescription medication costs exceeded \$234 billion by 2008, an annual rate of increase of over 10 % (Kaiser Family Foundation 2010). Some of the most expensive oral cancer drugs are used to treat patients with breast cancer, such as everolimus, which can cost \$100,000 or more per year. The financial burden borne by patients prescribed these drugs can be very high, with co-pays running from hundreds up to thousands of dollars per month. It is known that as out of pocket costs increase, the likelihood of compliance with medications decreases, which can adversely affect survival outcomes. It is well-known that adherence to hormonal therapy is a large problem in breast cancer, and co-payment amount has an independent effect on adherence and early discontinuation of hormone therapy (Neugut et al. 2011). Furthermore, the cost of oral supportive care medications, such as anti-emetic therapies, can be prohibitive for some patients, resulting in unnecessary toxicity and decreased quality of life. Not surprisingly, out-of-pocket expenses are the largest in countries of low and lower-middle income, despite the fact that people in these countries have the lowest resources to cover these extra costs (Anderson et al. 2011).

A major challenge as the number of cancer survivors increases will be to provide cost effective follow-up care by reducing overuse of unnecessary tests and procedures so that access to effective medications can be preserved. Public health efforts, such as the Cancer Treatment Fairness Act, which requires insurance to cover oral cancer treatment medications the same as they cover intravenously and injected cancer treatment medications, may increase drug price transparency, improve access and reduce out of pocket costs for life-saving cancer treatments. Efforts at decreasing economic disparities in breast cancer care are especially important given the rapid increase of expensive oral cancer therapies.

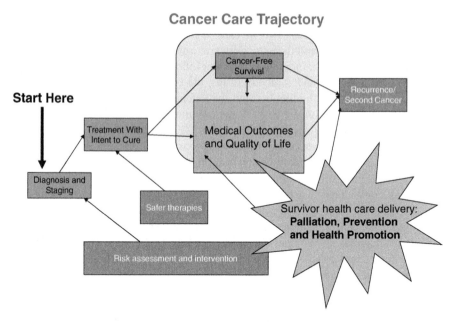

Fig. 17.2 Model depicting the role cancer survivorship care and the cancer care trajectory

Disparities in Breast Cancer Treatment and Outcome

Patient, provider, and systems barriers contribute to delays in cancer care, lower quality of care, and poorer outcomes in vulnerable populations, including low income, underinsured, and racial/ethnic minority populations (Fig. 17.2). Compared to non-Hispanic white women, overall breast cancer incidence is lower among black women but breast cancer mortality is higher (about 40 %) with trends that vary depending on age and location (American Cancer Society 2011). The racial difference in outcome has increased over time, and may reflect disparities in diagnosis and treatment. Despite the fact that nationally the use of mammography is nearly equivalent for blacks and whites (American Cancer Society 2013), black women have a much higher rate of incidence before the age of 40 years, are more likely to be diagnosed with larger tumors (>5.0 cm), and have higher rates of distant-stage disease at diagnosis (American Cancer Society 2011). Differences between blacks and whites also exist with regard to access to clinical trials and innovative cancer treatments (Sateren et al. 2002; Tejeda et al. 1996); receipt of biomarker testing, follow-up care post-treatment, and surveillance mammography (Shavers and Brown 2002).

The factors contributing to the striking difference in mortality between blacks and whites (Li et al. 2003; Wheeler et al. 2013) are likely to be multi-factorial and complex, and have been attributed to differences in tumor biology (Bowen et al. 2006; O'Brien et al. 2010; Carey et al. 2006; Lund et al. 2009), psychological, behavioral factors, and social factors and access to care (Magai et al. 2008; Gerend and Pai 2008; O'Brien et al. 2010; Du et al. 2007, 2008), and access to and response to new adjuvant treatments including hormonal therapy (Menashe et al. 2009; Jatoi et al. 2003; Caudle et al. 2010). Interestingly, when you look at differences in survival between races over time, the separation began in the 1980s and has continued since that time, as white women have had improvements in breast cancer survival and black women have not. This separation coincides with an increased understanding of the importance of adjuvant treatment, and suggests that this disparity is modifiable (2010). Also of interest, recent studies suggest that the evolution of racial disparities in breast cancer survival are different in different cities in the US, which may be a reflection of state level screening programs, access and public health education (Hunt et al. 2014).

Recent studies have suggested that black women more often did not receive timely treatment compared to other women (Shavers and Brown 2002); are less likely to receive optimal systemic adjuvant therapy than white women (Hassett and Griggs 2009; Bickell et al. 2006); and are more likely to have delays in the initiation of adjuvant chemotherapy and radiotherapy, which are all associated with worse survival (Hershman et al. 2006a, b). Despite the fact that black women are more likely to have triple negative breast cancer, the racial disparities gap is greatest among the hormone-sensitive subtypes of breast cancer and because non-adherence to anti-estrogen treatment has been shown to adversely impact survival, differences in the utilization of this treatment may well explain some of the black-white breast cancer mortality disparity (Shavers and Brown 2002).

In low and middle-income countries advanced stages at presentation and poor diagnostic and treatment access contribute to lower breast cancer survival than in higher income countries (Harford et al. 2011). In 2010 the Breast Health Global Initiative reported an executive summary of their consensus meeting. Challenges for improving outcomes include little community awareness that breast cancer is treatable, inadequate pathology services for diagnostics, fragmented treatment options and establishment of data registries to show progress with interventions (Anderson et al. 2011).

Much work has been done to define the problem and establish modifiable factors that may contribute. Efforts going forward will need to focus on interventions and public policy changes to reduce the disparity in outcome by intervening in factors that can easily be modified.

Research Underway to Address These Issues and Future Strategies/Policy

Reduce Overdiagnosis and Over Treatment

With the expansion of population based mammography screening described earlier, there has been a stage shift to earlier stage breast cancer, as well as an explosion in the detection of non-invasive ductal cancers or ductal carcinoma in situ (DCIS).

In 2013, there were expected to be 64,640 DCIS cases and 232,340 cases of invasive cancer (DeSantis et al. 2014). The continued increase in diagnosis of DCIS has not reduced the number of invasive cases of breast cancer and is felt to be overdiagnosis of precancerous disease that would not likely become invasive or not be detected and cause death (Esserman et al. 2009, 2013; Esserman and Thompson 2010). This also leads to over treatment, as patients with DCIS are subjected to the same local therapy approaches (i.e., surgery and radiation therapy) that are applied to patients with invasive cancer. Moreover, the psychological distress associated with the diagnosis of DCIS is substantial (Ganz 2010).

Reduction in the age of initiation of screening mammography to the 40–50 years age group, as well as the interval frequency for mammography screening in women over 50 years remains controversial, in spite of evidence based reviews that suggest that starting at age 50 years is sufficient, and that the interval can be less frequent than annually. Among the biggest challenges with DCIS is the identification of high risk disease that would in fact lead to significant morbidity and mortality, or the converse, those women who need minimal if any treatment. In the case of stage I hormone receptor positive breast cancer, where low risk disease patients can avoid chemotherapy, there have been only a few trials that have looked at the omission of radiation therapy, and the uptake of avoiding this therapy has been limited (Giordano 2012). The NRG clinical trials group is hoping to do a large simple trial to address this question in early stage patients. This will reduce both morbidity and cost if treatment can be avoided. Future trials will hopefully be able to incorporate genomic and molecular markers to identify high and low risk patients and to tailor the intensity of treatment to the tumor characteristics.

Among the many challenges we face in this area is changing the beliefs of women regarding the value of mammographic screening, given the 30 years campaign by various health professional organizations supporting the use of this technique for early detection of breast cancer (Welch and Passow 2014). Women and their physicians are reluctant to give up the idea that earlier detection of a cancer will make a difference. Translating data from the population to the individual patient is challenging, and patients do not want to be denied a procedure that they think might be lifesaving. The same applies to other imaging technologies that may be used for screening, staging or monitoring of breast cancer, such as breast MRI and PET-CT scans. These currently have no role in the management of breast cancer, with exception of breast MRI in women at high risk for breast cancer (e.g., *BRCA1/2* gene carriers), but their use is widespread, and in fact, the use of breast MRI may be contributing to the recent increase in bilateral mastectomy, even when unilateral breast conserving treatment would be appropriate. Whether these choices are rational, or driven by overzealous treatment recommendations of physicians, is uncertain. The ability to perform immediate breast reconstruction at the time of initial treatment, and the advances in cosmetic results (e.g., nipple sparing surgery), have encouraged both patients and physicians to opt for this therapy. The misunderstanding and confusion about the appropriateness of this extreme therapy for high risk gene carriers (e.g., Angelina Jolie) and not for the general population of women with breast cancer has increased the demand for this treatment. Unfortunately, many physicians go along with these approaches, and it is uncertain whether these recommendations are independent of financial considerations. Finally, in the post-treatment phase, many women cannot accept the fact that surveillance testing for recurrence is unproven (Khatcheressian et al. 2013), and it is easier for physicians to offer testing, than to spend time discussing the lack of value in these assessments. Everyone feels better when the blood work and scans come back normal, but when the tumor marker or imaging provides a false positive result, much anxiety and additional testing results. ASCO and other professional societies are participating in the ABIM Foundation Choosing Wisely campaign, which have identified these types of services as being of low value and a target for quality improvement efforts.

Survivorship Care Plans: Assessment and Referral to Appropriate Clinicians

One of the recently promoted means of improving the coordination of care for breast cancer survivors has been the use of survivorship care planning (Ganz and Hahn 2008), and a care plan document, as a means of summarizing what treatments have been received, what surveillance is needed to identify recurrence, and how to manage persistent symptoms that do not resolve in the post-treatment period, as well as be on the lookout for rare but important late effects of treatment. With the IOM report on adult cancer survivors in 2005 (Hewitt and Ganz 2006; Hewitt et al. 2006), there was a flurry of activity to try to move forward with the idea of care plans. Sadly, it has had relatively modest uptake in clinical practice, but the most widely studied cancer has been breast cancer (Tevaarwerk et al. 2014; Birken et al. 2014; Haq et al. 2013). It was not until the recent decision by the American College of Surgeons Commission on Cancer to set survivorship care planning as a standard for accreditation in 2015 that clinical cancer delivery settings have identified strategies to make this happen. One of the authors has been extensively involved in the dissemination of care plans during the past decade, and it is good that we are finally seeing some uptake. Nevertheless, the care plan document, which has been the focus of many studies, is not really the issue. It is the communication and coordination of care that is critically important as part of the post-treatment care planning. With the anticipated work shortages for all oncology health professionals and the increasing number of cancer cases expected in the next decade (Institute of Medicine 2013), medical and surgical oncologists will have limited space in their practices to provide ongoing care for early stage, low risk breast cancer patients, and they must develop strategies to share the care with primary care providers who can continue the monitoring of these patients while addressing age-related comorbid conditions as well as persistent cancer treatment related symptoms such as fatigue, menopausal symptoms, depression and others. As called for in the recent IOM report on the delivery of high quality cancer care (Institute of Medicine 2013), coordination of care will be absolutely essential to deliver high-quality cancer care. Breast cancer patients are an ideal target for innovations in the delivery of quality care.

In addition to post-treatment care planning and coordination of care, we need to emphasize the importance of psychosocial care services and palliative care in breast cancer survivors. This is extensively called out in the recent IOM report on quality of care (Institute of Medicine 2013) as being an essential component of high quality cancer care from the time of diagnosis. Among the breast cancer survivors that present for consultation at UCLA, almost all have had superb and technically appropriate medical care. However, few if any have had their psychosocial needs addressed and many are seeking help for severe and debilitating symptoms (e.g., fatigue, cognitive dysfunction, neuropathy) that are not being addressed in the routine follow-up care they are receiving, usually by at least 2–3 oncology specialists. Some research (see Chaps. 5, 6, 7, 8, 9 on various symptoms), is beginning to identify genetic or behavioral risk profiles that may allow us to identify patients at high risk for persistent post-treatment symptoms. Possible strategies in the future may include a battery of questionnaires and blood tests that will facilitate risk profiling and allow tailoring of treatments and/or early interventions to reduce the risk of persistent problems. Much more prospective observational, biopsychosocial data collection will be necessary. Ideally this should be conducted within the setting of clinical trials, but might be feasible within the learning health care systems of the future (Abernethy et al. 2010; Institute of Medicine 2013).

To accomplish these goals, we must build and develop a knowledge base as well as improve the self-efficacy among primary care providers who have not been heavily engaged in the follow-up care of cancer patients for several decades (Cheung et al. 2013; Han et al. 2013; Potosky et al. 2011; Blanch-Hartigan et al. 2014). Primary care providers would like to share the care of cancer patients with oncologists and find the idea of care plans very attractive and helpful to them (Shalom et al. 2011; Hewitt et al. 2007). Here again, breast cancer is an excellent model for this type of shared care. There are many women's health primary care providers who have large numbers of breast cancer survivors in their practices. These physicians often have an interest in menopause-related issues, such as vasomotor symptom management and bone health. This makes them excellent primary care providers for the follow-up of the post-treatment, low risk breast cancer patient. With specific recommendations about which cancer surveillance tests are necessary, and when the oncologist needs to re-engage in care, these providers can manage breast cancer survivors very competently, as has been shown in several randomized trials (Grunfeld et al. 1996, 2006). Oncology professional societies must lead the way in working with other health care provider professional groups to develop curricula and educational strategies to enhance the competencies of all care providers who will be following breast cancer survivors in the post-treatment period (2013).

Improving Quality and Reducing Health Care Disparities

In recent years there has been progress in increasing screening rates for breast cancer, however, despite this, the gap between white and black breast cancer mortality rates is still widening because early detection does not reduce mortality unless those diagnosed are subsequently treated in a timely and effective way. One interventional approach has been through patient navigation. Patient navigation refers to the individualized assistance offered to patients, families and caregivers to help overcome healthcare systems barriers and facilitate timely access to quality medical care (Freeman and Wasfie 1989). Patient navigation has repeatedly been shown to improve rates and timeliness of follow-up of cancer screening abnormalities in various populations (Paskett et al. 2011). Less is known about treatment adherence, satisfaction with care and survival. The challenge will be to figure out the best implementation among patients with the greatest need in a cost-efficient manner. Other interventions are currently being tested to improve adherence to hormone therapy for breast cancer such text messaging and email reminders.

To improve outcomes of breast cancer survivors it will be necessary to focus on interventions to improve the quality of care. To do this requires the development of breast cancer specific quality indicators. Based on the work done by the National Initiative on Cancer Care Quality, ASCO and NCCN developed several quality indicators, three of which were specifically for the treatment of breast cancer patients. They have advocated for the use of radiation therapy following breast conservation therapy for women under the age of 70, adjuvant hormonal therapy for women hormone sensitive breast cancer and combination chemotherapy for women with tumors that are not hormone sensitive. The establishment of ASCO's Quality Oncology Practice Initiative and the Commission on Cancer reporting standards have impacted physician behavior, and research has shown that, for the most part, physicians are compliant with these quality indicators. The problem is that these measures are very limited in providing measurement of complex care delivery for a disease such as breast cancer. Research has shown consistency where the information is clear-cut i.e. high level evidence, and more deviations in care where the treatment or management scenarios are not as well defined. Much work is being done to identify quality indicators, and the expectation is that physician reimbursement, financial incentives and practice certification requirements will continue to ensure that the most beneficial treatments are offered to all patients.

Summary

The quality of cancer care delivery in the US varies substantially, with patients at risk for too little or too much care, and with a cost that is exploding. Eliminating wasteful variability in care and focusing on pathway or guideline consistent care is an important goal. Other international health care systems (e.g., Canada, UK, Australia) tend to have more consistent evidence-based care, where treatments and diagnostic tests that are not recommended are less often used. A priority in breast cancer is guaranteeing everyone life-saving treatment in a timely way and eliminating modifiable factors that contribute to healthcare disparities. As payment reform occurs in the US health care system, moving to bundled payments or reimbursement for episodes of care, the incentives to utilize low value procedures are expected to diminish, as the fee for service payment system does little to discourage over-utilization. With the plethora of new, and often expensive cancer treatments, attention will need to be paid to the cost-effectiveness of new treatment strategies compared to existing, less expensive strategies. However, the need for more care that enhances patient engagement in self-management and decision-making will require adequate educational and informational strategies, as well as clinical staff to work with breast cancer patients from the time of diagnosis through the post-treatment phase. With the expected growth in the numbers of new breast cancer patients as the population ages, better use of team-based care, and coordination of care between oncology specialists and primary care providers will be required. No longer can cancer care be isolated from general medical care to the extent that it has been during the past 50 years. Risk stratification will be necessary to ensure that those patients in greatest need of oncology clinicians on an ongoing basis will remain in those practice settings, while low risk patients can resume care in settings where health promotion and chronic disease prevention are more generally managed, including access to psychosocial services. Understanding the challenges and opportunities in delivering high-quality cancer care is one of the most critical issues of the day. Breast cancer, because of its large numbers of patients, and because of the tremendous advances in our understanding of the disease and treatments, will likely be the focus of new models for the delivery of better and more efficient cancer care.

References

Abernethy AP, Etheredge LM, Ganz PA et al (2010) Rapid-learning system for cancer care. J Clin Oncol 28:4268–4274
American Cancer Society (2010) Cancer facts and figures 2010. Atlanta, GA: American Cancer Society
American Cancer Society (2011) Breast cancer facts and figures, 2011–2012. American Cancer Society, Atlanta
American Cancer Society (2013) Cancer prevention & early detection facts & figures 2013. American Cancer Society, Atlanta
Anderson BO, Cazap E, El Saghir NS et al (2011) Optimisation of breast cancer management in low-resource and middle-resource countries: executive summary of the breast health global initiative consensus, 2010. Lancet Oncol 12:387–398
Benson R, Wilson C, Williams MV (1998) Comments on costs of treating advanced colorectal cancer, Ross et al., Eur J Cancer 1996, 32A, S13-S17. Eur J Cancer 34:593–594
Berry DA, Cronin KA, Plevritis SK et al (2005) Effect of screening and adjuvant therapy on mortality from breast cancer. N Engl J Med 353:1784–1792
Bickell NA, Wang JJ, Oluwole S et al (2006) Missed opportunities: racial disparities in adjuvant breast cancer treatment. J Clin Oncol 24:1357–1362
Birken SA, Deal AM, Mayer DK et al (2014) Determinants of survivorship care plan use in US cancer programs. J Cancer Educ 29:720–727
Blanch-Hartigan D, Forsythe LP, Alfano CM et al (2014) Provision and discussion of survivorship care plans among cancer survivors: results of a nationally representative survey of oncologists and primary care physicians. J Clin Oncol 32:1578–1585
Bowen RL, Stebbing J, Jones LJ (2006) A review of the ethnic differences in breast cancer. Pharmacogenomics 7:935–942

Carey LA, Perou CM, Livasy CA et al (2006) Race, breast cancer subtypes, and survival in the Carolina breast cancer study. JAMA 295:2492–2502

Caudle AS, Gonzalez-Angulo AM, Hunt KK et al (2010) Predictors of tumor progression during neoadjuvant chemotherapy in breast cancer. http://www.cms.gov/Research-Statistics-Data-and-Systems/Statistics-Trends-and-Reports/NationalHealthExpendData/index.html?redirect=/nationalhealthexpenddata/ J Clin Oncol 28:1821–1828

Centers for Medicare and Medicaid Services: National Health Expenditure Data: Historical

Cheung WY, Aziz N, Noone AM et al (2013) Physician preferences and attitudes regarding different models of cancer survivorship care: a comparison of primary care providers and oncologists. J Cancer Surviv 7:343–354

DeSantis C, Ma J, Bryan L et al (2014) Breast cancer statistics, 2013. CA Cancer J Clin 64:52–62

Du XL, Fang S, Vernon SW et al (2007) Racial disparities and socioeconomic status in association with survival in a large population-based cohort of elderly patients with colon cancer. Cancer 110:660–669

Du XL, Fang S, Meyer TE (2008) Impact of treatment and socioeconomic status on racial disparities in survival among older women with breast cancer. Am J Clin Oncol 31:125–132

Early Breast Cancer Trialists' Collaborative Group (2005) Effects of chemotherapy and hormonal therapy for early breast cancer on recurrence and 15-year survival: an overview of the randomised trials. Lancet 365:1687–1717

Esserman L, Thompson I (2010) Solving the overdiagnosis dilemma. J Natl Cancer Inst 102:582–583

Esserman L, Shieh Y, Thompson I (2009) Rethinking screening for breast cancer and prostate cancer. JAMA 302:1685–1692

Esserman LJ, Thompson IM Jr, Reid B (2013) Overdiagnosis and overtreatment in cancer: an opportunity for improvement. JAMA 310:797–798

Freeman HP, Wasfie TJ (1989) Cancer of the breast in poor black women. Cancer 63:2562–2569

Ganz PA (2010) Quality-of-life issues in patients with ductal carcinoma in situ. J Natl Cancer Inst Monogr 2010:218–222

Ganz PA, Hahn EE (2008) Implementing a survivorship care plan for patients with breast cancer. J Clin Oncol 26:759–767

Ganz PA, Rowland JH, Desmond K et al (1998) Life after breast cancer: understanding women's health-related quality of life and sexual functioning. J Clin Oncol 16:501–514

Ganz PA, Kwan L, Somerfield MR et al (2006) The role of prevention in oncology practice: results from a 2004 survey of American society of clinical oncology members. J Clin Oncol 24:2948–2957

Ganz PA, Casillas J, Hahn EE (2008) Ensuring quality care for cancer survivors: implementing the survivorship care plan. Semin Oncol Nurs 24:208–217

Ganz PA, Kwan L, Stanton AL et al (2011a) Physical and psychosocial recovery in the year after primary treatment of breast cancer. J Clin Oncol 29:1101–1109

Ganz PA, Land SR, Geyer CE Jr et al (2011b) Menstrual history and quality-of-life outcomes in women with node-positive breast cancer treated with adjuvant therapy on the NSABP B-30 trial. J Clin Oncol 29:1110–1116

Gerend MA, Pai M (2008) Social determinants of black-white disparities in breast cancer mortality: a review. Cancer Epidemiol Biomarkers Prev 17:2913–2923

Giordano SH (2012) Radiotherapy in older women with low-risk breast cancer: why did practice not change? J Clin Oncol 30:1577–1578

Grunfeld E, Mant D, Yudkin P et al (1996) Routine follow up of breast cancer in primary care: randomised trial. BMJ 313:665–669

Grunfeld E, Levine MN, Julian JA et al (2006) Randomized trial of long-term follow-up for early-stage breast cancer: a comparison of family physician versus specialist care. J Clin Oncol 24:848–855

Han PK, Klabunde CN, Noone AM et al (2013) Physicians' beliefs about breast cancer surveillance testing are consistent with test overuse. Med Care 51:315–323

Haq R, Heus L, Baker NA et al (2013) Designing a multifaceted survivorship care plan to meet the information and communication needs of breast cancer patients and their family physicians: results of a qualitative pilot study. BMC Med Inform Decis Mak 13:76

Harford JB, Otero IV, Anderson BO et al (2011) Problem solving for breast health care delivery in low and middle resource countries (LMCs): consensus statement from the breast health global initiative. Breast 20(Suppl 2):S20–S29

Hassett MJ, Griggs JJ (2009) Disparities in breast cancer adjuvant chemotherapy: moving beyond yes or no. J Clin Oncol 27:2120–2121

Hershman DL, Wang X, McBride R et al (2006a) Delay in initiating adjuvant radiotherapy following breast conservation surgery and its impact on survival. Int J Radiat Oncol Biol Phys 65:1353–1360

Hershman DL, Wang X, McBride R et al (2006b) Delay of adjuvant chemotherapy initiation following breast cancer surgery among elderly women. Breast Cancer Res Treat 99:313–321

Hershman D, Kushi L, Shao T et al (2010) Early discontinuation and non-adherence to adjuvant hormonal therapy in a cohort of 8900 early stage breast cancer patients. J Clin Oncol

Hershman DL, Shao T, Kushi LH et al (2011) Early discontinuation and non-adherence to adjuvant hormonal therapy are associated with increased mortality in women with breast cancer. Breast Cancer Res Treat 126:529–537

Hewitt M, Ganz PA (2006) From cancer patient to cancer survivor – lost in transition: an American society of clinical oncology and institute of medicine symposium. National Academies of Press, Washington, DC

Hewitt M, Greenfield S, Stovall E (2006) Lost in transition. The National Academies Press, Washington, DC

Hewitt ME, Bamundo A, Day R et al (2007) Perspectives on post-treatment cancer care: qualitative research with survivors, nurses, and physicians. J Clin Oncol 25:2270–2273

Hunt BR, Whitman S, Hurlbert MS (2014) Increasing black: white disparities in breast cancer mortality in the 50 largest cities in the United States. Cancer Epidemiol 38:118–123

Institute of Medicine (IOM) (2013) Delivering high-quality cancer care: charting a new course for a system in crisis. The National Academies Press, Washington, DC

Jatoi I, Becher H, Leake CR (2003) Widening disparity in survival between white and African-American patients with breast carcinoma treated in the US department of defense healthcare system. Cancer 98:894–899

Kahn KL, Schneider EC, Malin JL et al (2007) Patient centered experiences in breast cancer: predicting long-term adherence to tamoxifen use. Med Care 45:431–439

Kaiser Family Foundation (2010) Prescription drug trends. Kaiser Family Foundation, Washington, DC

Khatcheressian JL, Hurley P, Bantug E et al (2013) Breast cancer follow-up and management after primary treatment: American society of clinical oncology clinical practice guideline update. J Clin Oncol 31:961–965

Li CI, Malone KE, Daling JR (2003) Differences in breast cancer stage, treatment, and survival by race and ethnicity. Arch Intern Med 163:49–56

Loren AW, Mangu PB, Beck LN et al (2013) Fertility preservation for patients with cancer: American society of clinical oncology clinical practice guideline update. J Clin Oncol 31:2500–2510

Lund MJ, Trivers KF, Porter PL et al (2009) Race and triple negative threats to breast cancer survival: a population-based study in Atlanta, GA. Breast Cancer Res Treat 113:357–370

Magai C, Consedine NS, Adjei BA et al (2008) Psychosocial influences on suboptimal adjuvant breast cancer treatment adherence among African American women: implications for education and intervention. Health Educ Behav 35:835–854

Menashe I, Anderson WF, Jatoi I et al (2009) Underlying causes of the black-white racial disparity in breast cancer mortality: a population-based analysis. J Natl Cancer Inst 101:993–1000

Mullan F (1985) Seasons of survival: reflections of a physician with cancer. N Engl J Med 313:270–273

National Institutes of Health (NIH) (2001) Consensus Development Conference statement: adjuvant therapy for breast cancer, November 1–3, 2000. J Natl Cancer Inst Monogr 5–15

Neugut AI, Subar M, Wilde ET et al (2011) Association between prescription co-payment amount and compliance with adjuvant hormonal therapy in women with early-stage breast cancer. J Clin Oncol 29:2534–2542

Neuss MN, Malin JL, Chan S et al (2013) Measuring the improving quality of outpatient care in medical oncology practices in the United States. J Clin Oncol 31:1471–1477

O'Brien KM, Cole SR, Tse CK et al (2010) Intrinsic breast tumor subtypes, race, and long-term survival in the Carolina breast cancer study. Clin Cancer Res 16:6100–6110

Paik S, Shak S, Tang G et al (2004) A multigene assay to predict recurrence of tamoxifen-treated, node-negative breast cancer. N Engl J Med 351:2817–2826

Paik S, Tang G, Shak S et al (2006) Gene expression and benefit of chemotherapy in women with node-negative, estrogen receptor-positive breast cancer. J Clin Oncol 24:3726–3734

Paskett ED, Harrop JP, Wells KJ (2011) Patient navigation: an update on the state of the science. CA Cancer J Clin 61:237–249

Perou CM, Sorlie T, Eisen MB et al (2000) Molecular portraits of human breast tumours. Nature 406:747–752

Potosky AL, Han PK, Rowland J et al (2011) Differences between primary care physicians' and oncologists' knowledge, attitudes and practices regarding the care of cancer survivors. J Gen Intern Med 26:1403–1410

Romond EH, Perez EA, Bryant J et al (2005) Trastuzumab plus adjuvant chemotherapy for operable HER2-positive breast cancer. N Engl J Med 353:1673–1684

Sateren WB, Trimble EL, Abrams J et al (2002) How sociodemographics, presence of oncology specialists, and hospital cancer programs affect accrual to cancer treatment trials. J Clin Oncol 20:2109–2117

Schnipper LE, Smith TJ, Raghavan D et al (2012) American society of clinical oncology identifies five key opportunities to improve care and reduce costs: the top five list for oncology. J Clin Oncol 30:1715–1724

Shalom MM, Hahn EE, Casillas J et al (2011) Do survivorship care plans make a difference? A primary care provider perspective. J Oncol Pract 7:314–318

Shavers VL, Brown ML (2002) Racial and ethnic disparities in the receipt of cancer treatment. J Natl Cancer Inst 94:334–357

Siegel R, DeSantis C, Virgo K et al (2012) Cancer treatment and survivorship statistics, 2012. CA Cancer J Clin 62:220–241

Smith TJ, Hillner BE (2011) Bending the cost curve in cancer care. N Engl J Med 364: 2060–2065

Sorlie T, Perou CM, Tibshirani R et al (2001) Gene expression patterns of breast carcinomas distinguish tumor subclasses with clinical implications. Proc Natl Acad Sci USA 98:10869–10874

Tejeda HA, Green SB, Trimble EL et al (1996) Representation of African-Americans, Hispanics, and whites in national cancer institute cancer treatment trials. J Natl Cancer Inst 88:812–816

Tevaarwerk AJ, Wisinski KB, Buhr KA et al (2014) Leveraging electronic health record systems to create and provide electronic cancer survivorship care plans: a pilot study. J Oncol Pract 10:e150–e159

Vanchieri C (2005) When will the U.S. flinch at cancer drug prices? J Natl Cancer Inst 97: 624–626

Welch HG, Passow HJ (2014) Quantifying the benefits and harms of screening mammography. JAMA Intern Med 174:448–454

Wheeler SB, Reeder-Hayes KE, Carey LA (2013) Disparities in breast cancer treatment and outcomes: biological, social, and health system determinants and opportunities for research. Oncologist 18:986–993

Wyatt GE, Desmond KA, Ganz PA et al (1998) Sexual functioning and intimacy in African American and white breast cancer survivors: a descriptive study. Womens Health 4:385–405

Index

© Breast Cancer Research Foundation 2015   271
P.A. Ganz (ed.), *Improving Outcomes for Breast Cancer Survivors*,
Advances in Experimental Medicine and Biology 862,
DOI 10.1007/978-3-319-16366-6

CPSIA information can be obtained at www.ICGtesting.com
Printed in the USA
LVOW05*1435120615

442274LV00001B/2/P